American Public Health Association

VITAL AND HEALTH STATISTICS MONOGRAPHS

EPIDEMIOLOGY OF NEUROLOGIC AND SENSE ORGAN DISORDERS

CONTRIBUTORS

NUNG WON CHOI, M.D., Ph.D.
Department of Social and Preventive Medicine
University of Manitoba
Winnipeg, Manitoba, Canada

IRVING D. GOLDBERG, M.P.H.
National Institute of Mental Health
Health Services and Mental Health Administration
Department of Health, Education, and Welfare
Rockville, Maryland

HYMAN GOLDSTEIN, Ph.D.
Maternal and Child Health Program
School of Public Health
University of California
Berkeley, California

LEONARD T. KURLAND, M.D., Dr.P.H.
Department of Medical Statistics and Epidemiology
Mayo Clinic and Mayo Foundation, and
Mayo Graduate School of Medicine (University of Minnesota)
Rochester, Minnesota

JOHN F. KURTZKE, M.D.
Department of Neurology and Department of Community Medicine and
  International Health
Georgetown University School of Medicine, and
Neurology Service, Veterans Administration Hospital
Washington, D. C.

FRANCES A. REEDER, M.D. (deceased)
Bureau of Medical Rehabilitation
New York State Department of Health
Albany, New York

JEROME D. SCHEIN, Ph.D.
Deafness Research and Training Center
New York University School of Education
New York, New York

GAIL R. WILLIAMS, M.D.
Department of Human Genetics
University of Michigan
Ann Arbor, Michigan

EPIDEMIOLOGY OF NEUROLOGIC AND SENSE ORGAN DISORDERS

LEONARD T. KURLAND, JOHN F. KURTZKE,
and IRVING D. GOLDBERG

1973 / HARVARD UNIVERSITY PRESS
Cambridge, Massachusetts

©Copyright 1973 by the President and Fellows of Harvard College. All rights reserved.

This material has been copyrighted to ensure its accurate quotation and use. Permission to reprint may be granted upon presentation of an adequate statement concerning the material to be used and the manner of its incorporation in other texts.

Library of Congress Catalog Card Number 72-90644
SBN 674-25875-4
Printed in the United States of America

11502

PREFACE

This monograph on the epidemiology of neurologic and sense organ disorders by Doctors Kurland, Kurtzke, Goldberg, and their associates is the first comprehensive study on the subject.

Great advances have been made with regard to the etiology and treatment of infectious and nutritional diseases by the epidemiologist, and it was natural to expect that similar results could be obtained by a study of noninfectious diseases involving the various organ systems of man. The American Public Health Association therefore decided to sponsor the publication of monographs on such studies. They were fortunate indeed in being able to entrust this volume on diseases of the nervous system to men who have been trained in both epidemiology and diseases of the nervous system.

Until recently there has been little interest in the incidence, prevalence, and geographic distribution of diseases of the nervous system. The results of a few studies on multiple sclerosis were reported in the first part of this century, but an intensive analysis of this relatively common and serious affliction was made only in recent years by Dr. Kurland and his associates. The report by Limburg in 1950 indicating that the incidence of this disease was perhaps related to climatic factors was the springboard which led Kurland to conduct a more thorough study with the aim of finding some factor related to climate which would be of etiologic significance. He was soon joined in this endeavor by Kurtzke, Dean, and others. The results of their investigations now raise the possibility that multiple sclerosis is caused by a virus, perhaps a slow-acting one, that is acquired at an early age under certain climatic conditions, but the onset of symptoms may be delayed for a number of years in the exposed subject regardless of the climatic conditions of the place of residence at the time symptoms develop. Time will tell us whether or not this hypothesis is correct.

The specialty of neuroepidemiology also received a great stimulus by the phenomenal developments in genetics. The discovery that genetically conditional defects were caused by a disturbance in one or more enzyme systems resulting from a defect in the genes gave promise of obtaining methods of treating or preventing such diseases.

The publication of this monograph could be considered as marking the birth and early development of neuroepidemiology as a specialty in the field of medicine. The authors state in their conclusions that their studies have raised more questions than they have provided answers. This is to be expected in view of the paucity of our knowledge of noninfectious diseases of the nervous system. It is important, however, that these questions be raised in order that answers may be obtained.

Pertinent information is available mainly from mortality statistics and scattered, and sometimes fragmentary, reports of the incidence and prevalence of the various diseases in certain localities. The authors emphasize that the value of these reports is determined to a great extent by the completeness of the records with regard to age, sex, and nationality of the patients studied—and to a greater extent by the accuracy of the diagnosis. Diagnosis, in particular, leaves much to be desired because of both the inadequate number of physicians trained in the study of diseases of the nervous system and the lack of specific diagnostic tests for most of the diseases under study.

The authors comment that this monograph is directed toward the medical practitioner in order to make him cognizant of the problems involved and thus make him better equipped to record the data in his cases and correctly codify the diagnosis. If this result is achieved, future studies by epidemiologists and neurologists will give information which may make it possible to determine the cause of a particular disease of the nervous system and thereby discover a method of prevention or an effective cure.

A vast amount of information derived from research in various parts of the world is presented in this book. The authors have carefully evaluated these data, pointing out possible errors that have resulted from the biases inherent in the work. The conclusions they were able to reach with regard to etiologic factors are limited, but more valid conclusions will be possible in a second edition if medical practitioners, neurologists, ophthalmologists, and otolaryngologists study this volume and follow its precepts in reporting their studies.

H. HOUSTON MERRITT, M.D.

Henry L. and Lucy Moses Professor Emeritus of Neurology
Dean Emeritus and Vice-President Emeritus
Faculty of Medicine
Columbia University College of Physicians and Surgeons

ACKNOWLEDGMENTS

We thank the American Association of Neurological Surgeons for permission to reprint Tables 3.1 through 3.6 and A.3.2 which are modified from G. R. Williams, L. T. Kurland, and I. D. Goldberg, "Morbidity and mortality with parkinsonism," *Journal of Neurosurgery*, 24:138-143, 158 (1966).

We thank Grune & Stratton, Inc., for permission to reprint Tables 5.3 through 5.8, A.5.1 through A.5.3, and A.5.5 which are modified from L. T. Kurland, N. W. Choi, and G. P. Sayre, "Implications of incidence and geographic patterns on the classification of amyotrophic lateral sclerosis," in F. H. Norris, Jr., and L. T. Kurland, eds., *Motor neuron diseases: research on amyotrophic lateral sclerosis and related disorders* (New York: Grune & Stratton, Inc., 1969), pp. 28-50.

We thank the National Society for the Prevention of Blindness, Inc., for permission to reprint Table 12.1 which is modified from E. M. Hatfield, "Causes of blindness in school children," *Sightsaving Review*, 33:218-233 (1963).

We acknowledge the previous publication of Table 5.9 which is modified from L. T. Kurland, "Amyotrophic lateral sclerosis: a reappraisal," in D. C. Gajdusek, J. C. Gibbs, Jr., and M. Alpers, eds., *Slow, latent, and temperate virus infections* (NINDB Monograph No. 2, Public Health Service Publication No. 1378) (Washington, D. C.: Government Printing Office, 1965), pp. 13-22; of Tables 12.2 through 12.8 and A.12.1 through A.12.7 which are modified from the National Institute of Neurological Diseases and Blindness, *Statistics for 1966 on blindness in Model Reporting Area [MRA]*, Public Health Service Publication (Washington, D. C.: Government Printing Office, 1969), 63 pp.; and of Tables 8.5, 8.6, A.8.4, 9.1, 9.19, 9.20, 9.23, and A.9.11 which are derived from A. C. Stevenson, H. A. Johnston, M. I. P. Stewart, and D. R. Golding, "Congenital malformations: a report of a study of series of consecutive births in 24 centres," *Bulletin of the World Health Organization,* 34 Suppl:1-108 (1966).

Dr. Frances A. Reeder assisted in the early development and preparation of the chapter on convulsive disorders in 1966. Despite a recurrent illness she continued to review material on this chapter until her untimely death on September 18, 1972.

The authors wish to acknowledge the invaluable assistance in the preparation of manuscript and review of proof by members of the Section of Publications of the Mayo Clinic—in particular the editorial assistance of Marc A. Shampo and Mrs. Deanna Servick.

We further recognize the valuable contributions in organization and typing of manuscript and tabulation of statistical data by many dedicated members of our secretarial and statistical staffs. Among those whose efforts we particularly wish to acknowledge are the following:

- Mrs. Carol A. Dobbs and Mrs. Norma Bulger, Department of Medical Statistics and Epidemiology, Mayo Clinic.
- Mrs. Mary O. McAllister, Neurology Section, Veterans Administration Hospital, Washington, D.C.
- Mrs. Mote Dann, Mrs. Inez Roberts, Mrs. Aileen Edelin, and Mrs. Alma Barclay of the National Institute of Neurological Diseases and Blindness; also Mrs. Warnilla Cook and Miss Constance Burtoff of the National Institute of Mental Health, Public Health Service, Bethesda, Maryland.

The Rochester, Minnesota, data source referred to in many sections of this volume is supported in part by the National Institutes of Health program project grant, GM-14231.

CONTENTS

Preface by H. Houston Merritt, M.D.   v

Foreword by James R. Kimmey, M.D.   xxvii

Notes on Tables and Figures   xxx

1 / Introduction to Epidemiology   1

2 / Convulsive Disorders   15

3 / Parkinsonism   41

4 / Multiple Sclerosis   64

5 / Amyotrophic Lateral Sclerosis and Other Motor Neuron Diseases   108

6 / Muscular Dystrophy and Other Myopathies   128

7 / Myasthenia Gravis   144

8 / Down's Syndrome   153

9 / Congenital Malformations of the Nervous System   169

10 / Other Specific Neurologic Disorders   210

11 / Cerebral Palsy   232

12 / Blindness   246

13 / Hearing Disorders   276

14 / Neuroepidemiology—A Summation   305

Appendix Tables 335

References 400

Index 431

TABLES

2.1 Average annual crude and age-adjusted death rates per 100,000 population for epilepsy by age, color and sex: United States, 1959-61 ... 19

2.2 Average annual age-adjusted death rates per 100,000 population for epilepsy by color and sex: United States and census regions, 1959-61 ... 21

2.3 Prevalence rates per 1,000 population for convulsive disorders: selected studies, various years, 1955-68 ... 30

2.4 Age-specific prevalence rates per 1,000 population for epilepsy: Rochester, Minnesota; Carlisle, England; Iceland; and Jerusalem, Israel, 1955-61 ... 31

2.5 Average annual age-specific incidence rates per 100,000 population for epilepsy: Rochester, Minnesota; Iceland; Carlisle, England; and Jutland, Denmark, 1935-64 ... 32

2.6 Average annual incidence rates per 100,000 population for epilepsy by type: Rochester, Minnesota; Iceland; and Jutland, Denmark; various years, 1935-64 ... 35

3.1 Deaths and average annual death rates per 100,000 population for parkinsonism by age, color and sex: United States, 1959-61 ... 44

3.2 Average annual age-adjusted death rates per 100,000 population age 65 and over for parkinsonism by sex: United States and census regions, 1959-61 ... 45

3.3 Average annual age-adjusted death rates per 100,000 population age 65 and over for parkinsonism by color: United States and census regions, 1959-61 ... 48

3.4 Average annual age-adjusted death rates per 100,000 population age 65 and over for parkinsonism by color, sex and type of county: United States, 1959-61 ... 49

3.5 Average annual age-adjusted death rates per 100,000 population for parkinsonism by age, sex and marital status: United States, 1959-61 ... 50

3.6 Average annual age-adjusted death rates per 100,000 population for parkinsonism, white persons age 65 and over, by sex and nativity: United States, 1959-61 ... 50

3.7 Average annual age-specific incidence rates per 100,000 population for parkinsonism: Rochester, Minnesota, 1935-66 ... 53

3.8 Prevalence rates per 100,000 population for parkinsonism by type, with number of cases by sex: Rochester, Minnesota, 1965 and Iceland, 1963 ... 55

4.1 Death certificates listing multiple sclerosis as primary or secondary causes of death, with percent listed as primary cause: selected countries, various years, 1953-61 ... 66

4.2 Age-adjusted death rates per 100,000 population for multiple sclerosis: selected British Commonwealth countries and United States, various years, 1950-59 ... 67

xii / TABLES

4.3	Average annual age-adjusted death rates per 100,000 population for multiple sclerosis by sex: United States and census regions, 1959-61	69
4.4	Average annual age-adjusted death rates per 100,000 population for multiple sclerosis by color: United States and census regions, 1959-61	71
4.5	Deaths and average annual death rates per 100,000 population for multiple sclerosis among native born by residence at birth and death: northern tier and southern tier of United States, 1959-61	79
4.6	Average annual age-adjusted death rates per 100,000 population for multiple sclerosis by age, sex and marital status: United States, 1959-61	79
4.7	Average annual age-adjusted death rates per 100,000 population for multiple sclerosis, white persons, by age, sex and nativity: United States, 1959-61	80
4.8	Average annual death rates per 100,000 population for multiple sclerosis among immigrants to the United States by birthplace and reported rates for residents of their native countries: United States, 1959-61, and specified countries, various years, 1952-58	82
4.9	Prevalence rates per 100,000 population for multiple sclerosis: specified localities, various years, 1950-68	84
5.1	Death certificates listing motor neuron disease (MND) and amyotrophic lateral sclerosis (ALS) as primary or secondary causes of death, with percent listed as primary cause: selected countries, various years, 1953-61	110
5.2	Average annual age-adjusted death rates per 100,000 population for amyotrophic lateral sclerosis by race, age and sex: United States, 1959-61	113
5.3	Deaths and average annual age-adjusted death rates per 100,000 population for amyotrophic lateral sclerosis by sex, with male-female ratio of adjusted rates: United States and census regions, 1959-61	114
5.4	Deaths and average annual age-adjusted death rates per 100,000 population for amyotrophic lateral sclerosis by color, with white-nonwhite ratio of adjusted rates: United States and census regions, 1959-61	115
5.5	Average annual age-adjusted death rates per 100,000 population for amyotrophic lateral sclerosis by color, sex and type of county: United States and census regions, 1959-61	116
5.6	Average annual age-adjusted death rates per 100,000 population for amyotrophic lateral sclerosis by age, sex and marital status: United States, 1959-61	117
5.7	Average annual age-adjusted death rates per 100,000 population for amyotrophic lateral sclerosis, white persons, by sex and nativity: United States and census regions, 1959-61	117
5.8	Number of cases and average annual incidence rates per 100,000 population for motor neuron disease among residents: Rochester, Minnesota, 1925-64	119
5.9	Selected clinical and pathologic features of amyotrophic lateral sclerosis	122

TABLES / xiii

6.1	Average annual crude death rates per 100,000 population for inborn defect of muscle: selected countries, various years, 1951-58	131
6.2	Deaths and average annual death rates per 100,000 population for inborn defect of muscle by age, color and sex: United States, 1959-61	132
6.3	Average annual age-adjusted death rates and death rates under age 1 per 100,000 population for inborn defect of muscle by sex: United States and census regions, 1959-61	134
6.4	Average annual age-adjusted death rates per 100,000 population for inborn defect of muscle by color and age: United States and census regions, 1959-61	135
6.5	Average annual age-adjusted death rates per 100,000 population for inborn defect of muscle by sex and type of county: United States and census regions, 1959-61	136
6.6	Average annual age-adjusted death rates per 100,000 population for inborn defect of muscle by age, color, sex and type of county: United States, 1959-61	136
6.7	Average annual age-adjusted death rates per 100,000 population for inborn defect of muscle by age, sex and marital status: United States, 1959-61	137
6.8	Average annual age-adjusted death rates per 100,000 population for inborn defect of muscle, white persons, by age, sex and nativity: United States, 1959-61	138
6.9	Cases and prevalence rates per 100,000 population for muscular dystrophy: selected surveys, various years, about 1950-63	139
6.10	Cases and prevalence rates per 100,000 population for myotonic dystrophy: selected surveys, various years, about 1952-67	140
7.1	Average annual crude and age-adjusted death rates per 1,000,000 population for myasthenia gravis by age, color and sex: United States, 1959-61	147
7.2	Average annual age-adjusted death rates per 1,000,000 population for myasthenia gravis by color and sex: United States and census regions, 1959-61	148
7.3	Average annual age-adjusted death rates per 1,000,000 population for myasthenia gravis, white persons, by sex and nativity: United States and census regions, 1959-61	149
7.4	Cases and average annual incidence rates and point prevalence rates per 1,000,000 population for myasthenia gravis from population surveys: selected areas, various years, 1941-65	150
8.1	Average annual death rates per 100,000 population for Down's syndrome by age, color and sex: United States, 1959-61	155
8.2	Average annual death rates per 100,000 population under one year of age for Down's syndrome by color and sex: United States and census regions, 1959-61	157
8.3	Average annual death rates per 100,000 population under one year of age for Down's syndrome by color, sex and type of county: United States, 1959-61	157
8.4	Cases and incidence rates per 1,000 live births for Down's syndrome: selected surveys, various years, 1935-67	159
8.5	Cases and incidence rates standardized for maternal age per 1,000	

	total (live plus stillborn) single births for Down's syndrome: WHO study, 24 centers, 1961-64	162
8.6	Incidence rates per 1,000 total (live plus stillborn) single births for Down's syndrome by maternal age: WHO study of 24 centers, 1961-64	164
8.7	Male-female case ratios in Down's syndrome: selected surveys, various years, 1935-67	164
8.8	Concordance among twins with Down's syndrome according to zygosity, adapted from Øster's review of literature, 1899-1952	166
9.1	Percentage distribution of congenital malformations of the nervous system by type of malformation: WHO study of 24 centers, 1961-64	171
9.2	Death certificates listing congenital malformations of the nervous system as primary or secondary causes of death, with percent listed as primary cause, by type of malformation: selected countries, various years, 1953-61	173
9.3	Average annual age-adjusted death rates per 100,000 population for congenital malformations of the nervous system by type of malformation: selected countries, various years, 1951-58	174
9.4	Number of countries with specified male-female ratio of age-adjusted death rates for congenital malformations of the nervous system by type of malformation: selected countries, various years, 1951-58	175
9.5	Deaths and death rates per 100,000 population for congenital malformations of the nervous system by type of malformation: United States, 1959-61	178
9.6	Average annual death rates per 100,000 population under one year of age for congenital malformations of the nervous system by color, sex and type of malformation: United States, 1959-61	179
9.7	Age-specific death rates per 100,000 population for congenital malformations of the nervous system by type of malformation: United States, 1959-61	180
9.8	Male-female ratios of death rates under one year of age for congenital malformations of the nervous system by color and type of malformation: United States, 1959-61	181
9.9	White-nonwhite ratios of death rates under one year of age for congenital malformations of the nervous system by sex and type of malformation: United States, 1959-61	181
9.10	Average annual death rates per 100,000 population under one year of age for monstrosity by color and sex: United States and census regions, 1959-61	183
9.11	Average annual death rates per 100,000 population under one year of age for spina bifida and meningocele by color and sex: United States and census regions, 1959-61	185
9.12	Average annual death rates per 100,000 population under one year of age for congenital hydrocephalus by color and sex: United States and census regions, 1959-61	186
9.13	Average annual death rates per 100,000 population under one year of age for other malformations of the nervous system by color and sex: United States and census regions, 1959-61	188

9.14	Correlations of death rates under one year of age for specified types of congenital malformations of the nervous system occurring in the states: United States, 1959-61	189
9.15	Average annual death rates per 100,000 population under one year of age for monstrosity by color, sex and type of county: United States, 1959-61	192
9.16	Average annual death rates per 100,000 population under one year of age for spina bifida and meningocele by color, sex and type of county: United States, 1959-61	193
9.17	Average annual death rates per 100,000 population under one year of age for congenital hydrocephalus by color, sex and type of county: United States, 1959-61	193
9.18	Average annual death rates per 100,000 population under one year of age for other congenital malformations of the nervous system by color, sex and type of county: United States, 1959-61	194
9.19	Cases and incidence rates per 1,000 total (live plus stillborn) single births for congenital malformations of the nervous system by type of malformation: WHO study of 24 centers, 1961-64	196
9.20	Incidence rates per 1,000 total (live plus stillborn) births for major congenital malformations of the nervous system among single-born and twin-born infants by type of malformation: WHO study of 24 centers, 1961-64	196
9.21	Total number of cases and incidence rates per 1,000 births for congenital defects of the neural tube by type of defect: selected community surveys, various years, 1935-67	197
9.22	Correlations of incidence rates among total (live plus stillborn) single births for specified congenital malformations of the nervous system occurring alone in 24 areas: WHO study of 24 centers, 1961-64	201
9.23	Male-female ratios among total (live plus stillborn) births with neural tube defects by type of defect: selected surveys, various years, 1935-67	202
9.24	Peak years in secular trends of incidence rates among total (live plus stillborn) births for anencephaly: selected surveys, various years, 1920-65	204
10.1	Cases and average annual incidence and point prevalence rates per 100,000 population for dorsolateral sclerosis with or without pernicious anemia: Rochester, Minnesota, and Carlisle, England, various years, 1945-61	213
10.2	Percentage distribution of cases according to age at onset for Japanese myeloneuropathy by sex, with male-to-female ratio of the cases: Nagoya, Japan, 1956-69	214
10.3	Cases and average annual incidence rates per 100,000 population for Bell's palsy by sex: selected surveys, various years, 1955-67	216
10.4	Cases and average annual incidence rates per 1,000 population for herpes zoster by sex: selected surveys, various years, 1945-62	219
10.5	Cases and average annual incidence rates per 1,000 population for herpes zoster by age and sex: Hawick, Scotland, 1948-55, and Rochester, Minnesota, 1945-54	220
10.6	Cases and average annual incidence rates per 100,000 population	

	for Guillain-Barré syndrome: selected surveys, various years, 1935-67	222
10.7	Average age at onset and average duration of illness for Huntington's chorea: selected surveys, various years to 1965	224
10.8	Cases and prevalence rates per 100,000 population for Huntington's chorea: selected surveys, various years, about 1951-65	226
10.9	Age at onset for dystonia musculorum deformans by mode of transmission and ethnic origin, with number of cases by sex: selected areas and years, United States	231
11.1	Deaths and average annual death rates per 100,000 population for infantile cerebral palsy (cerebral spastic infantile paralysis) by age, color and sex: United States, 1959-61	236
11.2	Average annual age-adjusted death rates per 100,000 population under 15 years of age for infantile cerebral palsy (cerebral spastic infantile paralysis) by color and sex: United States and census regions, 1959-61	237
11.3	Deaths and average annual death rates per 100,000 population under one year of age and all ages for neonatal cerebral palsy (intracranial and spinal injury at birth) by color and sex: United States, 1959-61	239
11.4	Average annual death rates per 100,000 population under one year of age for neonatal cerebral palsy (intracranial and spinal injury at birth) by color and sex: United States and census regions, 1959-61	240
11.5	Cases and average annual incidence rates per 1,000 live births for cerebral palsy: selected surveys, various years, 1925-63	242
11.6	Cases and prevalence rates per 1,000 population, all ages and childhood ages, for cerebral palsy: selected surveys, various years, 1953-62	243
12.1	Estimated rates per 100,000 enrolled pupils for blindness among school-age children by cause: United States, selected residential schools for the blind, city school systems and state departments of education, specified years, 1933-59	252
12.2	Rates per 100,000 population for all additions to blindness register (reported incidence) and for total on register at end of year (reported prevalence): MRA by state, 1966	255
12.3	Rates per 100,000 population for all additions to blindness register (reported incidence) by age, color and sex: MRA, 1966	256
12.4	Percentage distribution of all additions to blindness register by degree of vision in better eye by color: MRA total, 1966	256
12.5	Percentage distribution of all additions to blindness register by degree of vision in better eye by age: MRA total, 1966	257
12.6	Percentage distribution of first additions to blindness register by selected major affection and cause groups: MRA total, 1966	261
12.7	Rates per 100,000 population for total on blindness register (reported prevalence) by color, sex and age as of end of year: MRA total, 1966	262
12.8	Percentage distribution of total on blindness register as of end of year by degree of vision in better eye by color: MRA total, 1966	263

13.1 Prevalence rates per 100,000 population for prelingual deafness (deaf mutism) by sex: censuses of various countries, 1930-56 — 281
13.2 Prevalence rates per 100,000 population for prelingual deafness by sex: United States, selected areas, various years, 1940-63 — 284
13.3 Prevalence rates per 100,000 children for deafness based on children enrolled in school and children of school age: various countries, 1957-58 — 286
13.4 Prevalence rates per 100,000 population for hearing impairments among children in schools as determined by audiologic surveys: various areas and years, 1951-63 — 288
13.5 Prevalence rates per 100,000 population for ability to hear at specified levels for speech in the better ear among persons 18 to 79 years of age, by age and sex: United States, 1960-62 — 290
13.6 Prevalence rates per 100,000 population for hearing impairment by estimated degree of loss, sex and age: United States, 1962-63 — 292
13.7 Prevalence rates per 100,000 population for prelingual deafness: United States, 1830-1930 — 302
13.8 Rate of enrollments in schools and classes for the deaf per 100,000 total school enrollments: United States, 1900-60 — 303
14.1 Approximate annual death rates per 100,000 population for various neurologic disorders reported as underlying cause of death among white populations: selected areas in the western hemisphere, about 1960 — 321
14.2 Approximate annual incidence rates per 100,000 population for various neurologic and sensory disorders from surveys of white populations: selected areas in the western hemisphere, about 1960 — 323
14.3 Approximate annual incidence rates per 1,000 births for various disorders of infancy: selected areas, about 1960 — 324
14.4 Approximate point prevalence rates per 100,000 population for various neurologic and sensory disorders from surveys of white populations: selected areas in the western hemisphere, about 1960 — 325
14.5 Average annual age-adjusted and crude death rates per 100,000 population for various neurologic disorders by color, sex and type of disorder: United States, 1959-61 — 326
14.6 Average annual death rates per 100,000 population under 1 year of age for various neurologic disorders present at or near birth by color, sex and type of disorder: United States, 1959-61 — 328

APPENDIX TABLES

A.2.1	Definition of convulsive disorders by clinical forms, ILAE, and modification used in Rochester, Minnesota, study	335
A.2.2	Deaths and average annual death rates per 100,000 population for epilepsy by age, color and sex: United States, 1959-61	336
A.2.3	Deaths and average annual age-adjusted death rates per 100,000 population for epilepsy, all ages: United States and each state, 1959-61	337
A.2.4	Average annual age-adjusted death rates per 100,000 population for epilepsy by color, sex and type of county: United States and census regions, 1959-61	338
A.2.5	Deaths and average annual age-adjusted death rates per 100,000 population for epilepsy by age, sex and marital status: United States, 1959-61	339
A.2.6	Average annual age-adjusted death rates per 100,000 population for epilepsy, white persons, by sex and nativity: United States and census regions, 1959-61	340
A.2.7	Average annual age-adjusted death rates per 100,000 population for epilepsy by sex: selected countries, various years, 1951-58	341
A.3.1	Deaths and average annual age-adjusted death rates per 100,000 population for parkinsonism: United States and each state, 1959-61	342
A.3.2	Average annual age-adjusted death rates per 100,000 population for parkinsonism by sex: selected countries, various years, 1951-58	343
A.4.1	Average annual age-adjusted death rates per 100,000 population for multiple sclerosis with male-to-female ratios: selected countries, various years, 1951-58	344
A.4.2	Deaths and average annual death rates per 100,000 population for multiple sclerosis by age, color and sex: United States, 1959-61	345
A.4.3	Average annual death rates per 100,000 population for multiple sclerosis among native born by state of birth and color: United States and each state, 1959-61	346
A.4.4	Average annual age-adjusted death rates per 100,000 population, all ages and 65 and over, for multiple sclerosis by color: United States and census regions, 1959-61	346
A.4.5	Average annual crude death rates per 100,000 population for multiple sclerosis by region of birth and death, native born: United States and census regions, 1959-61	347
A.4.6	Deaths from multiple sclerosis, 1959-61, among native born by region of birth and region of death, and 3-year total populations (in thousands) in each region by birthplace based on 1960 census: United States and census regions	348
A.4.7	Average annual age-adjusted death rates per 100,000 population	

	for multiple sclerosis by sex and type of county: United States and census regions, 1959-61	348
A.4.8	Deaths and average annual crude death rates per 100,000 population for multiple sclerosis, foreign-born white residents, by country of birth: United States, 1959-61	349
A.5.1	Average annual age-adjusted death rates per 100,000 population for motor neuron disease by sex: selected countries, various years, 1951-58	350
A.5.2	Death rates per 100,000 population for amyotrophic lateral sclerosis and for progressive muscular atrophy by color and sex: United States, selected years, 1949-64	351
A.5.3	Deaths and average annual death rates per 100,000 population for amyotrophic lateral sclerosis by age, color and sex: United States, 1959-61	352
A.5.4	Deaths and average annual age-adjusted death rates per 100,000 population, all ages and age 65 and over, for amyotrophic lateral sclerosis: United States and each state, 1959-61	353
A.5.5	Deaths and average annual death rates per 100,000 population for motor neuron disease by place of birth for foreign-born residents by sex, with male-female ratio of rates: United States, 1959-61	354
A.7.1	Deaths and average annual death rates for myasthenia gravis per 1,000,000 population by age, color and sex: United States, 1959-61	355
A.7.2	Average annual age-adjusted death rates per 1,000,000 population for myasthenia gravis by color, sex and type of county: United States and census regions, 1959-61	355
A.7.3	Average annual age-adjusted death rates per 1,000,000 population age 65 and over for myasthenia gravis by color, sex and type of county: United States and census regions, 1959-61	356
A.8.1	Deaths and average annual death rates per 100,000 population for Down's syndrome by age, color and sex: United States, 1959-61	357
A.8.2	Deaths from Down's syndrome by age, color and sex: each census region, United States, 1959-61	358
A.8.3	Deaths and average annual death rates per 100,000 population under one year of age and deaths all ages for Down's syndrome: United States and each state, 1959-61	359
A.8.4	Composition of 24-center WHO cooperative study on congenital malformations among births, 1961-64	360
A.9.1	Average annual age-adjusted death rates per 100,000 population for monstrosity by sex: selected countries, various years, 1951-58	361
A.9.2	Average annual age-adjusted death rates per 100,000 population for spina bifida and meningocele by sex: selected countries, various years, 1951-58	362
A.9.3	Average annual age-adjusted death rates per 100,000 population for congenital hydrocephalus by sex: selected countries, various years, 1951-58	363

A.9.4	Average annual age-adjusted death rates per 100,000 population for other congenital malformations of the nervous system by sex: selected countries, various years, 1951-58	364
A.9.5	Deaths and average annual death rates per 100,000 population for monstrosity by age, color and sex: United States, 1959-61	365
A.9.6	Deaths and average annual death rates per 100,000 population for spina bifida and meningocele by age, color and sex: United States, 1959-61	366
A.9.7	Deaths and average annual death rates per 100,000 population for congenital hydrocephalus by age, color and sex: United States, 1959-61	367
A.9.8	Deaths and average annual death rates per 100,000 population for other congenital malformations of the nervous system by age, color and sex: United States, 1959-61	368
A.9.9a	Number of deaths under one year of age from congenital malformations of the nervous system by type of malformation: United States and each state, 1959-61	369
A.9.9b	Average annual death rates per 100,000 population under one year of age for congenital malformations of the nervous system by type of malformation: United States and each state, 1959-61	370
A.9.10	Number of deaths under one year of age from congenital malformations of the nervous system by color, sex and type of malformation: United States and census regions, 1959-61	371
A.9.11	Cases and incidence rates per 1,000 total (live plus stillborn) single births, standardized for maternal age, for major neural tube defects by type of defect: WHO study, by center, 1961-64	372
A.11.1	Average annual age-adjusted death rates per 100,000 population for infantile cerebral palsy (cerebral spastic infantile paralysis) by sex: selected countries, various years, 1951-58	373
A.11.2	Average annual death rates per 100,000 population under 5 years of age for neonatal cerebral palsy (intracranial and spinal injury at birth) by sex: selected countries, various years, 1951-58	374
A.11.3	Average annual crude death rates per 100,000 population, all ages, for neonatal cerebral palsy (intracranial and spinal injury at birth) by sex: selected countries, various years, 1951-58	375
A.11.4	Death certificates listing cerebral spastic infantile paralysis (ICP) and intracranial and spinal injury at birth (NCP) as primary or secondary causes of death, with percent listed as primary cause: selected countries, various years, 1953-61	376
A.11.5	Deaths and average annual age-adjusted death rates per 100,000 population under 15 years of age for infantile cerebral palsy (cerebral spastic infantile paralysis): United States and each state, 1959-61	377
A.11.6	Average annual age-adjusted death rates per 100,000 population under 15 years of age for infantile cerebral palsy (cerebral spastic infantile paralysis) by color, sex and type of county: United States and census regions, 1959-61	378

A.11.7	Average annual death rates per 100,000 population under 1 year of age for neonatal cerebral palsy (intracranial and spinal injury at birth) by color, sex and type of county: United States and census regions, 1959-61	379
A.12.1	Percentage distribution of first additions to blindness register by major affection groups, by color and sex: MRA total, 1966	380
A.12.2	Percentage distribution of first additions to blindness register by major affection groups, by age: MRA total, 1966	381
A.12.3	Percentage distribution of first additions to blindness register by degree of vision in better eye, by major affection groups: MRA total, 1966	382
A.12.4	Percentage distribution of first additions to blindness register by major cause groups, by color and sex: MRA total, 1966	383
A.12.5	Percentage distribution of first additions to blindness register by major cause groups, by age: MRA total, 1966	384
A.12.6	Percentage distribution of first additions to blindness register by degree of vision in better eye, by major cause groups: MRA total, 1966	385
A.12.7	Percentage distribution of total on blindness register as of end of year by degree of vision in better eye, by age: MRA total, 1966	386
A.12.8	Prevalence rates per 100,000 population for blindness by definition of blindness: selected countries, various years, 1940-65	387
A.12.9	Prevalence rates per 100,000 population for blindness by definition of blindness, age and sex: selected countries, various years, 1941-65	391
A.12.10	Number of blind persons and percentage distribution by site and by type of affection, by definition of blindness: selected countries, various years, 1944-68	394
A.12.11	Number of blind persons and percentage distribution by cause of blindness, by definition of blindness: selected countries, various years, 1944-68	397

FIGURES

2.1	Crude death rates per 100,000 population for epilepsy by year: United States, 1939-67	18
2.2	Average annual age-specific death rates per 100,000 population for epilepsy by color and sex: United States, 1959-61	20
2.3	Average annual age-adjusted death rates per 100,000 population for epilepsy by state: United States, 1959-61	21
2.4	Average annual age-specific death rates per 100,000 population for epilepsy by marital status: United States, 1959-61	23
2.5	Average annual age-adjusted death rates per 100,000 population for epilepsy: selected countries, various years, 1951-58	25
2.6	Average annual age-specific incidence rates per 100,000 population for primary grand mal plotted on a square-root scale against age: Jutland, Denmark, 1959-61, and Iceland, 1959-64	33
2.7	Average annual incidence rates per 100,000 population for primary convulsive disorders by type and age at onset: Rochester, Minnesota, 1945-54	34
2.8	Average annual incidence rates per 100,000 population for secondary convulsive disorders by type and age at onset: Rochester, Minnesota, 1945-54	35
3.1	Average annual age-specific death rates per 100,000 population for parkinsonism by color and sex: United States, 1959-61	45
3.2	Average annual age-adjusted death rates per 100,000 population for parkinsonism by state: United States, 1959-61	46
3.3	Average annual age-adjusted death rates per 100,000 population for parkinsonism: selected countries, various years, 1951-58	51
3.4	Average annual age-specific incidence rates per 100,000 population for parkinsonism: Rochester, Minnesota, 1935-66; Carlisle, England, 1955-61; and Iceland, 1954-63	54
3.5	Age-specific prevalence rates per 100,000 population for parkinsonism: Rochester, Minnesota, January 1, 1965	55
3.6	Mean age at onset for parkinsonian patients, according to calendar intervals when first seen at Massachusetts General Hospital, 1875-1960, compared with the proportion of elderly among United States white adults	59
4.1	Average annual age-adjusted death rates per 100,000 population for multiple sclerosis: selected countries, various years, 1951-58	66
4.2	Crude death rates per 100,000 population for multiple sclerosis by year: United States, 1949-67	68
4.3	Average annual age-specific death rates per 100,000 population for multiple sclerosis by color and sex: United States, 1959-61	70
4.4	Average annual age-adjusted death rates per 100,000 population for multiple sclerosis by state of residence at death: United States, 1959-61	72
4.5	Average annual crude death rates per 100,000 population for	

multiple sclerosis among native born by state of birth: United States, 1959-61 73

4.6 Average annual crude death rates per 100,000 population for multiple sclerosis, white persons whose state of birth was state of residence at death, by state: United States, 1959-61 73

4.7 Average annual crude death rates per 100,000 population for multiple sclerosis, persons whose census region of birth was region of residence at death, by census region: census regions except Mountain and Pacific, United States, 1959-61 75

4.8 Average annual crude death rates per 100,000 population for multiple sclerosis, persons whose place of birth and residence at death were in same tier (northern or southern), by census region of death: census regions except Mountain and Pacific, United States, 1959-61 76

4.9 Average annual crude death rates per 100,000 population for multiple sclerosis, persons whose place of birth and residence at death were in *opposite* tiers (northern or southern), by census region of *birth:* census regions except Mountain and Pacific, United States, 1959-61 76

4.10 Average annual crude death rates per 100,000 population for multiple sclerosis, persons whose place of birth and residence at death were in *opposite* tiers (northern or southern), by census region of residence at *death*: census regions except Mountain and Pacific, United States, 1959-61 77

4.11 Average annual crude death rates per 100,000 population for multiple sclerosis among foreign-born white residents of the United States by country of birth: United States, 1959-61 81

4.12 Prevalence rates per 100,000 population for multiple sclerosis. *a.* By geographic latitude, selected surveys, United States and Canada, various years, 1950-60. *b.* By geographic latitude of birthplace for immigrants to Israel, 1960 87

4.13 Prevalence rates per 100,000 population for multiple sclerosis by geographic latitude 88

4.14 Case-control ratios for multiple sclerosis cases in United States Army males in World War II versus controls matched by age, sex, color, date of induction, and length of service, by latitude of place of birth 90

4.15 Prevalence rates per 100,000 population for multiple sclerosis: Norway and Denmark (counties), Finland (hospital districts), and Sweden (small administrative units), various years, 1925-64 92

4.16 Average annual age specific incidence rates per 100,000 population for multiple sclerosis by sex: Denmark, based on prevalence survey of 1949 93

4.17 Percent survival among patients with multiple sclerosis by years after onset: Rochester, Minnesota, and United States Army males ... 95

5.1 Average annual age-adjusted death rates per 100,000 population for motor neuron disease: selected countries, various years, 1951-58 111

xxiv / FIGURES

5.2	Crude death rates per 100,000 population for amyotrophic lateral sclerosis, progressive muscular atrophy, and motor neuron disease by year: United States, 1949-64	112
5.3	Average annual age-specific death rates per 100,000 population for amyotrophic lateral sclerosis by color and sex: United States, 1959-61	113
5.4	Average annual age-adjusted death rates per 100,000 population for amyotrophic lateral sclerosis by state: United States, 1959-61	115
6.1	Average annual age-specific death rates per 100,000 population for inborn defect of muscle by sex: United States, 1959-61	133
6.2	Average annual age-specific death rates per 100,000 population for inborn defect of muscle, persons age 15 and over, by marital status: United States, 1959-61	138
8.1	Average annual death rates per 100,000 population under 1 year of age for Down's syndrome by state: United States, 1959-61	158
9.1	Birth rates per 1,000 population and crude death rates per 100,000 population accumulated for monstrosity, spina bifida, congenital hydrocephalus, and other congenital neural defects by year: United States, 1950-67	177
9.2	Average annual death rates per 100,000 population under 1 year of age for monstrosity by state: United States, 1959-61	182
9.3	Average annual death rates per 100,000 population under 1 year of age for spina bifida by state: United States, 1959-61	184
9.4	Average annual death rates per 100,000 population under 1 year of age for congenital hydrocephalus by state: United States, 1959-61	186
9.5	Average annual death rates per 100,000 population under 1 year of age for other congenital malformations of the nervous system by state: United States, 1959-61	188
9.6	Average annual death rates per 100,000 population under 1 year of age for all congenital malformations of the nervous system by state: United States, 1959-61	191
9.7	Rates per 1,000 total births for anencephaly by year: selected surveys, various years, 1920-65	205
10.1	Average annual age-specific incidence rates per 1,000 population for herpes zoster: Cirencester, England, 1947-62; Hawick, Scotland, 1948-55; and Rochester, Minnesota, 1945-54	221
10.2	Cumulative percentage frequency for Huntington's chorea by age at onset, and by age at death: Victoria, Australia, various years to 1963	225
11.1	Death rates per 100,000 population under 1 year of age for neonatal cerebral palsy (intracranial and spinal injury at birth) by year: United States, 1949-67	235
11.2	Average annual age-specific death rates per 100,000 population for infantile cerebral palsy (cerebral spastic infantile paralysis) by color: United States, 1959-61	237
11.3	Average annual age-adjusted death rates per 100,000 population under 15 years of age for infantile cerebral palsy (cerebral spastic infantile paralysis) by state: United States, 1959-61	238

13.1 Number of persons per 100 adult population having hearing levels better than "normal," and with some hearing handicap in the better ear, at specified cycles per second, by color   294
13.2 Number of persons per 1,000 population with binaural hearing loss by family income, educational attainment of individual, and age   297

FOREWORD

Rapid advances in medical and allied sciences, changing patterns in medical care and public health programs, an increasingly health-conscious public, and the rising concern of voluntary agencies and government at all levels in meeting the health needs of the people necessitate constant evaluation of the country's health status. Such an evaluation, which is required not only for an appraisal of the current situation, but also to refine present goals and to gauge our progress toward them, depends largely upon a study of vital and health statistics records.

Opportunity to study mortality in depth emerges when a national census furnishes the requisite population data for the computation of death rates in demographic and geographic detail. Prior to the 1960 census of population there had been no comprehensive analysis of this kind. It therefore seemed appropriate to build up for intensive study a substantial body of death statistics for a three-year period centered around that census year.

A detailed examination of the country's health status must go beyond an examination of mortality statistics. Many conditions such as arthritis, rheumatism, and mental diseases are much more important as causes of morbidity than of mortality. Also, an examination of health status should not be based solely upon current findings, but should take into account trends and whatever pertinent evidence has been assembled through local surveys and from clinical experience.

The proposal for such an evaluation, to consist of a series of monographs, was made to the Statistics Section of the American Public Health Association in October 1958 by Mortimer Spiegelman, and a Committee on Vital and Health Statistics Monographs was authorized, with Mr. Spiegelman as Chairman, a position he held until his death on March 25, 1969. The members of this committee and of the Editorial Advisory Subcommittee created later are:

Committee on Vital and Health Statistics Monographs

Carl L. Erhardt, D.Sc., Chairman
Paul M. Densen, D.Sc.
Robert D. Grove, Ph.D.
Clyde V. Kiser, Ph.D.
Felix Moore

George Rosen, M.D., Ph.D.
William H. Stewart, M.D.
  (withdrew June 1964)
Conrad Taeuber, Ph.D.
Paul Webbink
Donald Young, Ph.D.

Editorial Advisory Subcommittee

Carl L. Erhardt, D.Sc., Chairman
Duncan Clark, M.D.
E. Gurney Clark, M.D.
Jack Elinson, Ph.D.

Eliot Freidson, Ph.D.
(withdrew February 1964)
Brian MacMahon, M.D., Ph.D.
Colin White, Ph.D.

The early history of this undertaking is described in a paper presented at the 1962 Annual Conference of the Milbank Memorial Fund.* The Committee on Vital and Health Statistics Monographs selected the topics to be included in the series and also suggested candidates for authorship. The frame of reference was extended by the committee to include other topics in vital and health statistics than mortality and morbidity, namely fertility, marriage, and divorce. Conferences were held with authors to establish general guidelines for the preparation of the manuscripts.

Support for this undertaking in its preliminary stages was received from the Rockefeller Foundation, the Milbank Memorial Fund, and the Health Information Foundation. Major support for the required tabulations, for writing and editorial work, and for the related research of the monograph authors was provided by the United States Public Health Service (Research Grant CH 00075, formerly GM 08262). Acknowledgment should also be made to the Metropolitan Life Insurance Company for the facilities and time that were made available to Mr. Spiegelman before his retirement in December 1966, after which he devoted his major time to administer the undertaking and to serve as general editor. Without his abiding concern over each monograph in the series and his close work with the authors, the completion of the series might have been in grave doubt. The published volumes will be a fitting memorial to Mr. Spiegelman even though his name does not appear as an author.

The New York City Department of Health allowed Dr. Carl L. Erhardt to allocate part of his time to administrative details for the series from April to December 1969, when he retired to assume a more active role. The National Center for Health Statistics, under the supervision of Dr. Grove and Miss Alice M. Hetzel, undertook the

---

*Mortimer Spiegelman, "The Organization of the Vital and Health Statistics Monograph Program," *Emerging Techniques in Population Research (Proceedings of the 1962 Annual Conference of the Milbank Memorial Fund;* New York: Milbank Memorial Fund, 1963), p. 230. See also Mortimer Spiegelman, "The Demographic Viewpoint in the Vital and Health Statistics Monographs Project of the American Public Health Association," *Demography*, 3:574 (1966).

sizable tasks of planning and carrying out the extensive mortality tabulations for the 1959-61 period. Dr. Taeuber arranged for the cooperation of the Bureau of the Census at all stages of the project in many ways, principally by furnishing the required population data used in computing death rates and by undertaking a large number of varied special tabulations. As the sponsor of the project, the American Public Health Association furnished assistance through Dr. Thomas R. Hood, its Deputy Executive Director.

Because of the great variety of topics selected for monograph treatment, authors were given an essentially free hand to develop their manuscripts as they desired. Accordingly, the authors of the individual monographs bear the full responsibility for their manuscripts, and their opinions and statements do not necessarily represent the viewpoints of the American Public Health Association or of the agencies with which they may be affiliated.

James R. Kimmey, M.D.
Executive Director
American Public Health Association

NOTES ON TABLES AND FIGURES

1. Regarding 1959-61 mortality data:
    a. Deaths relate to those occurring in the United States, including Alaska and Hawaii;
    b. Deaths are classified by place of residence at death, unless otherwise stated;
    c. Fetal deaths are excluded;
    d. Deaths of unknown age, marital status, nativity, or other characteristics have not been distributed into the known categories, but are included in their totals;
    e. Deaths were classified by cause according to the *Seventh Revision of the International Statistical Classification of Diseases, Injuries, and Causes of Death* (Geneva: World Health Organization, 1957);
    f. Unless otherwise specified, all death rates are average annual rates per 100,000 population in the category specified, as recorded in the United States census of April 1, 1960;
    g. Age-adjusted rates were computed by the direct method using the age distribution of the total United States population in the census of April 1, 1940, as a standard.* The mortality tabulations prepared especially for this series included age-adjusted death rates for all ages, under 15 years, and 65 years and over. In tabulations by marital status, the age-adjusted groupings were 15 years and over, 15 to 64 years, and 65 years and over.
2. Regarding "crude" and "adjusted" rates:
    Unless otherwise specified, all rates are "crude" (unadjusted). However, in some instances crude rates have been so labeled intentionally for clarity, emphasis, or to avoid confusion with other similar tables or figures in which age-adjusted data are used.
3. Symbols used in tables of data:
    - - - Data not available;
    . . . Category not applicable;
    -     Quantity zero;
    0.0   Quantity more than zero but less than 0.05;
    *   Figure does not meet the standard of reliability or precision:
        a) Rate or ratio based on less than 20 deaths;
        b) Percentage or median based on less than 100 deaths;
        c) Age-adjusted rate computed from age-specific rates where more than half of the rates were based on frequencies of less than 20 deaths. For disorders sharply delimited by age, this criterion may give a spurious impression of imprecision; where feasible in such instances, numbers of deaths are also entabled.

---

*Mortimer Spiegelman and H. H. Marks, "Empirical Testing of Standards for the Age Adjustment of Death Rates by the Direct Method," *Human Biology*, 38:280 (September 1966).

4. Geographic classification:†
    a. Standard Metropolitan Statistical Area (SMSA): except in the New England states, "an SMSA is a county or a group of contiguous counties which contains at least one city of 50,000 inhabitants or more or 'twin cities' with a combined population of at least 50,000 in the 1960 census. In addition, contiguous counties are included in an SMSA if, according to specified criteria, they are (a) essentially metropolitan in character and (b) socially and economically integrated with the central city or cities." In New England, the Division of Vital Statistics of the National Center for Health Statistics uses, instead of the definition just cited, Metropolitan State Economic Areas (MSEA's) established by the Bureau of the Census, which are made up of county units.
    b. Metropolitan and nonmetropolitan: "Counties which are included in SMSA's, or, in New England, MSEA's are called metropolitan counties; all other counties are classified as nonmetropolitan."
    c. Metropolitan counties may be separated into those containing at least one central city of 50,000 inhabitants or more or "twin cities" as specified previously, and into metropolitan counties without a central city.
    d. Census regions: Nine geographic divisions of the United States as utilized by the Bureau of the Census, each region comprising a group of states (without reference to SMSA's), including as appropriate the District of Columbia, Alaska, or Hawaii.
5. The following sources in the Public Health Service, U.S. Department of Health, Education, and Welfare, were used in preparing the figures, text tables, and appendix tables referable to mortality data for the United States. Any additional sources are specified in the text tables and figures.
    a. National Center for Health Statistics, special tabulations of deaths and death rates for the period 1959-61 for the American Public Health Association.
    b. National Center for Health Statistics, *Vital Statistics of the United States*, Washington, D.C., issued annually.

†National Center for Health Statistics, *Vital Statistics of the United States, 1960* (Washington, D. C.: Public Health Service, 1963), vol. 2, *Mortality*, pt. A, sec. 7, p. 8.

American Public Health Association

VITAL AND HEALTH STATISTICS MONOGRAPHS

EPIDEMIOLOGY OF NEUROLOGIC AND SENSE ORGAN DISORDERS

1 / INTRODUCTION TO EPIDEMIOLOGY

Leonard T. Kurland
John F. Kurtzke

Planning began in 1958 for the American Public Health Association to sponsor a series of Vital and Health Statistics Monographs based on the 1960 census of the United States population and, for most of the series, 1959-61 mortality data. The monographs were intended to "be of use in schools of medicine and public health; and be useful to social scientists, students, research workers, medical care program workers, practicing physicians to some extent, and to market analysts and drug houses" (Spiegelman 1963). Ten of the volumes were to deal with individual diseases (tuberculosis) or types of disease based on pathogenesis (neoplasms) or organ systems involved (digestive). Among the last group was to be a volume on neurologic and sense organ disorders.

For neurology, this afforded an excellent opportunity to provide a full-length treatment of the population characteristics of disorders of the nervous system. Accordingly, the United States mortality data of 1959-61 have been used as a springboard for the incorporation of morbidity and mortality information from various lands and times. Not all disorders of the nervous system are considered. For some, no useful epidemiologic information exists. For others, the topics have been incorporated in other monographs of this series: cerebrovascular disease is encompassed by the volume on cardiovascular diseases (Moriyama et al. 1971) and is also the subject of an unrelated work (Kurtzke 1969b). Brain tumor is to be found in the monograph on cancer (Lilienfeld et al. 1972); the inflammatory disorders in the one on infectious diseases (Dauer et al. 1968); and neurosyphilis in the work on venereal diseases (Brown et al. 1970).

Since this volume is directed to the "practicing physician" as well as the public health worker, perhaps the latter will bear with us as we go into some degree of detail as to what is properly subsumed under the mantle of "epidemiology" and particularly as it applies to neurologic diseases in "neuroepidemiology."

Epidemiology—Scope and Definition

The main role of epidemiology is the investigation of disease characteristics in populations to provide new information concerning etiology and, as an important by-product, to develop and test new methods of disease control and prevention (Fox et al. 1970). There are three commonly identified aspects of epidemiology: descriptive, analytic, and experimental (MacMahon et al. 1960). The *descriptive* aspect of epidemiology refers to the identification of the persons affected and unaffected in a population, and the circumstances (time and place) under which the disease occurs. Results from descriptive studies may generate specific hypotheses as an *analytic* aspect of epidemiology. Studies under conditions that permit the investigator to control relevant factors constitute the *experimental* aspect of epidemiology.

Perhaps because of mistaken etymology, many equate the field of epidemiology with the investigation of epidemic diseases. Modern practices, however, have renovated its literal translation as the discourse or study (*logos*) upon (*epi*) people (*demos*). As Paul (1966) has stated, this is the field "concerned with measurements of the circumstances under which diseases occur, where diseases tend to flourish, and where they do not." In the context of this definition is the consideration of the frequency of a disorder based on comparisons of the affected with the unaffected in the population under study or "at risk," together with any notable predilections for geography and population characteristics such as sex, age, and race. It also includes spatial distributions at levels from family groups to entire countries, and temporal relations for diurnal, seasonal, annual, or even centennial epochs. For the individual as well as the community, factors associated with the manifestation of the illness are sought in the inherent characteristics of affected persons as well as in their environment.

Interrelated with the frequency of a disease and its recognition are its severity and clinical course.

To whom and for what purposes is this information of value? While the major goal is clarifying etiology which influences health care at many levels, various groups and governmental and voluntary agencies may also benefit from the collection of epidemiologic data. Planners of health and social programs need these data for valid estimates as to the cost of illness, not only in terms of the diseased person and the expense of his care, but also in terms of its influence on his family and productivity. In addition, the construction and staffing of health care facilities are dependent on an accurate estimate of the frequency and outcome of disease.

The public health worker needs epidemiologic data to determine the extent and nature of illness in the community, to establish departures from the base-line experience (epidemics), to project past experience into future trends, and to devise and carry out whatever environmental control or genetic counseling measures are appropriate or feasible to attack the problems at hand.

The medical practitioner is not only the major source of epidemiologic information on disease, but also one of its principal users. It is his role to define the disease in groups of patients; it is his role to determine what happens in these patients during the course of illness; and it is his role to seek ways to alter this course with the establishment of preventive or treatment measures.

Historical Note

Almost ninety years ago, Hirsch (1883) of Berlin in his *Handbook of Geographical and Historical Pathology* stated:

> In these considerations lie the germs of a science, which, in an ideally complete form, would furnish a *medical history of mankind* [and] will give: firstly, a picture of the occurrence, the distribution, and the types of the diseases of mankind, in distinct epochs of time, and at various points of the earth's surface; and, secondly, will render an account of the relations of those diseases to the external conditions surrounding the individual and determining his manner of life. And this science I have named, from the dominating point of view, the science of *geographical and historical pathology.*

Although much of Hirsch's collection was clinical and anecdotal because few quantitative studies were available, it was an important step forward in an era when knowledge of cause of even the common infectious disorders was just emerging. The impression that beri-beri was related to nutritional deficiency is well documented; but the association of climate, soil, race, occupation, or customs with the distribution of chorea, epilepsy, or apoplexy only rarely seems pertinent to our current understanding of etiology and pathogenesis. However, Hirsch's expression (1886) of the problems of diagnosis and case ascertainment is appropriate even today to large areas of neuroepidemiology:

> Apart from a few diseases . . . what we find in the ancient and mediaeval writings upon nervous diseases, as well as in those of the modern period . . . is that great

aggregate of symptoms ... behind which lie concealed all sorts of diseases of the nervous system.

No less appropriate even today is his reference to a dearth of accurate mortality and morbidity statistics.

The early advances in epidemiology occurred when infectious and nutritional disorders were concentrated in time and place (for example, cholera, scurvy, and goiter) and when affected persons could be readily distinguished from unaffected. The remarkable population surveys and experiments by Goldberger and his associates (1920) on pellagra about fifty years ago still serve as a classic illustration of epidemiology and illustrate how such studies could lead to preventive measures even before pathogenesis or specific biochemical defects are identified. Goldberger's studies on pellagra included a *descriptive* aspect of mortality, morbidity, seasonal distribution, and selection by age, sex, and socioeconomic status; an *analytic* aspect which led to the nutritional deficiency hypothesis; and an *experimental* program in human populations which confirmed this hypothesis.

The elucidation of the natural history of deficiency and infectious diseases of the nervous system was largely dependent on advances in laboratory-oriented sciences, as well as in clinical and population studies. Even as these problems were being clarified, interest was directed toward neurologic diseases of unknown cause, such as lathyrism in India, subacute combined degeneration in Scandinavia, and multiple sclerosis in the Northern Hemisphere. Charcot (1879), in his lectures of 1868, had suggested that there was a variation in the geographic distribution of multiple sclerosis, as its recognition in France and Germany contrasted with its apparent absence in England. However, as the literature on multiple sclerosis became more widely dispersed, the disease was found to be of relatively high frequency throughout northern Europe, Great Britain, Canada, and the northern United States. It is of interest that in 1905, before the serologic test for syphilis, multiple sclerosis was reportedly rare in New York compared to New Orleans (Van Wart 1905), which is contrary to more recent evidence (Kurland 1952). The population surveys for multiple sclerosis in Europe by Allison (1931), Bing and Reese (1926), and Ackermann (1931) were an important development in the study of the incidence and distribution of chronic neurologic disease. From these beginnings and with international efforts to provide comparable statistics, systematic studies of mortality and morbidity of neurologic disorders have gradually evolved.

The Interrelation of Genetics and Epidemiology

It was long ago recognized that many diseases of the nervous system occurred in familial aggregations and were presumably hereditary. The classic studies by Huntington (1872; 1910) on hereditary chorea in New York, by Thomsen (1892) on myotonia congenita, and by Osler (1880) on progressive spinal muscular atrophy are examples of the elucidation of dominant traits responsible for neurologic disease.

Even where a hereditary factor is deemed critical to the expression of disease, environmental conditions may affect the time of onset of the disease, the rapidity of its progression, and perhaps even the development of new mutations. The interplay of the complex elements of environment on the genetic background of the individual may determine the manifestation of disease to the extent that it often becomes difficult to distinguish "genetic" from "nongenetic" conditions (Myrianthopoulos 1959). The relative roles of heredity and environment in some of the diseases occurring in familial aggregation will be considered later in this monograph. An excellent survey of the genetic aspects of neurology has been published by Pratt (1967).

Geographic Isolates

A geographic isolate in the context of this monograph refers to a population that is inbred, isolated, or otherwise distinct and is characterized by high frequency of a new or rare disease or unusual prevalence of a well-known disease. Such isolates are avidly sought since they may demonstrate ecologic associations that otherwise might not be appreciated. Large numbers of an ordinarily uncommon disease may also more readily demonstrate the full clinical spectrum of the disease. The studies of Andrade (1952) on amyloid neuropathy in Portugal may be cited as an example.

Factors of chance or "genetic drift" and balanced polymorphism* may influence the development of these isolates. The presence of a dominant form of progressive muscular dystrophy in one of the early Mormon settlers who sired more than thirty children accounts for

---

*A genetic term used to describe the situation in which a trait in the heterozygous condition has beneficial influence or reproductive superiority over the dominant and recessive homozygotes.

the high incidence of this disease in the Salt Lake City area (Tyler and Stephens 1950). Recessive genetic traits often become prevalent in small inbred populations in spite of adverse selection pressures. The foci that come to medical attention can range from ruling dynasties which perpetuate inbreeding to religious, national, or racial minorities who choose to reside apart or are restricted from integrating with the general population. The isolates in which intensive neuropsychiatric studies have been carried out include various islands and such places as villages in the Alps or in remote parts of Scandinavia (Vogel 1964).

In recent years in neurology, a number of studies in circumscribed populations have included such exotic names as Minamata disease in Japan (Kurland et al. 1960), kuru in New Guinea (Gajdusek 1965), progressive neuropathy in Jamaica (Cruickshank 1961), and lytico (Kurland and Mulder 1954) and bodig on Guam (Lessell et al. 1962*a*). All have the following features: a high incidence of a serious and generally fatal nervous system disease; an isolated geographic setting; some familial aggregation of cases; and, early in the investigation, uncertainty as to the role of heredity. Although several of these foci will be referred to later, our primary concern in this work will be to provide some useful "base-line statistics" that will facilitate our recognition of unusual rates of disease occurrence when we encounter them.

Diagnosis of Disease

The identification of diseases or syndromes—basic to epidemiologic study of an illness—is influenced by many factors such as the presence of pathognomonic physical signs or specific laboratory test results, current nomenclature, diagnostic fashions, medical standards, and the frequency of the disease. The disease state may vary in intensity from the "subclinical" or clinically inapparent (where only a test such as an immunologic skin reaction identifies the affected) to the clinically apparent case (with mild to severe or even fulminating features) to the initial recognition as the cause of death or as an incidental finding at autopsy. Certain diseases such as amyotrophic lateral sclerosis are usually correctly labeled when clinically diagnosed, whereas others such as multiple sclerosis are more subject to appreciable misdiagnosis.

Diagnostic criteria are of special import in assessing mortality statistics. In this country only a small proportion of those who die are autopsied. Attempts at validation of mortality statistics with autopsy material have of course been made (Swartout and Webster 1940; Munck 1952; James et al. 1955; Waaler and Grimstvedt 1958; Hamtoft and Mosbech 1961; Heasman 1962; Stazio et al. 1964; Zschoch 1964; Heasman and Lipworth 1966; Jablon et al. 1966), often with rather discouraging results. But where the majority of deaths are not subject to pathologic verification, one might well expect to find a factitiously high rate of error in clinical diagnosis, as generally it is the unusual or the uncertain cause of death for which autopsy is performed. Still, even for such a common disorder as cerebrovascular disease, as many as one of four deaths so listed may be in error (Kurtzke 1969b).

Aside from autopsy verification, one may seek to validate death data by review of clinical records (Moriyama et al. 1958; 1966); this, however, is diagnostic consensus rather than diagnostic proof. One ordinarily questions diagnostic validity in prevalence surveys, as there is then available for diagnosis only the clinical impression with whatever laboratory support exists. But in such a setting diagnostic scrutiny is ordinarily intensive, and one might with justification believe the clinical entity in question to be thereby much better defined than is often the case with mortality data.

In sum, therefore, a considerable amount of the information utilized in population studies rests on the diagnostic impressions of the practicing physician.

Types of Epidemiologic Data

Discussions of the frequency of disease commonly are based on case series, relative frequencies, and rates.

Case Series

This is a consecutive list of cases observed in a hospital, clinic, or physician's practice. The term "consecutive" is supposed to imply the absence of bias in selection; but such a series may not relate the subjects to any clearly defined population base and serves only to identify the presence of the disease. Because of selective factors in hospitalization or clinic care, such a series is rarely representative of any identifiable population.

Those intrigued with "controls" drawn from hospital registrations should remember that they too are subject to input bias, and not necessarily in the same manner as the patients for whom they are the comparison group.

Autopsy series not only are but a fraction of hospital cases with their potential biases, but also are limited to further selection among those who die; they therefore may not be representative of all who have been affected with the disease in question.

Unfortunately, the tendency persists for pathologists and clinicians to compare two or more clinical or autopsy series and to speculate on reasons for observed differences, often without considering that the cases might have been drawn from different populations. Another misinterpretation common in medical analysis is the assumption that the most frequent age group of persons in the series represents the age of greatest risk for that disease. Without a basis of reference, such as the population from which the cases arose, it may be impossible to determine from the distribution of cases alone whether a disease is really more common in one age, sex, or group than another. In spite of these shortcomings, it is the case series and the studies of relative frequency (referred to next) that generally provide the basis for hypotheses as to cause or risk factors, and lead to intensive, refined, and (hopefully) more definitive population-oriented studies.

Relative Frequency

If, for a given disease, one relates the number of clinical cases, hospital deaths, or autopsies to the total of admitted patients, deaths, or autopsies performed, this provides a ratio which is a measure of relative frequency. However, the relative frequency varies not only with the number of diagnosed or verified cases in the numerator, but also with the number and character of cases, deaths, or autopsies in the denominator. The type of practice or admission policies of the hospital, the combined influences leading to all causes of death, and the social as well as the medical factors influencing autopsy practices affect the denominator as well as the numerator, but not necessarily in the same way in different studies.

Population-Oriented Studies

Although it would be preferable to screen by a test procedure or examine the entire population to identify those affected with the disease under study, this is usually impractical and one must generally resort to review of records of all known sources of medical information including physicians, hospitals, and insurance, disability, or pension rolls. This may give the total of those known or thought to be affected in the community, but will of course miss the asymptomatic persons and those cases which are diagnosable but have not come to medical attention.

Of those who are under care for the disease, a portion may die because of the disease. The disease should then be listed on the death certificate as the underlying cause of death. This is the manner in which routine mortality data are compiled to give the death rates as officially published in most lands. There may be an additional proportion of the affected who die for reasons unrelated to the disease. If the diagnosis has been made, however, it should be cited on the death certificate under the section pertaining to complications or contributory causes. In selected instances these deaths can be retrieved under schemes allowing for multiple causes of death and on occasion are part of the corpus of official mortality statistics.

At all levels of information, then, some proportion of the affected population may be overlooked; this proportion increases (but in an unpredictable fashion) the farther we get from a survey of the population or a representative sample of it.

As stated, we want to get as close as possible to the ascertainment of all cases (numerator) in a defined population (denominator). What are these population-based rates?

Population-Based Rates

In this monograph we shall be dealing with three types of rates: incidence, prevalence, and mortality. Each of these has a numerator and a denominator—each of which is subject to some error—and each of which can be expressed in appropriate units:

Incidence rate: $\dfrac{\text{cases occurring during a stated interval of time}}{\text{population at risk}}$,

Prevalence rate: $\dfrac{\text{Cases present on a given date}}{\text{population at risk}}$, and

Mortality rate: $\dfrac{\text{deaths during a stated interval of time}}{\text{population at risk}}$.

The *incidence* or *attack rate* is defined as the number of new cases that develop in an interval of time per unit of population and is usually expressed as cases per 100,000 population per year. It is preferably concerned with the time of *onset* of the disease, and since the association of some factor responsible for the disease may be sufficiently recent to be discerned, it is the preferred measure for etiologic studies. The denominator or population at risk may be the entire population, or both the cases and denominator may refer only to a specified segment with respect to age, sex, and the like within the total population. In conditions with an insidious or uncertain onset, it is at times more practical to measure "incidence" based on the earliest date of diagnosis, even though this obviously varies with the individual's readiness to seek medical services as well as the availability and quality of such services.

The *point prevalence rate*, strictly speaking, is a *ratio* of the affected to the population at risk at a given time. For a relatively uncommon disease with an insidious onset and a prolonged course, prevalence may be a more useful statistic than incidence for population comparisons. The prevalence (rate) of a chronic disease such as multiple sclerosis represents the accumulation of cases over several years and provides a larger and more stable numerical value for comparisons than does annual incidence. This rate, too, is expressed as cases per unit of population.

Prevalence reflects the number of patients alive with the disease and residing in the specified geographic area; it includes affected immigrants and excludes former residents who emigrated before prevalence day. With the assumption of no migration or change in annual incidence or survival over time, the interrelation of incidence and prevalence for a chronic disease can be expressed as:

$$\text{Prevalence rate} = \text{average duration (in years)} \times \text{average annual incidence rate.}$$

Mortality or *death rate* is a type of incidence rate in which "death" is substituted for "case"; it is usually expressed as the number of persons who die each year from the specified disease per 100,000 population. For a uniformly fatal disease, especially one of short duration, the death rate is also a reflection of the incidence rate. Again sex-, age-, and race-specific rates can be used. The *case-fatality* rate defines the frequency of death among the afflicted. If 40 of 100 patients with tuberculous meningitis die in a year, the case-fatality rate is 40 percent, whereas if these 40 were part of a community of 10,000,000 people, the annual mortality rate for this disease would be 0.4 per 100,000 population.

Rates of morbidity and mortality vary with such characteristics as age and, for some ailments, race or sex. One must take into account the population "at risk" in developing suitable comparisons. This is particularly important if one is comparing the frequency of a disease in two populations with different age distributions. For example, the crude (unadjusted) death rate, all ages combined, for amyotrophic lateral sclerosis is twice as high in England as in Japan. However, if one adjusts for the differences in age distribution between the populations of these countries, and these age-adjusted rates, all ages, are compared—or if the death rates by smaller age groups are compared (age-specific rates)—most of the difference disappears, suggesting that the incidence of this fatal illness is similar in the two countries.

Several items determine the choice of rates in population studies. As has been pointed out, most of the neurologic disorders have such a low incidence that case finding through individual examinations of the population is impractical, as are prospective studies comparing the subsequent development of a disease among those exposed to some hypothetical risk factor. Most information on population size and composition is derived from the census; the cases in most studies are obtained from surveys of populations or from records of physicians and other medical resources in the community. Census information is subject to error, usually of underenumeration that may vary with age, sex, ethnic group, and marital status of the population under study.

In most epidemiologic studies, however, it is the numerator that is subject to greater error. Among the possible inadequacies of numerator data are failure of the physician to record or recall the diagnosis of all patients he has observed, inaccuracies of diagnosis, and variations among physicians in diagnostic criteria or definition of a disease or syndrome. The published mortality rates are useful if the disease has a high case-fatality rate, is likely to be reported as the underlying cause of death, and is properly coded through the International Statistical Classification of Diseases, Injuries, and Causes of Death (ISC) (World Health Organization 1957). The Seventh Revision of the ISC is used for the 1959-61 deaths in this report, although it has since been revised appreciably in the Eighth Revision adopted in 1968.

Incidence and prevalence data provide different measures of the impact of the disease on a population; both are useful if properly applied. Incidence implies recognition of a date of onset, or if this is vague as is often true in chronic neurologic diseases, a date of diagnosis. Prevalence for a disease of long duration is a more stable rate and particularly useful in comparing the frequency of a slowly progressive disease whose duration does not vary appreciably in different populations. Therefore the selection of a particular rate depends on the clinical characteristics of the disease under study, the source of information, the delineation of the population "at risk," and the point the investigator is trying to present or stress. As a general rule, the clear identification of each affected person in the population is desired, if not essential.

Most epidemiologic studies are observational and seldom attain the status of a carefully controlled experiment. In such circumstances, when differences in results are statistically significant at a given probability level, we can safely conclude that *either* a rare event has occurred, *or* the series are truly different, *or* there is hidden bias so that the series are not truly comparable.

In a carefully controlled experiment, when our observed results are not significantly different, we can only conclude that any true difference which exists is not sufficiently large to have been detected by an experiment of this size and precision. In observational studies, we conclude similarly that there is no difference, or that our sample size was too small to detect whatever true difference existed, or that noncomparability of the two series has masked the difference.

In the chapters that follow, we give confidence intervals for incidence and prevalence rates. The confidence intervals tell us how much information our study has given us. For example, if there are 64 cases in a population of 50,000, we estimate the incidence rate as $\frac{64}{50,000} \times 100,000 = 128$ per 100,000. By using an approximate 95-percent confidence level, we feel that we have enough information to pin the rate down as $128 \pm 2 \left[\frac{\sqrt{64}}{50,000} \right]$, or between 96 and 160 per 100,000.*

Detailed procedures for analyzing and presenting statistics in retrospective and prospective studies have been well reviewed by Dorn (1955), and by Fox and his colleagues (1970). The reader is

---

*Corrections for asymmetry and use of 1.96 instead of 2 would provide limits of 99 and 163, as confirmed from tables of the Poisson distribution (Pearson and Hartley 1954).

also referred to standard textbooks of statistics for a description of test procedures (Hill 1962; Dunn 1964; Dixon and Massey 1969).

Source Material Utilized

In this work, we shall be concerned primarily with the descriptive and analytic epidemiology of chronic, progressive, and particularly noninfectious neurologic or neuromuscular diseases or syndromes. The following sources provide the statistics in our chapters on neurologic and neuromuscular disorders.

(1) An international comparison of mortality rates for a series of diseases of the nervous system (Goldberg and Kurland 1962).

(2) A detailed analysis of mortality rates from 1959 through 1961 in the United States, specially prepared for this and other monographs in the APHA series. The sum of the deaths in the three years divided by three times the population derived from the 1960 United States census provides the appropriate death rates. Age adjustment is done to the 1940 United States population by the direct method.

(3) The study of neurologic diseases in the population of Rochester, Minnesota, for 1945-54 inclusive (Kurland 1958a), which is now being extended to provide incidence, trends, prevalence, and survival data for several decades through 1969. Data are derived from the records of the Mayo Clinic and other sources. Although the main advantage of this ongoing study is a high level of case ascertainment and diagnostic accuracy, it is recognized that a major justification for the extrapolation from a relatively small population (30,000 in 1950; 50,000 in 1965) of limited ethnic and socioeconomic composition to the population of the United States as a whole is the paucity of information from other sources.

(4) A recent study from Carlisle, England (Brewis et al. 1966) (population about 70,000), for 1955-61 inclusive. This was based on a survey of reports from local hospitals, general practitioners, private consultants, and the Medical Officer of Health.

(5) The studies based on the experience of selected general

practitioners in Great Britain as reported by Logan and Cushion (1958) and the Research Committee of the Council of the College of General Practitioners (1962).
(6) Studies by the Gudmundssons (1966; 1967b; 1968b) on the frequency of various neurologic diseases in Iceland.
(7) Other sources, such as the Selective Service, the military forces, and health insurance institutions, whose data generally relate to segments of the population and are not necessarily representative of the population at large.
(8) Cancer registries and special surveys on multiple sclerosis and other conditions.
(9) A recent study of neurologic diseases in Guam (Chen et al. 1968).
(10) Special surveys of blindness and deafness in selected populations—for example, the Model Reporting Area for Blindness Statistics (National Institute of Neurological Diseases and Blindness 1963).

2 / CONVULSIVE DISORDERS

John F. Kurtzke
Leonard T. Kurland
Irving D. Goldberg
Nung Won Choi
Frances A. Reeder*

Known since antiquity, the epilepsies or convulsive disorders have yet to be classified to the satisfaction of all. According to Robb (1965):

Epilepsy has been defined as a group of conditions characterized by recurring convulsions [or] a group of disorders in which the common factor is a paroxysmal, excessive, neuronal discharge within the brain ... accompanied by a sudden disturbance of function of body or mind.

Alternatively, according to Kurland and Kurtzke (1972):

Convulsive disorders are states characterized by sudden, brief, repetitive, and stereotyped alterations of behavior which are presumed to be due to a paroxysmal discharge of cortical or subcortical neurons.

The equivalence of "epilepsy" and "convulsive disorders" is generally accepted, although some workers would limit the former to seizure states wherein no obvious cause can be ascribed. Most would agree, however, that single seizures should not be classed as "epilepsy" and that "febrile seizures" likewise should be omitted.

One of the recent efforts to classify convulsive disorders has been that of the Commission on Terminology of the International League against Epilepsy (ILAE). The preliminary classification of seizures was published in 1964 (Commission on Terminology) and slightly modified in 1969 (Gastaut). However, this is a classification of seizures rather than a classification of epilepsy and is based upon both clinical and electroencephalographic (EEG) criteria. A modification of this classification limited to the clinical characteristics of seizure disorders has been employed in a current study in Rochester, Minnesota (Hauser et al., unpublished data) and may prove satisfactory for epidemiologic inquiry in the future.

The usual clinical classification of seizures as grand mal, petit mal, focal, psychomotor, and other or unclassified has been applied in most population studies. "Grand mal," the best-recognized pattern clinically, is the generalized tonic-clonic seizure. In studies of

*Deceased September 18, 1972.

patients with focal seizures, categories such as "temporal" or "psychomotor" are variably included with the "jacksonian" and "focal motor or sensory" seizures. The category of "petit mal" or simple *absences* refers to frequent but brief episodes of impairment of consciousness with or without myoclonic jerks or postural alterations, but always without aura or postictal features. In Table A.2.1, we have attempted to relate the categories in these several schemata to the clinical forms of seizures.

Clinically, focal and psychomotor seizures are considered to be effects of local cerebral lesions and therefore can be classified as secondary seizures. Petit mal seizures are ordinarily present with no demonstrable structural or metabolic defect and can thus be considered primary (essential, idiopathic) seizures. Grand mal may be either primary or secondary, and even petit mal in rare instances may be a sign of underlying disease. In any given circumstance, the frequency with which grand mal is considered "primary" or "secondary" will be greatly dependent on the intensity and accuracy of the diagnostic measures employed.

The definition of an underlying lesion will be dependent on the degree of scrutiny as well as on the characterization of the seizure itself. A seizure may be misidentified as "grand mal" if a focal onset is unwitnessed or unreported. The fact that any focal seizure may become generalized has long led clinicians to seek focal phenomena in the preictal and postictal periods. Even classic *absences* have been shown by careful cinematographic studies (Penry, unpublished data) to consist of complex behavior.

An excellent discussion of the pathophysiology of seizures, and one that is not outdated, is that of Gastaut and Fischer-Williams (1959). Their contention that 95 percent of all epilepsy is "organic" (secondary), however, does not appear warranted, as may be seen later in this chapter.

Mortality Data

Mortality statistics, because they are readily available for large populations in which demographic features are known, can serve as a guide in evaluating geographic characteristics of many diseases. They are of limited value in epilepsy; nevertheless, mortality rates have been evaluated in some depth to determine whether new geographic, racial, or other characteristics may be discerned.

When convulsive disorders result from tumor, trauma, or other diseases, they should not be included in deaths from epilepsy because the cause of death is supposed to be assigned to the underlying disease process, when known. Therefore statistics based on underlying cause of death can be expected to reveal only that proportion of the epilepsies likely to be fatal and unassociated with other diseases—in essence, primary grand mal. Furthermore, since the case-fatality rate for grand mal is low, those dying of this disorder may well be unrepresentative of all those with the disease. In addition, deaths attributed to primary grand mal will incorrectly include those in which an underlying disorder that caused the fits was known but not reported or went undetected for lack of proper diagnosis during life or at autopsy.

Retrieval of epilepsy as an "associated condition" on death certificates will provide *some* cases of primary grand mal in which death was from unrelated diseases, as well as *some* cases in which there were secondary seizure disorders. In Norway for 1956-60 (Statistisk Sentralbyrå 1961), the Netherlands for 1953-61 (Central Bureau of Statistics 1961), and the United States for 1955 (National Center for Health Statistics 1965) on approximately half of the death certificates on which epilepsy was recorded, it was classified as the primary cause of death and on half it was assigned to one of the secondary causes.

United States Mortality Data

Mortality data for epilepsy in the United States for 1959-61 were prepared in order to compare the rates for epilepsy with rates in other countries and with rates of previous years in this country. In the United States, the crude rate for epilepsy as the primary cause of death was about 1.1 per 100,000 population (Tables 2.1 and A.2.2).

Trend. Figure 2.1 shows annual death rates for epilepsy from 1939 through 1967 for the United States (Grove and Hetzel 1968). The crude rate rose from 1.7 in 1939-41 to nearly 2.0 during the next four years. It then declined to 1.5 by 1950 and 1.1 for 1959-61, after which it maintained a level of 1.0 during 1963-67. Age adjustment of these rates to the 1940 population produces little change: 1.6 per 100,000 in 1949-51 and 1.2 in 1959-61. The alterations in coding consequent to the several revisions of the International Statistical Classification also would change this trend only slightly; if the rules of the later revisions had applied, the

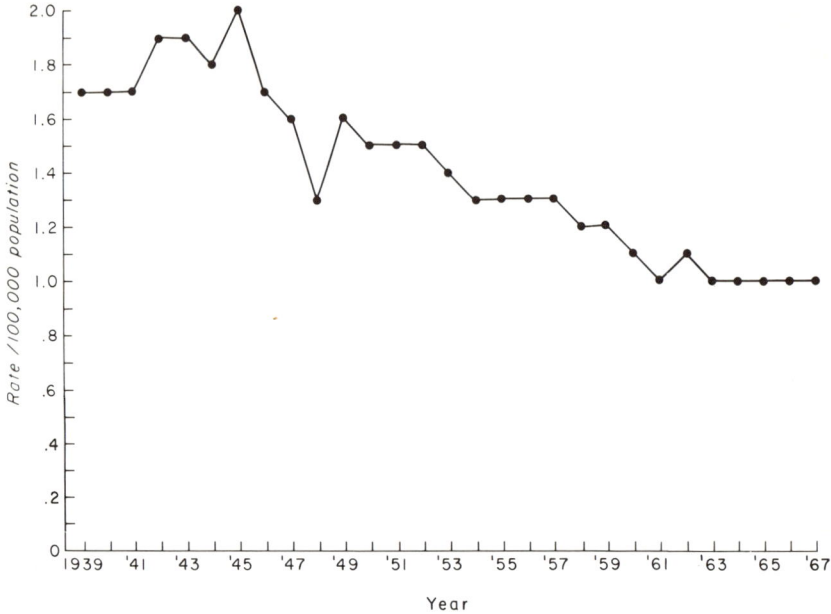

Figure 2.1 Crude death rates per 100,000 population for epilepsy by year: United States, 1939-67

1939-41 rates would have been 2.0 and those of 1949-51 would have been 1.6.

Accordingly, the recorded death rate for epilepsy has declined to nearly half its 1940 level during the ensuing twenty years. This degree of change seems too great to attribute to artifacts of diagnostic coding, and does correlate well in time with the introduction of effective anticonvulsant therapy.

Age, sex, and color. Age-specific death rates according to color and sex for epilepsy in the United States, 1959-61, are presented in Table 2.1 and Fig. 2.2. There were 5,961 death certificates that listed epilepsy as the primary cause of death during this period. The mortality rates were lowest for white females, followed by white males, nonwhite females, and nonwhite males, in that order. For the white population, the rate increased gradually to about age 40, then gradually declined to age 70, followed by an increase in the oldest age groups. For the nonwhite population, a similar pattern is seen, except that the magnitude of the increase in young adults is much greater, particularly for males. The secondary rise in the senium for all groups is based on small numbers of deaths.

Table 2.1 Average annual crude and age-adjusted death rates per 100,000 population for epilepsy by age, color and sex: United States, 1959-61[a]
(ISC code 353)

Color and sex	Crude rate	Age-adjusted rate		
	All ages	All ages	Under 15	65 & over
Total				
Total	1.1	1.2	0.5	1.3
Male	1.4	1.4	0.6	1.5
Female	0.9	0.9	0.4	1.0
White				
Total	0.9	1.0	0.4	1.1
Male	1.1	1.2	0.5	1.3
Female	0.8	0.8	0.3	1.0
Nonwhite				
Total	2.5	2.8	0.9	2.7*
Male	3.4	3.9	1.0	3.7*
Female	1.6	1.7	0.8	1.8*

[a] Detail in Table A.2.2.

Mortality data on nonwhites in the United States must be considered with caution, however, not only because of questions as to the quality and quantity of medical care available but also because of the likelihood of serious population undercount. Sirken (1967) has estimated that the net error from underenumeration and age misreporting in the 1960 census was as high as 26 to 46 percent for Negroes 45-64 years old; for those 25-44 years old, the degree of net underestimation was 18 percent for males and 6 percent for females. Among whites, the maximal error for any age was given as 5 percent. Correction for this bias would reduce the reported excess for nonwhites.

Despite the unreliability in the completeness of the census for nonwhites by age, the nonwhite-white excess was noted in the age-adjusted rates for all ages, being 2.3 to 1 for those less than 15 years old and 2.5 to 1 for those 65 or older (Table 2.1). It is largely this consistency of the excess that requires an explanation. Excess of males in both color groups also must be considered. Perhaps trauma and alcohol, which presumably affect more males than females, are direct factors in these higher death rates.

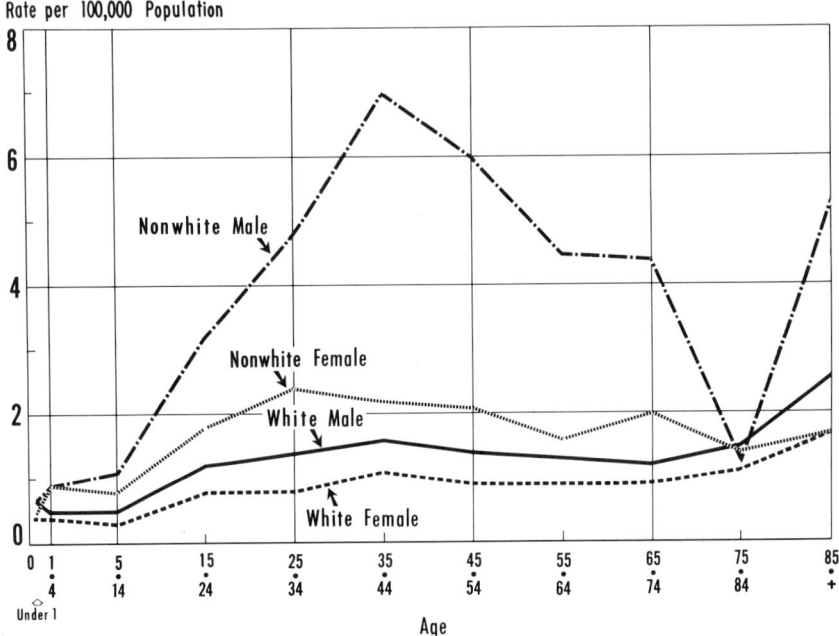

Figure 2.2 Average annual age-specific death rates per 100,000 population for epilepsy by color and sex: United States, 1959–61

The observed differences in mortality rates by color are really not explicable with the available information. Possibly the differences reflect socioeconomic conditions as they relate to cerebral injury, differences in medical care, and sensitivity of the physician to reporting the cause of death in fatal status epilepticus; they may also reflect true differences in the incidence of epilepsy by color. These matters require further evaluation.

Geographic distribution. In the U.S. the age-adjusted annual mortality rates per 100,000 population for epilepsy among the fifty states and the District of Columbia ranged from 0.3 in Nevada (where only 3 deaths were reported) to 2.2 for Wyoming and 2.7 for the District of Columbia (see Table A.2.3). For all other states, the range was appreciably less—from 0.7 to 1.8. For the United States as a whole, the rate was 1.2.

There was no clear-cut pattern to the distribution of the rates by state, although the Pacific states were all in the low range (below the national rate) and many of the southern "cotton belt" states were in

CONVULSIVE DISORDERS / 21

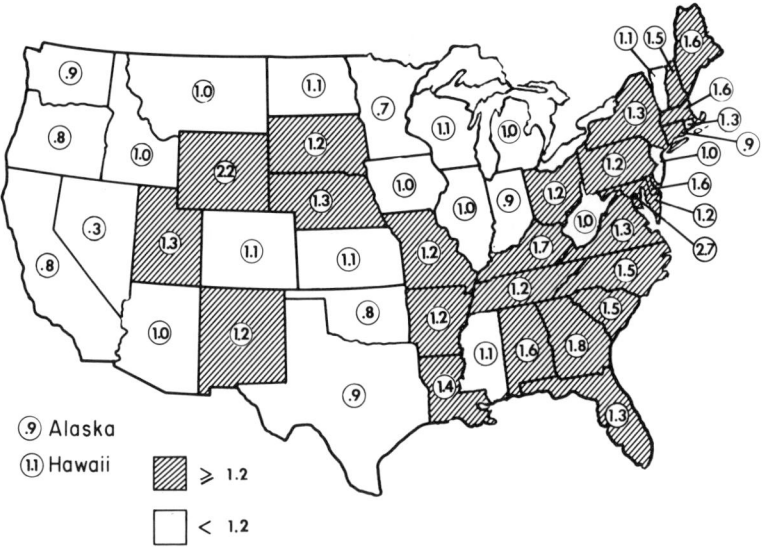

Figure 2.3 Average annual age-adjusted death rates per 100,000 population for epilepsy by state: United States, 1959–61. Rates that do not meet the standard of reliability or precision as defined in Notes on Tables and Figures are indicated by an asterisk (*) in Table A.2.3.

the high range, largely because of the greater Negro populations in the southern states, as shown in Fig. 2.3. Investigation of this aspect requires grouping of the states to provide rates based on a sufficient number of deaths. Table 2.2 shows the death rates among the nine

Table 2.2   Average annual age-adjusted death rates per 100,000 population for epilepsy by color and sex: United States and census regions, 1959-61
(ISC code 353)

Region	Total			White			Nonwhite		
	Total	M	F	Total	M	F	Total	M	F
United States	1.2	1.4	0.9	1.0	1.2	0.8	2.8	3.9	1.7
New England	1.4	2.0	0.9*	1.4	1.9	0.9*	3.7*	6.7*	0.8*
Mid. Atlantic	1.2	1.5	0.9	1.0	1.3	0.8	3.1*	4.7*	1.8*
E. No. Central	1.1	1.3	0.8	1.0	1.2	0.8	1.9*	2.8*	1.0*
W. No. Central	1.0	1.3	0.8*	1.0	1.2	0.8*	2.7*	3.5*	1.9*
So. Atlantic	1.4	1.9	1.0	0.9	1.1	0.7*	3.6	5.1	2.2*
E. So. Central	1.4	1.7	1.2*	1.0	1.1*	1.0*	3.0	4.2*	2.0*
W. So. Central	1.0	1.2	0.8*	0.8	0.9*	0.7*	2.4*	3.2*	1.7*
Mountain	1.2	1.3*	0.9*	1.1	1.2*	0.9*	2.8*	3.9*	1.6*
Pacific	0.8	1.0*	0.7*	0.8	0.9*	0.6*	1.4*	1.9*	1.0*

geographic census regions of the United States. The range of rates was appreciably less than that observed for the distribution by state. In each region a male preponderance was seen for both whites and nonwhites. Also in each region, the excess for nonwhites persisted; it was least in the Pacific region and greatest in the South Atlantic. Rates for nonwhites were highest in the New England and South Atlantic regions; the rates for whites also were high in New England.

Type of county. Age-adjusted mortality rates by metropolitan and nonmetropolitan counties are shown in Table A.2.4. The rates per 100,000 population for both sexes combined varied from 0.8 to 1.5 in metropolitan counties and from 1.0 to 1.5 in nonmetropolitan counties. The nonmetropolitan rates were slightly higher in the western part of the United States (Pacific, Mountain, West South Central, and West North Central) and elsewhere were essentially equal. For further analysis the metropolitan counties were subdivided into those with and without a central city. If there were a population-density gradient, or an urban-rural difference in each region of the country, then the greatest difference in rates should be between metropolitan counties with central cities (most urban) and the nonmetropolitan counties (most rural). As may be seen in Table A.2.4, this was not the case; the greatest differences generally were found between the metropolitan areas with central cities and those without central cities. The reason for the difference is not clear. Possibilities include overreporting in more rural regions of the West or preferential migration of the affected to western nonmetropolitan areas from either the neighboring cities or as part of the general westward movement in the United States. It may also indicate that the chronically ill may not be moving from the farm to the city to the same extent as the healthy. Comparison of rates according to birthplace would help resolve some of these points. That urban-rural differences were not consistently found, however, suggests the existence of some artifact, or at least the inference that ruralization is not a factor directly related to epileptic deaths.

Marital status. Age-adjusted death rates by marital status are shown in Table A.2.5. The rates were highest for single persons, followed by divorced, widowed, and married persons in that order. The death rate per 100,000 for single persons 15 years old or older was 6.5, whereas that for the married was 0.6. In Fig. 2.4, the uniformly low rates at all ages for married people contrast with the higher and fluctuating

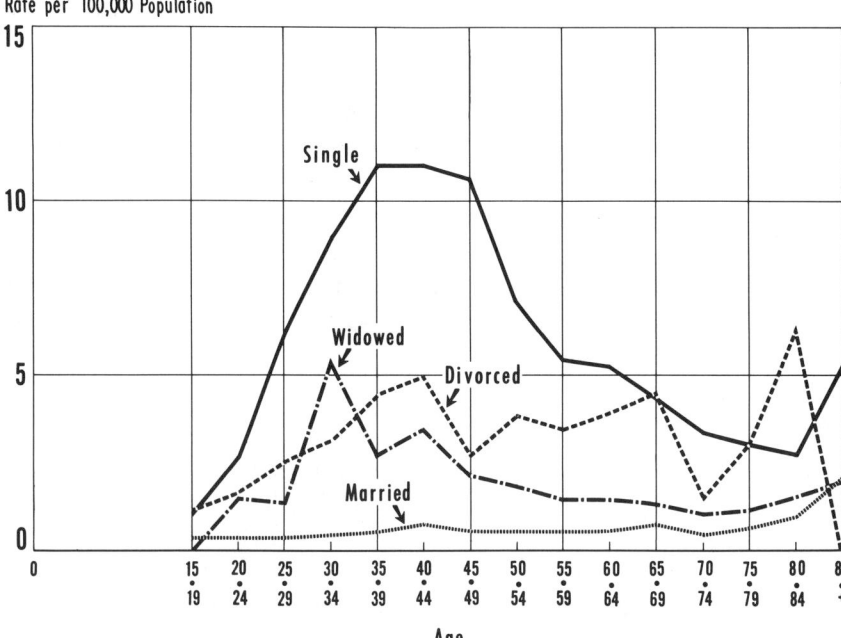

Figure 2.4 Average annual age-specific death rates per 100,000 population for epilepsy by marital status: United States, 1959–61

rates by age for single persons. The most striking difference occurred at ages 35-49 years, where the rate was about 11 per 100,000 for single people and 0.7 for the married. The age-specific rates for the widowed and divorced were based on relatively small numbers of deaths. For those of each marital condition, the rates tended to peak at age 40-44. Rates at the oldest ages are based on too few cases to permit critical comparisons. In terms of the *numbers* of deaths, males predominated in the single and divorced, females in the widowed, and neither in the currently married. However, the death *rate* for males was about twice the rate for females in each of the nonmarried groups. In those presently married, there was no significant difference between the sexes in epilepsy death rates.

The excess rates for single people may be explained by selection against marriage for epileptics, but also may be attributable to the leading of a more regular life, with less trauma and alcohol and greater readiness to seek and follow medical advice, by the married group. That such factors may be operant is suggested by the higher rates among the divorced and widowed, as well as the higher rates for males in all the nonmarried groups.

Nativity. For whites of both sexes, the age-adjusted death rate for foreign born (0.6) was lower than that for native born (1.0) (Table A.2.6). Although rates were based on only a few deaths in some of the regions, the pattern of lower rates for the foreign born was reasonably consistent among the nine census regions and for both males and females. The overall lower mortality rates for foreign-born persons may be attributable to the laws that exclude epileptics from immigrating to the United States.

International Mortality Comparisons

The age-adjusted mortality rates for epilepsy from various countries are shown in Table A.2.7 and Fig. 2.5. The highest rates were for Colombia, Chile, Portugal, Mexico, nonwhites in the United States, and for the Maori population of New Zealand. The lowest were for Denmark, Poland, Sweden, United States whites, and Israel. In all countries reporting, except Israel, there was a male preponderance. The completeness of death reporting and the proportion of fatal cases in which epilepsy was certified as the primary cause of death varied from country to country and may account for some of the diversity of reported mortality by country.

There is some reason to suspect that the recorded rates tended to vary inversely with reporting adequacy in these lands. If the first five columns of Fig. 2.5 are exluded on this basis, the range was relatively narrow—from 2.5 to 1.1 per 100,000. Although some racial predilection might be suspected in the United States for nonwhites (the vast majority of whom are Negroes), there are no supporting data for this. The similar excess for the Maoris of New Zealand (Table A.2.7) represents different racial stock. The only other predominantly nonwhite population is that of Japan, whose rate is at the median in Fig. 2.5.

Population Surveys

Because death certificates identify only a small fraction of those with convulsive disorders, studies of the incidence and prevalence of fits must be used to establish patterns of distribution and population selectivity. Unfortunately, in the few population studies that have been conducted, there was not always uniformity of either definition

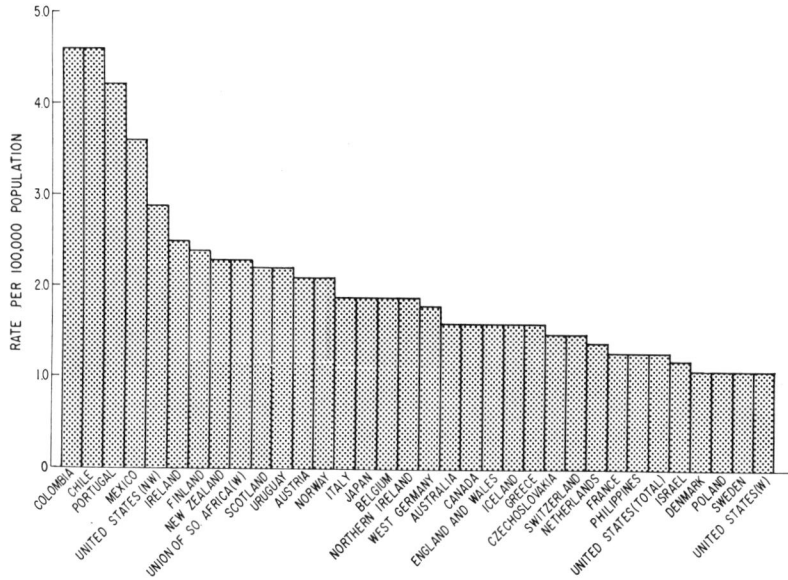

Figure 2.5 Average annual age-adjusted death rates per 100,000 population for epilepsy: selected countries, various years, 1951–58 (Source: Goldberg and Kurland 1962. By permission of Lancet Publications, Inc.)

or classification of epilepsy. Furthermore, methods of case finding differed so that studies from various parts of the world may be difficult to compare. Among the studies that have come to our attention and in which some evaluation of definition and methods was possible are the following.

(1) An early population survey of convulsive disorders covering the ten years 1945-54 was that of Kurland (1959). Prevalence rates were determined from the patients residing in Rochester, Minnesota, on January 1, 1955, and incidence rates from the patients whose first seizure occurred during the decade of study. All clinical data were derived from the Mayo Clinic files, which were considered a nearly complete record of serious illness in the resident population of Rochester. Only cases of recurrent seizures were included; those of febrile seizures were tabulated separately. The seizures were classified by predominant clinical type, as listed in Table A.2.1, except that cases of focal and psychomotor fits were combined.

(2) Crombie and his associates (1960) described the occur-

rence of fits in sixty-seven general practices from England and Wales during the year commencing October 1957. Patients who had repeated seizures or who were receiving regular anticonvulsant medication for the two years before the study were grouped under chronic epilepsies, and the incidence was determined from data on first fits in the study year. The rates were calculated from estimates of the England-Wales population distributions. Fits were divided only into "major" and "other," with the former used if both types were present.

(3) The frequency of convulsive disorders in the population of Carlisle, England, was studied by Brewis and her colleagues (1966). Persons who had had more than one "episode of cerebral origin" at any time in the past were included. Definition of epilepsy and classification by type were similar to those listed at the beginning of this chapter. However, convulsions secondary to cerebral-vascular disease or secondary to tumors were coded according to the known pathology and were not considered to be convulsive disorders. The study was part of a detailed survey of neurologic disease occurring between 1955 and 1961 in this city of 70,000. Sources of data were records of hospitals, general practitioners, consultants, and the Medical Officer of Health, plus death certificates and a sample interview of 12 percent of households.

(4) Three other British surveys were less complete. Pond and his co-workers (1960) reported on seizures in fourteen general practices of southeastern England chosen from among physicians volunteering to participate in the study. Detailed data were provided for only three practices; and the data from one of these were aberrant. Some patients were included whose fits "were not unequivocally epileptic," and patients with febrile fits and probably those with single seizures were also included.

Cooper (1965) described seizures in a longitudinal study of 5,000 children of the National Survey of Health and Development in Great Britain. Seizure disorders were defined by an answer of "yes" by the mother to the question whether "the child had ever had any sort of fit or convulsion" at age 2 years, or by a "yes" answer for the single year preceding an examination made at ages 6, 7, 11, and 15 years. The query at age 2 was by a lay home visitor; school medical officers requested the information at later ages.

Logan and Cushion (1958) reported on a survey of 106 general practices in England and Wales for the year commencing May 1955, and this included convulsive disorders (Research Committee of the Council of the College of General Practitioners 1962). Criteria for "epilepsy" were not stated.

(5) In a nationwide prevalence study in Iceland, Gunnar Gudmundsson (1966) described the occurrence of fits as of January 1, 1960. Diagnostic criteria were similar to Kurland's (1959), with an additional statement as to cause (unknown, probable, known). Patients considered as having "active" seizures were those with fits or those who were receiving regular medication within five years of prevalence day. After preliminary medical contacts, almost all patients were personally examined, or relatives were interviewed if the patient was deceased. With these data and the average duration of illness, Kurtzke (1968c) calculated average annual incidence rates.

(6) From the data of Juul-Jensen (1964), Kurtzke (1968c) also estimated incidence and prevalence rates for seizures in Jutland. Juul-Jensen's clinic at Aarhus was the only adult epilepsy clinic in Jutland, which is the peninsula containing thirteen of the twenty-three counties or *Amter* that comprise Denmark. His study covered twenty-six months from 1959 and concerned about 1,000 patients. Data for the first decade of life were discarded as incomplete. Diagnostic criteria were similar to those cited previously in this chapter.

(7) Krohn (1961) surveyed Northern Norway, chiefly from records of physicians and hospitals. Recently, this study has been updated (Henriksen and Krohn 1969; Henriksen 1969). An epileptic was defined as one who presently had recurrent seizures or who had had seizures and was currently receiving medication.

(8) Leibowitz and Alter (1968) investigated convulsive disorders in Jerusalem, Israel, for the four years 1958-61. Epilepsy was as defined previously in this chapter, but "all cases in which the seizures were due to a known cause or

were strongly suspected of being symptomatic ... or cases in which there was a definite neurological deficit on examination, were excluded." However, diagnoses such as "suspect epilepsy" and "questionable epilepsy" were included in the grand mal classification, and 54 patients with psychomotor seizures and 46 patients with focal seizures were tabulated among the 689 cases.

(9) A number of other studies have been performed. Lessell and his associates (1962b) used a retrospective history of seizures obtained from the population of the village of Merizo on Guam to estimate incidence rates for febrile seizures and epilepsy. Similar surveys, also in the Mariana Islands, were carried out in 1962 by Mathai and colleagues (1968) on Rota, Saipan, and in Umatac on Guam. Sato (1964) sought to determine the number of seizure patients in Niigata, Japan, from the records of hospitals and general practices and school authorities. Seizure types and exclusions were similar to those of the Israel series. Levy and his co-workers (1964) obtained histories of persons who had at least one fit (including febrile fits) among about 17,500 residents of the Semokive reserve in southern Rhodesia. The rates provided by Bird and his group (1962) were derived from male Bantu gold-mine workers in South Africa. Dada (1968) recorded the results of a randomized population sample survey of households in Lagos, Nigeria.

(10) An extension of the earlier study of epilepsy in Rochester, Minnesota, recently has been completed (Hauser et al., unpublished data). It covers 1935-64, with intensified case ascertainment methods, and includes sources not reviewed in the earlier study. Incidence rates were determined by decade and prevalence rates were also determined as of January 1 of each of the decennial census years and for January 1, 1965, since a special census was conducted for the community in that year. Classification of cases remained clinical, although the modification of the ILAE terminology (Table A.2.1) was used.

Prevalence of Convulsive Disorders

Based on the aforementioned studies, prevalence rates for seizures as defined have been calculated for a number of different locations and racial groups. The results are summarized in Table 2.3. The results were variable, and some may be dismissed because of poorly delineated case definition or methods of case ascertainment. The lowest rate (in Niigata, Japan) was derived from a study that did not include a systematic identification of patients of private physicians, who probably supplied most of the medical coverage for the population. The study with the highest rate (7.4 in Semokive, Africa) included any person with a history of one convulsion or more, including febrile seizures. Similar criticism may be leveled at some of the surveys in which the rates were about 3 or 4 per 1,000, because there may have been a combination of incomplete case ascertainment of the epileptics and broad definition of cases that may have included febrile seizures or even syncope.

The most complete survey utilizing intensive case-finding techniques and specific diagnostic criteria appears to be that of Hauser and colleagues (unpublished data), from which some results are available in a preliminary form. It will be noted here that the rate in Rochester of about 6 per 1,000 was appreciably higher than that reported for 1955 by Kurland for that community. The more recent study covers some of the same years as the earlier survey, but a more intensive case-finding procedure was instituted, sources outside the Mayo Clinic contributed some cases, and modifications of the census to exclude some nonresidents (such as patients of the Rochester State Mental Hospital) resulted in a population reduction that has affected incidence and prevalence rates, especially in the older age groups. In addition, some residents with onset outside Rochester were included.

The best evidence would indicate that the present international prevalence of convulsive disorders is about 4 to 6 per 1,000 population; the studies differed sufficiently to preclude assessment of differences by race, geography, or socioeconomic status. Interestingly, almost every author has stressed the point that his rates must be considered as minimal estimates. If from these studies we assume that a reasonable estimate of prevalence is 5 per 1,000, then in the 200,000,000 population of the United States there would be about 1,000,000 persons with epilepsy.

In Table 2.4 the age-specific prevalence rates in the earlier Rochester, the Iceland, and the Jerusalem studies appear similar, although reference has been made to a few items of difference in case definition and case ascertainment. The rates for Carlisle were generally higher than those from the three other studies, but the Carlisle

Table 2.3 Prevalence rates per 1,000 population for convulsive disorders: selected studies, various years, 1955-68

Source	Area	Year	Prevalence rate	Number of cases
Kurland (1959)	Rochester, Minnesota	1955	3.6	109
Hauser et al. (unpublished data)	Rochester, Minnesota	1960	6.2	242
Hauser et al. (1970)	Rochester, Minnesota	1965	5.7	268
Crombie et al. (1960)	England-Wales G.P.	1957	4.2	1,209
Brewis et al. (1966)	Carlisle, England	1961	5.5[a]	389
Pond et al. (1960)	S.E. England G.P.	1958 (?)	6.2[a]	245
Logan and Cushion (1958); Research Committee of the Council of the College of General Practitioners (1962)	England-Wales G.P.	1955	3.3	c. 1,260
Gudmundsson (1966)	Iceland	1960	3.6	642
Krohn (1961)	Northern Norway	1960 (?)	2.3	951
Henriksen (1969); with Krohn (1969)	Northern Norway	1968 (?)	3.7	1,750
Leibowitz and Alter (1968)	Jerusalem, Israel	1961	4.1	689
Lessell et al. (1962b)	Merizo, Guam	1961	3.7	5
Mathai et al. (1968)	Other Marianas	1962	3.4	24
Sato (1964)	Niigata, Japan	1958	1.5[b]	191
Levy et al. (1964)	Semokive, Africa	1964	7.4[a]	130
Bird et al. (1962)	Bantu miners	1961 (?)	3.7	1,347
Dada (1968)	Lagos, Nigeria	1967	3.1	8

[a] "Active" plus "inactive" seizure disorders.
[b] Review of limited sources of medical records.

Table 2.4 Age-specific prevalence rates per 1,000 population for epilepsy: Rochester, Minnesota; Carlisle, England; Iceland; and Jerusalem, Israel, 1955-61

Age	Rochester, Minnesota (Jan. 1, 1955)	Carlisle, England[a] (Jan. 1, 1961)	Iceland (Jan. 1, 1960)	Jerusalem, Israel[b] (1961)	Rochester, Minnesota[c] (Jan. 1, 1960)
All ages					
Crude	3.6	5.5	3.6	4.1	6.2
Age-adjusted[d]	3.8	5.6	3.7	3.3	6.3
0-9	5.8	3.3	2.4	3.9	4.4
10-19	3.4	6.3	4.4	5.0	6.6
20-29	3.5	7.9	4.6	4.1	4.4
30-39	4.3	8.2	4.2	4.5	7.6
40-49	3.4	5.1	4.2	3.5	6.4
50-59	3.6	4.6	4.2	3.2	8.2
60-69	1.2	4.5	2.7	2.8	8.2
70 & over	1.1	2.7	1.6	1.4[e]	7.8
(Number)	(109)	(389)	(642)	(689)	(242)

Sources: Kurland 1959; Brewis et al. 1966; Gudmundsson 1966; Leibowitz and Alter 1968; and Hauser et al. (unpublished data).
[a] "Active" plus "inactive" seizure disorders.
[b] Approximated for certain decades.
[c] Regardless of residence at onset.
[d] Adjusted to the 1950 census population of the United States.
[e] Age 65 years old or older.

study included both "active" and "inactive" cases. The preliminary results in the study recently completed in Rochester were higher in almost all age groups; this may be a result of improved case finding rather than any appreciable change in the incidence of the disease in the community, because the cross-index files on the Rochester population have been improved in the ongoing epidemiology program. However, if the rates were computed only for those residents with onset in Rochester, they would be in closer accord with other studies. The prevalence rates from practically all studies showed a slight preponderance in males (about 1.2 to 1 ratio).

Incidence of Convulsive Disorders

The incidence rates for epilepsy according to age are summarized in Table 2.5. The rates were similar for patients up to 50 years old in Iceland, Carlisle, Jutland, and Rochester. The rates from Rochester for the new study exceeded the others in the older age groups. Highest rates were found in the first decade of life; there was a tendency for the rates to decline irregularly thereafter, and in

Table 2.5 Average annual age-specific incidence rates per 100,000 population for epilepsy: Rochester, Minnesota; Iceland; Carlisle, England; and Jutland, Denmark, 1935-64

Age	Rochester, Minnesota (1945-54)	Iceland (1959-64)	Carlisle, England (1955-61)	Jutland, Denmark (1959-61)	Rochester, Minnesota (1935-64)
All ages	30	33	28	36[a]	45
0-9	102	62	57	80[a]	85
10-19	21	59	48	57	36
20-29	4	23	22	33	23
30-39	21	18	16	24	27
40-49	10	14	21	18	28
50-59	18	11	21	8[b]	37
60 & over	21	6	12	---	60[c]
(Number)	(89)	(987)	(141)	(1,500)[a]	(305)

Sources: Kurland 1959; Gudmundsson 1966; Brewis et al. 1966; Kurtzke 1968c and Juul-Jensen 1964; Hauser et al. (unpublished data).
[a] Estimated (Kurtzke 1968c).
[b] 50 years and over.
[c] 51 for age 60-69 years, 79 for age 70+ years.

Rochester to increase again among the elderly. Kurtzke (1968c) has suggested that the age-specific incidence rates for all convulsive disorders are the result of two main classes of seizures: primary grand mal and petit mal together, and all secondary seizures. As may be seen from Fig. 2.6, the rates for primary grand mal from Iceland and Jutland showed a geometric decline with age, from a peak in infancy to 0 by age 69. The rates for petit mal generally followed the same curve but became negligible by about age 20 or 25. However, the rates for secondary fits tended to be relatively high at both extremes of life and rather evenly distributed in between. To some extent, this concept is reinforced by the data from the earlier Rochester study, as seen in Fig. 2.7 (Kurland 1959).

On the basis of the results presented, particularly with the stated reservations regarding completeness of case ascertainment, it would appear that for all types of recurrent convulsive disorders combined, the annual incidence is conservatively about 40 per 100,000 population. On that basis there would be about 80,000 newly affected persons annually in the United States.

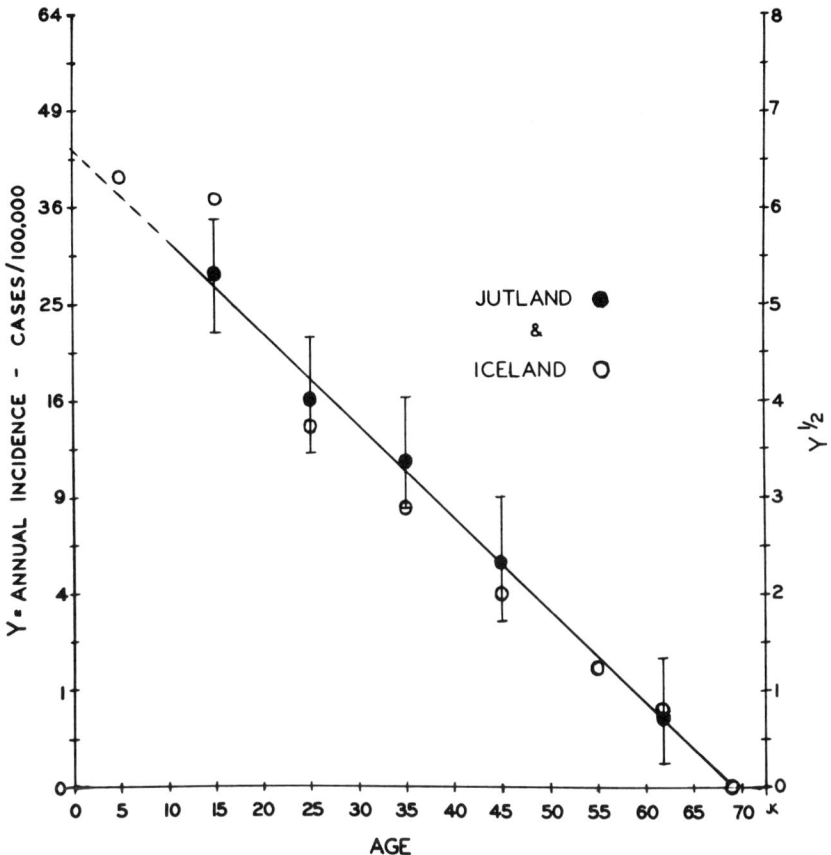

Figure 2.6 Average annual age-specific incidence rates per 100,000 population for primary grand mal plotted on a square-root scale against age: Jutland, Denmark, 1959–61, and Iceland, 1959–64. Vertical lines represent 95-percent confidence intervals for Jutland rates. (Source: Kurtzke 1968c. By permission of Pergamon Press Limited.)

Types of Seizures

In Fig. 2.7, the age-specific incidence rates of primary grand mal and petit mal are shown for the early Rochester material. The rates for secondary seizure disorders from the same study are presented in Fig. 2.8. The average annual incidence rates for the three main types of seizure as classified in early papers are indicated in Table 2.6, in which both Rochester series are compared with those of Iceland and Jutland. The apparent discrepancies between the early Rochester series and those of Iceland and Jutland are within chance variation,

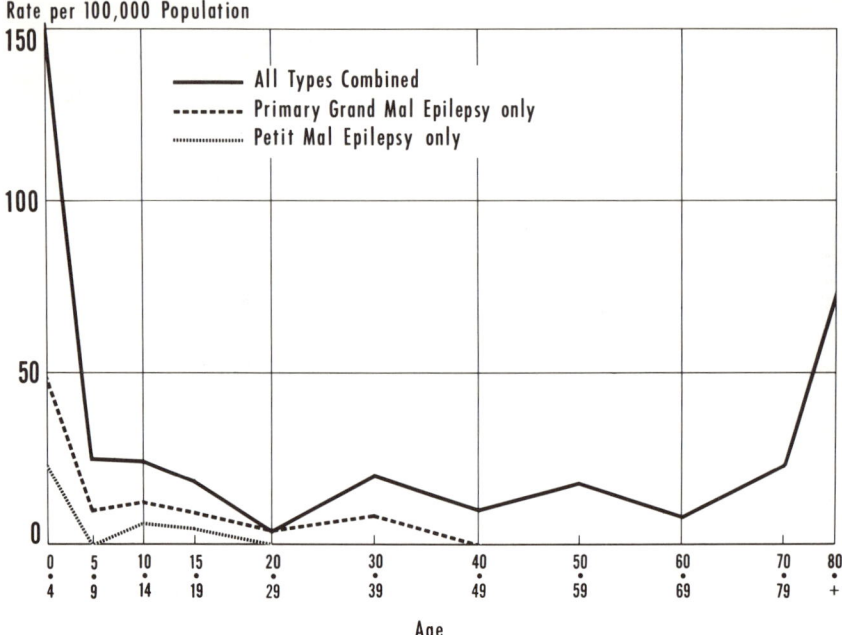

Figure 2.7 Average annual incidence rates per 100,000 population for primary convulsive disorders by type and age at onset: Rochester, Minnesota, 1945–54 (Source: Modified from Kurland 1959. By permission of Elsevier Publishing Company.)

considering the small numbers for some of the rates. However, the methods and results of the Rochester study suggest a finer diagnostic screen at the Mayo Clinic, and this possibility is reinforced by the more recent survey results that present an even higher proportion of all cases as either secondary (etiology presumably identified) or with a recognized focal onset.

From the clinical data, the male excess in mortality, incidence, and prevalence rates for seizure disorders would seem largely (if not entirely) a result of the male preponderance for secondary seizures. There seems little evidence for any major sex difference in primary grand mal or petit mal.

Febrile Seizures

Convulsions with fever are not uncommon. Hauser and his colleagues (1970) in a Rochester, Minnesota, study covering 1945-64 reported 427 cases; of these, only 11 were of patients more than 4

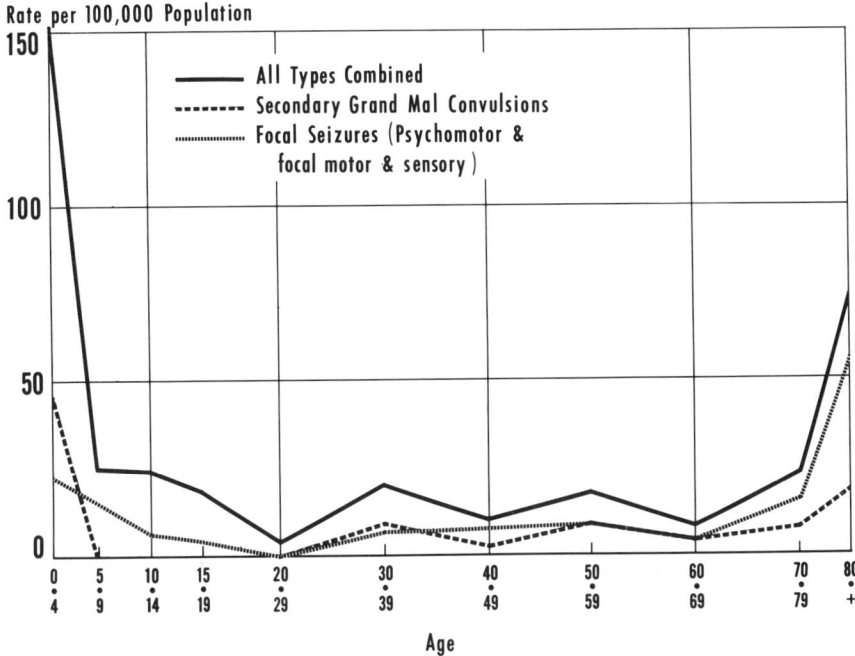

Figure 2.8 Average annual incidence rates per 100,000 population for secondary convulsive disorders by type and age at onset: Rochester, Minnesota, 1945-54 (Source: Modified from Kurland 1959. By permission of Elsevier Publishing Company.)

Table 2.6 Average annual incidence rates per 100,000 population for epilepsy by type: Rochester, Minnesota; Iceland; and Jutland, Denmark; various years, 1935-64

Survey area (source)	Total seizures	Primary grand mal	Petit mal alone	Secondary[a] seizures
Rochester (Kurland 1959)	30[b]	8	3	17
Rochester (Hauser et al., unpublished data)	45[c]	10	4	30
Iceland (Gudmundsson 1966)	33	19	1	13
Jutland (Kurtzke 1968c; Juul-Jensen 1964)	36	17	4	15

[a] Includes focal, psychomotor, and secondary (etiology known) generalized seizures.
[b] Includes 1 per 100,000 unclassified.
[c] Includes 2 per 100,000 unclassified.

years old. The average annual incidence rate was 4 per 1,000 for children less than 5 years old. The median age of onset was 18 months, and nearly 1 percent of the children in the community had a febrile convulsion during the second year of life. Almost 50 percent had recurrent febrile convulsions, but only 2.5 percent of the group, which was followed for an average of ten years, had subsequent recurrent afebrile convulsions. In Denmark, Frantzen and associates (1968) traced about 200 children who had febrile seizures to the age of 5 years and noted recurrent febrile seizures in 25 percent; the frequency of recurrence was inversely related to age at the first episode. They also found that only five (2.5 percent) had recurrent convulsions without fever during that period. The mean age at onset was also about 18 months, and nearly four-fifths were between 9 and 30 months old at the time of first seizure, only 3 percent being more than 48 months old. There was little difference by sex. Paroxysmal EEG discharges (spike or spike-wave) developed in almost a third of these patients (none in a control series), most after one and a half years or more had elapsed following the fit. However, these changes were not correlated with later clinical seizures.

Lessell and co-workers (1962b) reported that 14 percent of the children of the village of Merizo in Guam were said to have had febrile fits, whereas the cumulative figure from Rochester was about 2 to 3 percent. Yet the incidence and prevalence rates for nonfebrile convulsive disorders did not differ significantly in the Guam and Rochester populations.

The desirability of anticonvulsant treatment in febrile fits is dependent on the prognosis. Carter (1964) maintained that continuous prophylaxis is indicated after febrile convulsions, whereas Millichap (1968) thought the dangers of treatment outweighed the risk of later fits. These studies suggest that patients with one febrile convulsion are more likely to have recurrence of febrile seizures, but that the risk of subsequent development of epilepsy is only slightly higher than in the population at large.

Heredity and Seizures

Most clinical series of patients with seizures showed a high frequency of positive family histories. This was also noted for febrile convulsions (Kurland 1959; Frantzen et al. 1968) and for paroxysmal and temporal lobe abnormalities on EEG (Metrakos and Metrakos 1961; Rodin and Gonzalez 1966; Frantzen et al. 1968).

Evans (1962) also found family histories more often indicative of fits in patients with head injury who had seizures than in those with equivalent trauma without fits. The desirability of using sibships and parent populations of known size for both numerator and denominator (population at risk), rather than the ill-defined "family history," is well recognized in modern genetic research.

Twin studies are also of value, particularly if the bias for case reports of twins concordant for a disease is recognized and avoided by the study design. Vercelletto and Courjon (1969) noted concordance for epilepsy in ten of fourteen pairs of monozygotic twins, but in their series the twins seem to have been collected from two large clinics for epilepsy, and accordingly little detail is provided as to the genetic features or case-selection methods.

Harvald and Hauge (1965) have been following, since 1954, all available twins born in Denmark during the period 1870-1910. Almost 7,000 pairs had been traced to 1963 in terms of medical records, deaths, and questionnaires; and zygosity was determined in all but some 230 pairs. In 127 pairs of twins epilepsy was diagnosed, and this included "genuine and symptomatic epilepsy." Ten of the 27 monozygotes with epilepsy were concordant, as opposed to 6 of the 43 same-sexed dizygotes and 4 of the 57 opposite-sexed dizygotic twins. The difference between monozygotic (10 of 27) and dizygotic (10 of 100) twins was statistically significant. Pratt (1967), however, indicated the need for caution in accepting even these results as evidence of heredity as a primary factor in the etiology of epilepsy, because twins in general are more subject to perinatal trauma, including anoxia, and are more likely to be premature. However, monozygotic twins should not be that much more susceptible to such exogenous factors than dizygotic twins, and a hereditary predisposition to seizures of all types would seem a reasonable conclusion if there was no bias in the selection of the twin pairs for study.

Metrakos and Metrakos (1961) have contended that centrencephalic EEG abnormalities are the manifestation of a single autosomal dominant gene. It is likely that the predisposition to any variety of seizure disorder is inherited, but that the patterns and penetrances are varied.

A centrencephalic, 3-per-second, spike-wave discharge was found in 346 patients in Aarhus, Denmark (Dalby 1969). On the basis of *absence* states, 47 percent of the total number of patients were originally classed as having petit mal, but only one-third of the fits were free of focal or psychomotor components on close analysis of the attacks. Fits among the other 53 percent of the total patients included grand mal (16 percent), focal (16 percent), myoclonic (11 percent), and psychomotor (4 percent); 2 percent had no seizures. Thus, even the "purest" EEG pattern had little relation to the type of seizure.

Summary and Conclusions

This chapter is concerned with the incidence, prevalence, and mortality rates, and the population features of convulsive disorders. For the mortality studies, an epileptic was defined as one whose death was so coded. In the studies of incidence and prevalence rates, attention was paid primarily to studies dealing with recurrent convulsive disorders. The classification of seizures was primarily by clinical type. The studies that have been conducted have not had uniformity either of definition of epilepsy or of classification of epilepsy. Furthermore, case ascertainment differed so that studies from various parts of the world were difficult to compare.

Epilepsy is infrequently certified as a cause of death among patients with seizure disorders. When it is recorded on the death certificate, it is probably because the seizures had been a serious problem or because death was caused by status epilepticus. In about half the cases in which epilepsy was recorded on the death certificate, it was assigned as the underlying cause of death.

In the United States for 1959-61, the annual rate for epilepsy as a primary cause of death was 1.1 per 100,000 population. The mortality rates were lowest for white females, followed by white males, nonwhite females, and nonwhite males, in that order. With respect to age, the rates tended to increase from age 10 to about age 40, followed by a decline until about 70 years of age. In the oldest ages (with small numbers), the rates increased sharply. This pattern was found for both sexes and colors, but was most pronounced for nonwhite males.

The differences by color may reflect socioeconomic conditions as they affect the amount of cerebral injury, differences in medical care, and sensitivity of the physician to reporting the cause of death; however, they may also reflect true differences in the incidence of epilepsy by color. These matters require further evaluation.

There was no obvious pattern in the epilepsy mortality rates by state in the United States except that the "cotton belt" states tended to have higher rates, largely because of the higher rates for non-whites. Age-adjusted mortality rates by type of county (that is, nonmetropolitan vs metropolitan residence of the patient) showed a slightly higher rate for rural counties, but only in the western regions of the country. This may be attributable to differential migration (rural to urban, east to west) or to differential recording; the absence of similar differences in the eastern United States suggests that this factor itself is not directly related to epileptic deaths. Rates were lower for metropolitan counties without central cities than with such cities, in further support of this conclusion.

The death rates were highest for single persons, intermediate for the divorced or widowed, and lowest for the married. This is probably a reflection in part of the effect of prior epilepsy on marriage eligibility, but also of increased exposure to trauma and toxins and decreased likelihood of being under adequate medical control for those not currently married. The sex ratio for epileptic deaths among the married was about one-to-one; widows were twice as numerous as widowers, and among the single and divorced, there were about twice as many males as females. Death *rates*, however, were greater for males in all groups of the unmarried, by a factor of two or so.

The age-adjusted death rates were nearly twice as high for native born as for foreign born, presumably because the United States immigration laws exclude persons with known epilepsy.

Incidence and prevalence rates for seizure disorders were compared among the available population surveys which seemed to have appropriate methodology and roughly equivalent definitions. The studies included were from Rochester, Minnesota, and Carlisle, England; several surveys of general practices in England and Wales; Northern Norway; Iceland; Jutland, Denmark; Jerusalem, Israel; and various smaller studies from the Mariana Islands, Africa, and Japan.

Several of the studies reported prevalence rates for "active" seizure disorders as between 4 and 6 per 1,000 population. Three of the four studies that recorded higher rates (5.5 to 7.4) included "inactive" seizures—that is, patients who at any time in their life had had more than one fit, and the two highest of these rates also included febrile fits and single convulsions. However, the recent Rochester study in which the prevalence rate was also about 6 per 1,000 included only active cases. Incidence and prevalence rates for all types combined were generally somewhat higher for males than for females; the rates for the primary types were equal by sex, and the secondary forms tended to be more common in males.

Age-specific incidence rates were maximal in the first decade of life and declined thereafter, although there was an increase in the oldest ages in the Rochester study. On the basis of the population studies reviewed, it is estimated that in the United States population of 200,000,000, when all types of recurrent seizures are considered together, approximately 80,000 persons annually will be newly affected and that at any given time about 1,000,000 can be diagnosed as having recurrent convulsive disorders.

The proportions for given seizure types are partially dependent on the intensity of the diagnostic examination and follow-up; for example, the latest Rochester study had one of the lowest proportions of idiopathic generalized seizures and the highest of recognized secondary seizures and those with focal onset.

Febrile convulsions are disorders of early life in which the peak age of onset is about 18 months and onset almost always begins by the age of 4 years. Among children less than 5 years old, about 4 per 1,000 were newly afflicted each year; and in the Rochester study, about 1 percent of all children 1 to 2 years of age had had at least one febrile seizure. Among children with one febrile seizure, there were recurrent febrile convulsions in 25 to 50 percent. Among children with febrile seizures who were followed in prospective type studies, only about 2.5 percent subsequently had *afebrile* seizures. Although this is more than one might expect on the basis of the incidence rates for epilepsy in the population, it is sufficiently low to provide encouragement to the families of such children regarding the prognosis with respect to future episodes of epilepsy.

3 / PARKINSONISM

Leonard T. Kurland
John F. Kurtzke
Irving D. Goldberg
Nung Won Choi
Gail Williams

Paralysis agitans was first described in 1817 by James Parkinson, whose name has been attached to the symptom complex. Clinically, it is characterized chiefly by muscular rigidity, poverty of movement (bradykinesia), and tremor that is typically regular and rhythmic, maximal at rest, and mostly distal in the limbs. The major pathologic features are degenerative changes in the basal ganglia, especially the substantia nigra and corpus striatum, together with less prominent alterations in the cerebral cortex. Biochemical aberrations of monamine levels, particularly dopamine and serotonin, have assumed recent prominence with the advent of L-3, 4-dihydroxyphenylalanine (levodopa) as a promising therapeutic agent in this disorder.

Classification of the Parkinson syndrome has varied.

(1) There are a small number of patients in whom these features are associated with traumatic, vascular, or tumorous lesions of the brain, and a larger number in whom these features are of toxic origin (carbon monoxide, manganese, and phenothiazines among others). This group is considered to have "secondary parkinsonism," and will not be discussed in the present chapter.
(2) Postencephalitic parkinsonism, which was the early or late sequel of von Economo's type A encephalitis that followed the great influenzal pandemic after World War I, is characterized clinically by prominent autonomic and eye-movement disorders, in addition to the extrapyramidal features. This entity will be discussed further.
(3) The most common form of this syndrome is idiopathic parkinsonism or paralysis agitans.
(4) Some authors add another category, that of arteriosclerotic parkinsonism, which also is occasionally classified as a "secondary" form. In this chapter, parkinsonism will refer to the idiopathic and the arteriosclerotic varieties. When a differen-

tiation is made, the arteriosclerotic type will be referred to as "parkinsonism associated with arteriosclerosis." The clinical and pathologic basis for this subdivision is the presence of changes attributed to cerebral arteriosclerosis, in addition to the extrapyramidal symptom complex in question. We consider these cases as involving both parkinsonism and cerebral arteriosclerosis.

(5) There is another illness that may be mentioned, the disorder called the parkinsonism-dementia complex (P-D). This is highly prevalent in Guam and some of the other Mariana Islands, where it accounts for about 7 percent of the deaths in the local population. Clinically and pathologically, it is admixed with the Marianas' form of motor neuron disease (Kurland 1965; Kurland et al. 1969a). At the present time, the relationship of the P-D complex to classic parkinsonism seems to be remote, but this is an area that requires clinical, genetic, and epidemiologic inquiry. In this chapter, we shall not concern ourselves with the P-D complex.

Few epidemiologic studies have provided valid data on the distribution of parkinsonism, even though it ranks as one of the most prevalent primary disorders of the central nervous system. In its full manifestation, this disease is readily recognized by the general practitioner—and even by the layman. Its treatment in the past has been relatively unsatisfactory. In its milder forms, both patient and physician may accept parkinsonism as a concomitant of aging, not warranting special diagnostic studies. The insidious onset that is most characteristic also serves to delay if not obviate medical inquiry. These features undoubtedly influence the identification of cases for both prevalence studies and mortality data analysis.

Mortality Data

If mortality rates are used as a measure of the frequency of parkinsonism, there will be a gross underestimation. From a special study of all the Canadian death certificates in 1951, Kurland reported that of 529 certificates in which parkinsonism or paralysis agitans had been recorded, only 46 percent listed it as the underlying cause of death (Kurland 1958b). Similarly, it was recorded as the underlying cause in from one-third to one-half of the deaths in Norway for 1956-60, in the Netherlands for 1953-61, and in the United States for 1955 (Williams et al. 1966). When the death certificates of parkinsonian patients in Rochester, Minnesota, were reviewed, parkinsonism was certified as a cause of death in only one in five (Kurland 1958b). Among hospitalized patients in Baltimore who subsequently died, parkinsonism was certified as the underlying cause of death in 10 percent of the cases and as a contributing cause in an additional 28 percent (Kessler 1972). Omission of this label should not be taken as a diagnostic error, because the case-fatality rate of parkinsonism is not high. Conversely, it is probable that when parkinsonism is listed, it is the correct diagnosis and an important factor in the death of the patient.

Earlier Mortality Data of the United States and Canada

The crude death rates for parkinsonism in the United States for the years 1949-61 have remained fairly stable. The crude rate for 1949-51 was 1.4; the age-adjusted rate was 1.2 per 100,000, which is identical to the 1959-61 rate adjusted to the same 1940 population. When the death rates for each of six major geographic regions of the United States (1949-55) and Canada (1951) were computed, they varied from 1.3 to 1.9 per 100,000 population, but no specific pattern north to south or east to west was noted (Kurland 1958b; Goldberg and Kurland 1962; Williams et al. 1966; Grove and Hetzel 1968). In both the United States and Canada, there was a slight male excess at 1.3 to 1 in the United States and 1.2 to 1 in Canada. In the United States, the rates have been higher for whites than for nonwhites.

United States Mortality Data, 1959-61

Deaths attributed to parkinsonism as the underlying (primary) cause in the United States were collected for 1959-61. As shown in Table 3.1, the average annual mortality per 100,000 was 1.8 for males and 1.5 for females; for both sexes combined, the rate was 1.6, or 1.2 adjusted to the 1940 population.

Age. Of the 8,674 certificates listing parkinsonism as the underlying cause of death, 84 percent were for persons age 65 years or older and 96 percent were for those 55 or older. Age-specific death rates for the total United States (Table 3.1 and Fig. 3.1) were similar to those of the 1951 Canadian mortality experience (Kurland

Table 3.1 Deaths and average annual death rates per 100,000 population for parkinsonism by age, color and sex: United States, 1959-61
(ISC code 350)

Age	Total			White			Nonwhite		
	Total	Male	Female	Total	Male	Female	Total	Male	Female
	Number of deaths								
All ages	8,674	4,682	3,992	8,439	4,540	3,899	235	142	93
Under 25	8	5	3	7	5	2	1	-	1
25-34	4	3	1	4	3	1	-	-	-
35-44	39	25	14	34	24	10	5	1	4
45-54	265	159	106	247	148	99	18	11	7
55-64	1,087	617	470	1,030	582	448	57	35	22
65-74	3,612	2,051	1,561	3,529	1,999	1,530	83	52	31
75-84	3,120	1,591	1,529	3,060	1,554	1,506	60	37	23
85 & over	536	229	307	525	223	302	11	6	5
Unknown	3	2	1	3	2	1	-	-	-
	Crude death rate								
All ages	1.6	1.8	1.5	1.8	1.9	1.6	0.4	0.5	0.3
Under 25	0.0*	0.0*	0.0*	0.0*	0.0*	0.0*	0.0*	-	0.0*
25-34	0.0*	0.0*	0.0*	0.0*	0.0*	0.0*	-	-	-
35-44	0.1	0.1	0.0*	0.1	0.1	0.0*	0.1	0.0*	0.1*
45-54	0.4	0.5	0.3	0.4	0.5	0.4	0.3*	0.4*	0.2*
55-64	2.3	2.7	1.9	2.4	2.8	2.0	1.4	1.7	1.0
65-74	10.9	13.4	8.8	11.6	14.2	9.4	3.2	4.2	2.3
75-84	22.4	26.2	19.5	23.6	27.6	20.6	6.3	8.2	4.6
85 & over	19.2	21.1	18.0	20.4	22.5	19.1	5.1*	6.4*	4.1*
	Age-adjusted death rate								
All ages	1.2	1.5	1.0*	1.3	1.5	1.1*	0.4*	0.5*	0.3*
65 & over	14.1	16.9	11.9	15.0	17.9	12.6	4.1	5.3	3.0

1958*b*). Rates for those under 45 years of age were almost 0 but increased sharply and steadily for each age group thereafter to a peak at age 75-84 years.

Sex. Beginning with the age group 45 to 54 years, the death rate for parkinsonism was higher for males than for females (Fig. 3.1). The male-female ratio of the age-adjusted rates for persons 65 years old or older was 1.4 to 1 for the total United States and ranged from 1.2 to 1.5 among the nine geographic census regions of the United States (Table 3.2).

Geographic distribution. Age-adjusted death rates in the nine census regions of the United States for persons 65 or older are noted in Table 3.2. Similarly, death rates in each state are shown in Figs. 3.2*a, b,* and *c,* with the underlying data given in Table A.3.1. The only major deviations in the geographic distribution of parkinsonism mortality rates apparent from these data were the lower rates re-

PARKINSONISM / 45

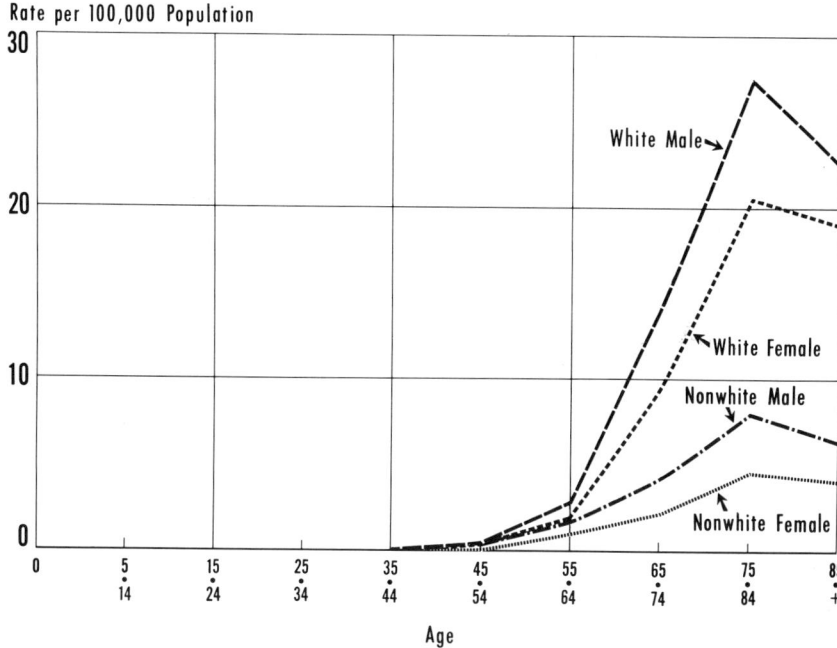

Figure 3.1 Average annual age-specific death rates per 100,000 population for parkinsonism by color and sex: United States, 1959–61

Table 3.2 Average annual age-adjusted death rates per 100,000 population age 65 and over for parkinsonism by sex: United States and census regions, 1959-61
(ISC code 350)

Region	Male	Female	M:F ratio
United States	16.9	11.9	1.4
New England	18.1	13.8	1.3
Middle Atlantic	17.3	12.5	1.4
East North Central	18.1	12.4	1.5
West North Central	22.8	15.4	1.5
South Atlantic	12.8	8.8	1.5
East South Central	11.4	7.7	1.5
West South Central	12.2	8.1	1.5
Mountain	16.2	13.3	1.2
Pacific	19.3	14.0	1.4

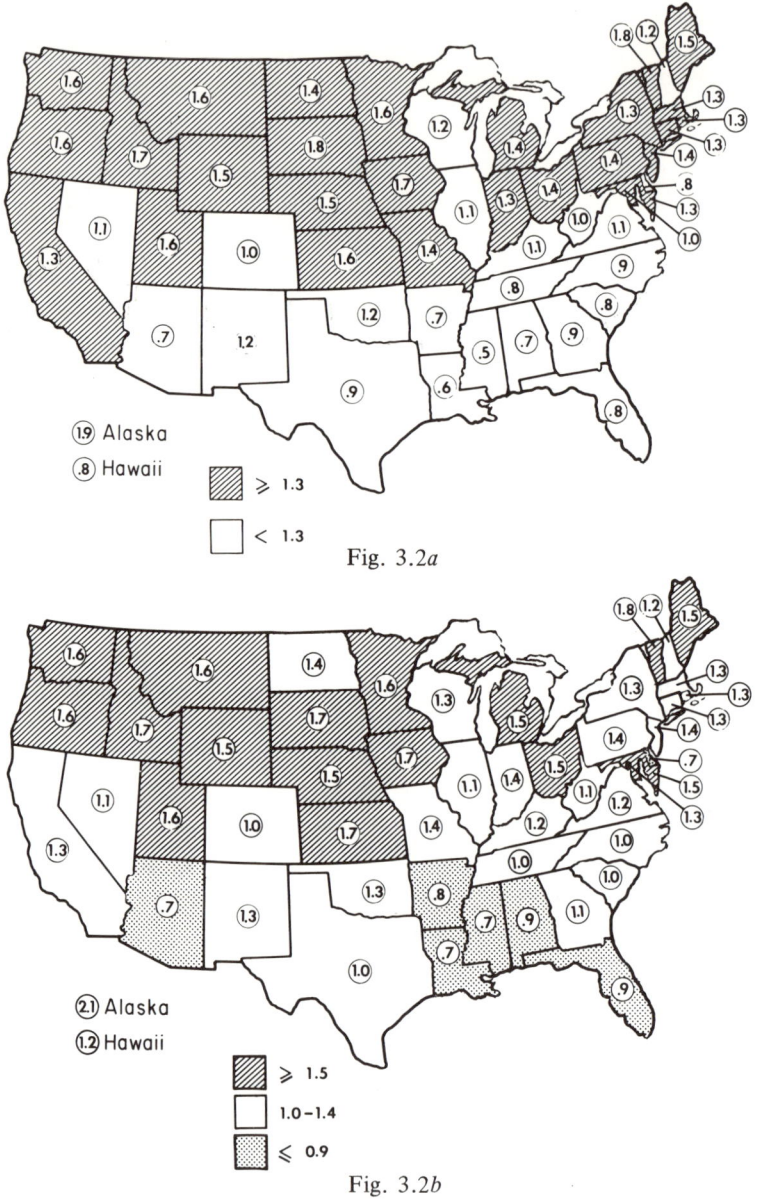

Figure 3.2 Average annual age-adjusted death rates per 100,000 population for parkinsonism by state: United States, 1959–61. *a.* All persons. None of the rates meets the standard of reliability or precision as defined in Notes on Tables and Figures. *b.* White persons, all ages. None of the rates meets the standard of reliability or precision. *c.* White persons, age 65 and over. Rates that do not meet the standard of reliability or precision are indicated by an asterisk (*) in Table A.3.1.

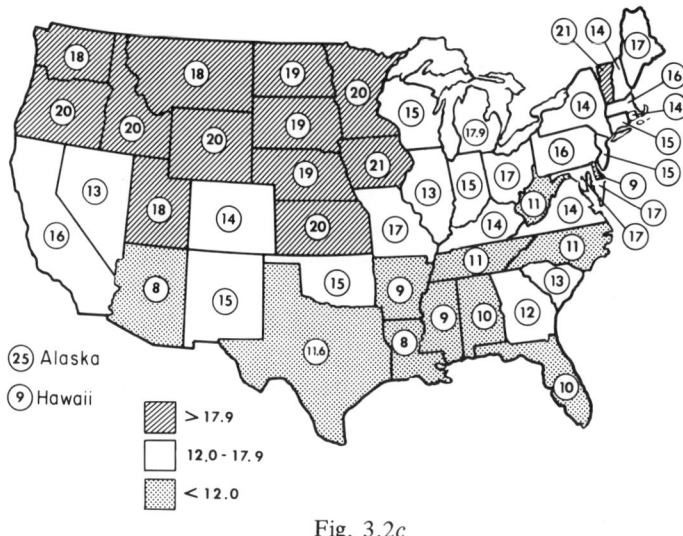

Fig. 3.2c

Fig. 3.2 (*continued*)

ported in the South; otherwise the regional differences were small. When whites and nonwhites were compared separately, the same regional difference was still noted, although it was more evident among the nonwhites, as seen in Table 3.3.

The death rates by state as in Fig. 3.2a suggest a "gradient," with increasing rates as latitude increases in the row of states across the nation. This, however, is largely the result of an admixture of differing rates by color. The effect of differences by race is brought out in the comparisons of Figs. 3.2a and b, where the same scale of rates is used for the different states. When we consider the rates for whites only (as in Figs. 3.2b and c), the gradient is less apparent, but the rates still appear to be about 20 percent lower in the cotton belt states of the southeastern United States than in other sections (Table 3.3). No other pattern emerges as one examines these rates on a state-by-state basis. (The Alaskan rate for those 65 or older was based on only 5 deaths.)

The extent of the geographic variation should be considered from the deaths among whites alone because of the small numbers of nonwhites. The geographic differences were not striking, and the regions of low frequency were those where the per-capita ratio of physicians was also low (Kurtzke 1969b). Accordingly, the geographic difference may be little more than a reflection of reporting adequacy.

Table 3.3 Average annual age-adjusted death rates per 100,000 population age 65 and over for parkinsonism by color: United States and census regions, 1959-61
(ISC code 350)

Region	White	Nonwhite	W:NW ratio
United States	15.0	4.1	3.7
New England	15.8	6.7*	2.4
Middle Atlantic	15.0	6.5*	2.3
East North Central	15.5	5.1*	3.0
West North Central	19.2	5.5*	3.5
South Atlantic	12.1	3.1*	3.9
East South Central	11.3	2.0*	5.7
West South Central	11.3	2.3*	4.9
Mountain	14.9	8.7*	1.7
Pacific	16.7	9.4*	1.8

Color. The ratio of age-adjusted death rates in the United States for all ages in 1953-57 was three times greater for whites than for nonwhites (Goldberg and Kurland 1962). The same ratio was present for 1959-61, with rates of 1.3 and 0.4 per 100,000 for whites and nonwhites, respectively. The ratio was 3.7 to 1 for persons 65 years old or older in 1959-61. The higher rates for whites were found in all nine subdivisions of the United States (Table 3.3), although the number of nonwhite deaths was small in all regions. The white-nonwhite ratio in the three subdivisions of the South was greater than in other regions where less of a difference in medical care between whites and nonwhites might be expected. Part of this difference then may also be attributed to reporting adequacy, but these data still raise a question regarding a possible predilection for parkinsonism by color.

Type of county. Age-adjusted mortality rates for metropolitan and nonmetropolitan counties are shown in Table 3.4. The rates by both sex and color were slightly higher in the metropolitan counties. The white-nonwhite ratio of age-adjusted rates was 3.4 to 1 in metropolitan counties, whereas it was 4.3 to 1 in nonmetropolitan counties. This difference would be consistent with the assumption that com-

Table 3.4 Average annual age-adjusted death rates per 100,000 population age 65 and over for parkinsonism by color, sex and type of county: United States, 1959-61
(ISC code 350)

Color and sex	Metropolitan counties	Nonmetropolitan counties
United States	14.5	13.8
White	15.2	14.7
Nonwhite	4.5	3.4
Male	17.6	16.0
Female	12.0	11.7

pleteness of reporting is a contributing factor to the variation by color.

Marital status. Age-adjusted rates by marital status are shown in Table 3.5. The division by age (that is, above and below 65 years) can be expected to add little to interpretation since less than 1 percent of all deaths occurred before age 45, by which time almost all who marry have done so, at least for the first time. Among those less than 65 years old, the rates are based on relatively small numbers of deaths; the rates for both males and females were lowest for those married. In the older patients, the rates were higher for males of each marital status, though the difference was slight among those never married. The observed differences probably are reflections of varied selection biases in the reporting of disease or the effects of disease on marital status, rather than a result of any intrinsic relationship between them.

Nativity. Age-adjusted death rates for native-born and foreign-born whites 65 or older are shown in Table 3.6. The rates in the two groups were essentially the same throughout the nine census regions in the United States (table not shown), except for the East South Central region, where the rates were more than twice as high among foreign-born whites than among native-born whites; however, their numbers were very small. The basic equality according to birthplace is a reflection of parkinsonism as a disease of the elderly and there-

Table 3.5   Average annual age-adjusted death rates per 100,000 population for parkinsonism by age, sex and marital status: United States, 1959-61
(ISC code 350)

Age and sex	Single	Married	Widowed	Divorced
15 & over				
Total	2.3	1.7	1.6*	1.9*
Male	2.7*	1.9	2.2*	2.3*
Female	1.9*	1.3	1.4*	1.5*
15-64				
Total	0.9*	0.3*	0.4*	0.7*
Male	1.3*	0.3*	0.7*	0.9*
Female	0.5*	0.2*	0.4*	0.5*
65 & over				
Total	16.0	15.6	13.1	13.6
Male	16.8	17.7	17.7	16.1
Female	15.3	12.0	11.8	11.2

Table 3.6   Average annual age-adjusted death rates per 100,000 population for parkinsonism, white persons age 65 and over, by sex and nativity: United States, 1959-61
(ISC code 350)

Nativity	Total	Male	Female	M:F ratio
Native born	15.1	18.1	12.9	1.4
Foreign born	15.8	19.3	12.4	1.6

fore not subject to appreciable immigration restrictions. One might surmise that the incidence of parkinsonism among foreign-born persons in the United States is little influenced by their place of birth.

International Mortality Data

Age-adjusted death rates for parkinsonism in the 1950s for twenty-four countries were presented by Goldberg and Kurland (1962).

Rates for both sexes combined varied from 0.5 to 3.8 per 100,000 population, with Japan, Mexico, Czechoslovakia, and United States nonwhites having the lowest rates. Highest rates were recorded for Australia, Israel, and Belgium (Fig. 3.3, data by sex in Table A.3.2). There was no apparent pattern to the rather wide geographic variations, and a suggestion only that nonwhites might be less susceptible to this disease.

In an extensive analysis of the parkinsonism mortality trend in Great Britain, Duvoisin and Schweitzer (1966) concluded:

> Mortality rates have been stationary for the past 40 years or more [1921-62] at most ages. ... The risk of dying with paralysis agitans is about the same today as it was in the 1920s and ... has not in fact changed since the 1890s. Whatever influence the epidemic of encephalitis lethargica may have had, no long-term residual effect is apparent. Nor have the profound environmental changes of the past half-century appeared to exert any influence upward or downward.

The age-specific death rates since 1920 in England and Wales have been stationary for persons less than 65 years of age; there has been

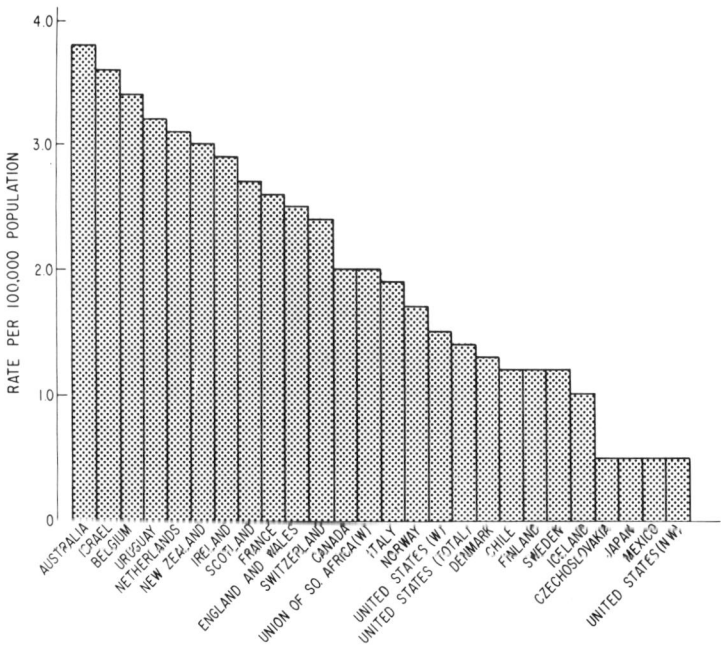

Figure 3.3 Average annual age-adjusted death rates per 100,000 population for parkinsonism: selected countries, various years, 1951-58 (Source: Goldberg and Kurland 1962. By permission of Lancet Publications, Inc.)

only a slight increase for those 65 through 74 years of age. In persons 75 or older, there has been an almost steady increase, and today the mortality rate in this group is about twice that of 1920. Since this eldest group is open-ended, the mortality rate is expected to increase with the aging population. Conversely, DeJong (1966) reported that mortality rates for parkinsonism seemed to be increasing with time, although the increase was not consistent. Unfortunately, further investigation for past trends of mortality is difficult and perhaps has already been fully exploited. The weight of the available evidence indicates an essentially stable death rate for parkinsonism.

Incidence and Prevalence Studies

Parkinsonism was included in a general neurologic survey conducted in Rochester, Minnesota (Kurland 1958a and b), for 1945-54. The average annual incidence rate for cases of newly diagnosed parkinsonism who were residents of Rochester at that time was 23 per 100,000. This study has now been extended to cover 1935-66 (Nobrega et al. 1967). In this interval, there were 191 patients who were residents of Rochester at the time of diagnosis. The incidence rate based on date of diagnosis showed no appreciable change in the last twenty-two years, being 21 and 19 per 100,000 population, respectively, in 1945-54 and 1955-66; in the 1935-44 decade, the rate was 11 per 100,000, presumably an underestimation. The overall average annual incidence for the entire period was 18 per 100,000. For 125 of these patients, an accurate date of onset after 1934 was ascertained. On the assumption that the distribution of those with known onset was the same as the distribution of those whose onset was uncertain, adjusted age-specific incidence rates were calculated from the date of onset and are indicated in Table 3.7. Although rates based on date of diagnosis are more accurate, they have an inherent delay of about four years: the mean age at diagnosis was 69 years, and at onset 65 years. For parkinsonism, however, this difference seems critical to the configuration of the age-specific attack-rate curve (see Fig. 3.4). The age-specific incidence rates from both methods are drawn in Fig. 3.4, where they are compared with those of other studies which will be considered.

Based on data from the 75 resident patients alive in Rochester, Minnesota, as of January 1, 1965, the prevalence rate for parkinsonism was 1.6 per 1,000, or 1.8 when age-adjusted to the 1960 United States white population. The rate increased markedly with

Table 3.7 Average annual age-specific incidence rates per 100,000 population for parkinsonism: Rochester, Minnesota, 1935-66

Age	Rate based on:	
	Date of diagnosis	Date of onset[a]
All ages	17.9[b]	17.9[b]
0-19	-	-
20-29	-	-
30-39	1	1
40-49	5	9
50-59	18	26
60-69	65	112
70-79	174	116
80 & over	167	52
(Number)	(191)	(125)[a]

[a] Rates based on 125 cases adjusted to N of 191.

[b] Rate of 18.5 when adjusted to 1960 white population of the United States.

age to 2.2 per 100 in the eldest group (see Fig. 3.5). Prevalence rate by type of parkinsonism was as noted in Table 3.8. About 7 percent had postencephalitic parkinsonism, about a third had parkinsonism associated with arteriosclerosis, and the rest had idiopathic parkinsonism. The sex ratio for the entire group was 1.2 males to 1 female, based on age-adjusted rates.

In a survey in Baltimore, Maryland, by Kessler (1972; unpublished data), patients with parkinsonism who had been hospitalized and patients with parkinsonism who were attended by a sample of practicing physicians in the community during a three-year period were identified. The prevalence of parkinsonism in the Baltimore metropolitan area was estimated as 128 per 100,000 for white males and 121 per 100,000 for white females, with a maximal prevalence in the age group 65 or older for whom it was about 1,000 per 100,000 (or 1 percent). These rates are appreciably less than those reported in the Rochester (Minnesota) study.

In the Baltimore study, the rate for Negroes was only about one-sixth that for whites for all ages combined, although for males 65 or older, the rate was only about twice as high for whites as for Ne-

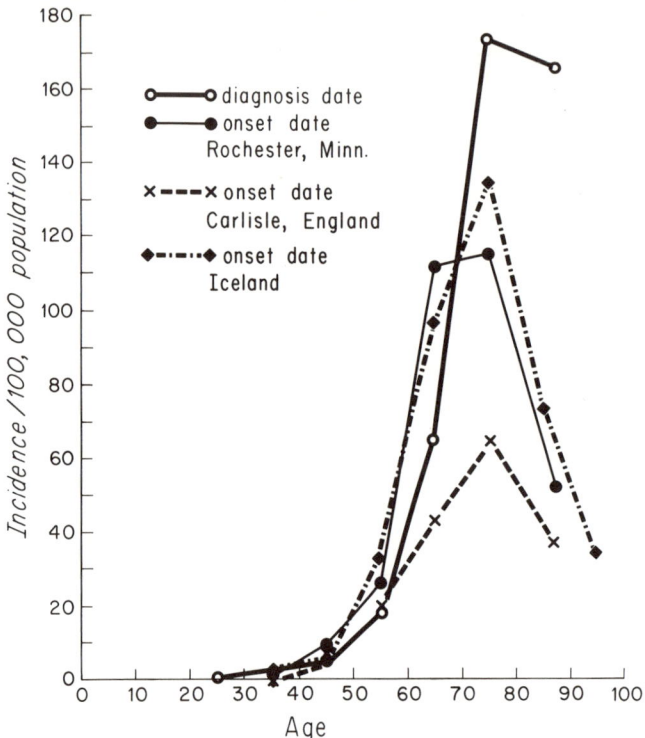

Figure 3.4 Average annual age-specific incidence rates per 100,000 population for parkinsonism: Rochester, Minnesota, 1935-66; Carlisle, England, 1955-61; and Iceland, 1954-63 (Source: Kurland and Kurtzke 1972. By permission of McGraw-Hill Book Company, Inc.)

groes. Some of the difference between whites and Negroes noted in Baltimore might result from reporting artifact, but the author believed that it was a real difference in the frequency of the disease by race. One possible explanation for the difference was postulated; the biogenic amine metabolic pathways involving tyrosine may affect the melanin content of the neurones of the substantia nigra, and this might be related to the melanin content of the skin.

It was also noted in a comparison of the cases and controls in the Baltimore study that patients with parkinsonism reported smoking less than did the controls. The authors speculated that nicotine somehow may also affect this same biogenic amine metabolic pathway (Kessler and Diamond 1971).

The prevalence study of Carlisle, England, by Brewis and her colleagues (1966) included parkinsonism. The discovery of 60 cases in

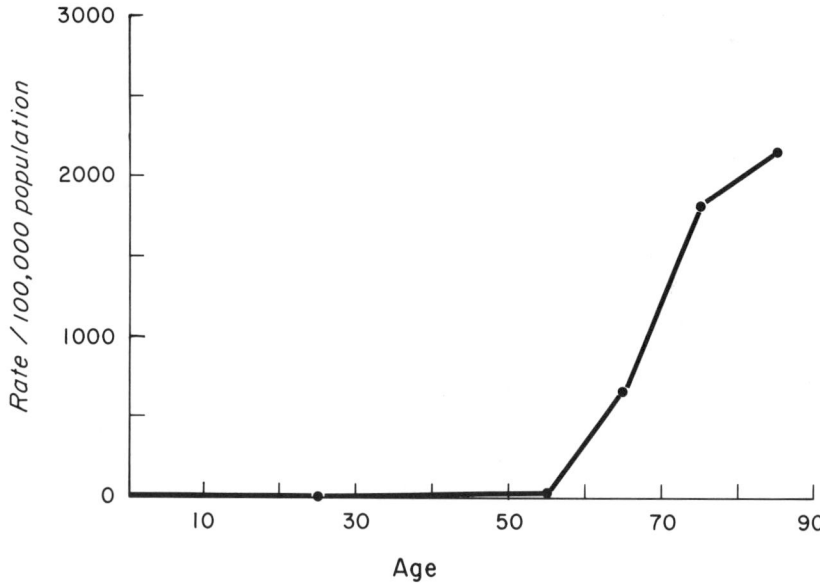

Figure 3.5 Age-specific prevalence rates per 100,000 population for parkinsonism: Rochester, Minnesota, January 1, 1954 (Source: Modified from Nobrega

Table 3.8 Prevalence rates per 100,000 population for parkinsonism by type, with number of cases by sex: Rochester, Minnesota, 1965 and Iceland, 1963

Area and type	Total rate	Number of cases		
		Total	Male	Female
Rochester				
All types	156.9[a]	75	30	45
Postencephalitic	10.5	5	2	3
With arteriosclerosis	48.1	23	9	14
Idiopathic	98.3	47	19	28
Iceland				
All types	169.0	316	170	146
Postencephalitic	6.4	12	5	7
With arteriosclerosis	17.1	32	16	16
Idiopathic	145.5	272	149	123

[a] 175.3 if age adjusted to 1960 white population of the United States.

the seven years surveyed gave an average annual incidence of 12 per 100,000. The age-specific rates are drawn in Fig. 3.4. Median age at onset was in the seventh decade. Prevalence as of January 1, 1961, was 1.1 per 1,000 population. The incidence and prevalence rates were considerably below those reported from Rochester. Although the difference may be real, the explanation probably lies with relative underdiagnosis or incomplete case ascertainment in the Carlisle study; the routine medical resources of the community provided the input in the Carlisle study. To support this impression, we note that the mortality rates for England and Wales were above the median in Fig. 3.3.

Kjartan Gudmundsson (1967b) identified 470 cases of parkinsonism in Iceland, two-thirds of which were his. He classified these cases as 82 percent idiopathic, 14 percent arteriosclerotic, and 4 percent postencephalitic. Incidence rates were based on the 272 cases of idiopathic parkinsonism with onset in 1954-63. This excluded only two patients (ages 33 and 16 years) who had the postencephalitic form. The age-specific incidence rates are drawn in Fig. 3.4. Average age of onset was 62.4 years. Prevalence as of December 31, 1963, with 316 patients was 1.7 per 1,000 and the distribution of rates by type is cited in Table 3.8. The mortality rate for parkinsonism was low in Iceland compared with other countries (Fig. 3.3).

Broman's survey (1963) of Göteborg, Sweden, based only on hospitalized patients, resulted in a prevalence rate of about 0.7 per 1,000; he estimated that the true rate was twice as high. Nine percent of his patients were encephalitic, and 15 percent were arteriosclerotic. The median age at onset was in the age group 55 through 59 years, which—like most hospital series—is probably biased toward younger patients. The mortality rate reported for Sweden is also relatively low (see Fig. 3.3).

In Victoria, Australia, Jenkins (1966) studied a neighboring area in detail and found 70 cases of parkinsonism, which provided a prevalence rate of 0.9 per 1,000 as of January 1, 1965. Seven percent were postencephalitic, and 14 percent were arteriosclerotic. The average age of onset was 61 years, excluding five patients who were postencephalitic. Age-specific incidence rates increased steadily with patient age, but the oldest group was the "70 and over" class, and the rates cannot be compared with those of Fig. 3.4. The average annual incidence rate was 7 per 100,000, conceded to be a "minimal" value. Australia had the highest mortality rate for parkinsonism in the 1950s of all countries analyzed (Fig. 3.3).

Wellington, New Zealand, was the site of a survey by Pollock and Hornabrook (1966). The prevalence rate as of December 1, 1962, was 1.1 per 1,000 population, based on 131 patients. Age of onset by type was identical with that reported for Rochester in the early study (Kurland 1958a). Eight percent of the patients were considered postencephalitic, and 29 percent were arteriosclerotic. New Zealand was found to rank relatively high in mortality rate (Fig. 3.3).

Logan and Cushion (1958) reported the results of a morbidity study from 106 general practices in England and Wales for the year commencing May 1955. The prevalence rate for parkinsonism was 0.9 per 1,000 population, with little noteworthy geographic variation. This rate is presumably low because of incomplete ascertainment. In its mortality rate, Britain ranked above the median of the lands reported (Fig. 3.3).

A survey of various illnesses, including Parkinson's disease, was made in 1950 by the Canadian government under the title *Canadian Sickness Survey* (1954). Trained lay interviewers visited approximately 10,000 randomly selected households and completed questionnaires for 33,000 persons distributed throughout each of the ten provinces of Canada. The prevalence rate based on reported cases of Parkinson's disease per 100,000 population was approximately 30 for all ages, and 150 for the group 65 or older (DeJong 1960). This low rate was presumably a result of underreporting and may reflect lack of recognition of the disease by the patient or lay informants. The mortality rate in Canada was comparable to that of the United States.

In summation, the studies that are most likely to approach complete case ascertainment (Rochester and Iceland) provided prevalence rates of nearly 2 per 1,000 population, with incidence rates of nearly 20 per 100,000, giving an estimated average duration of about ten years for this illness. Prevalence rates based on reports from general practices or the hospitals in a community were generally about half of these rates. Age-specific incidence rates increased from almost 0 for persons less than 40 years old to a peak at about age 75, and then appeared to decline. Prevalence rates increased steadily with age and among those 85 or older it exceeded 2 percent. Average annual death rates per 100,000 of nearly 2 for parkinsonism as the underlying cause contrasted with an incidence rate of nearly 20; this suggests appreciable underreporting on death certificates, or low case-fatality rates (about 10 percent), or a combination of both effects.

Encephalitis and Parkinsonism

It was early apparent after the influenza epidemic and the subsequent type A encephalitis of von Economo that many patients with encephalitis were left with or developed a parkinsonistic state. Dimsdale (1946) pointed out the young age of most patients with postencephalitic parkinsonism, their clinical differences from the typical paralysis agitans, and the less clear but still discernible clinical differences in the encephalitics with a later onset of parkinsonism. The mean age at onset was 55 years for 100 patients for whom paralysis agitans was recorded between 1900 and 1919, and 58 years for 52 patients with paralysis agitans recorded between 1931 and 1944. In this last period, there were also 24 encephalitics with delayed onset at an average age of 31 years and 42 with "indeterminate" parkinsonism whose mean age at onset was 36 years.

Schwab and colleagues (1956) noted that the mean age of parkinsonism patients at the Massachusetts General Hospital after 1945 was increasing. In part, this occurred because the same patients were being seen at later intervals, but even among new patients, there was a tendency for those seen in more recent years to be older than those seen in the preceding decade. On this basis, the authors contended that even in idiopathic parkinsonism, the encephalitis of von Economo might be an underlying cause. Later it was more definitely stated by Poskanzer and Schwab (1963) "that most cases of Parkinson's syndrome have a single etiology possibly related to subclinical infection in 1918 to 1920 resulting in the onset of Parkinson's syndrome up to 40 or more years later.... If the hypothesis is correct, then the cohort with Parkinson's syndrome will gradually disappear and the number of cases diminish [with] a precipitous drop . . . prior to 1980."

Duvoisin and his associates (1963; 1965) contested this hypothesis, stating that, first: "the age of onset of parkinsonism is now essentially what it was 50 to 75 years ago," since there was little change in the mean age of 52 years in a number of clinical series before 1923 and that noted at the Columbia Presbyterian Medical Center between 1950 and 1962, when it averaged 57 years; secondly, the Duvoisin group stressed the difference in the clinical picture of the postencephalitic group. Eadie and his colleagues (1965), Pollock and Hornabrook (1966), and Jenkins (1966) concluded that only a small proportion of parkinsonism could be attributed to encephalitis.

According to Poskanzer and Schwab (1963), the mean age of

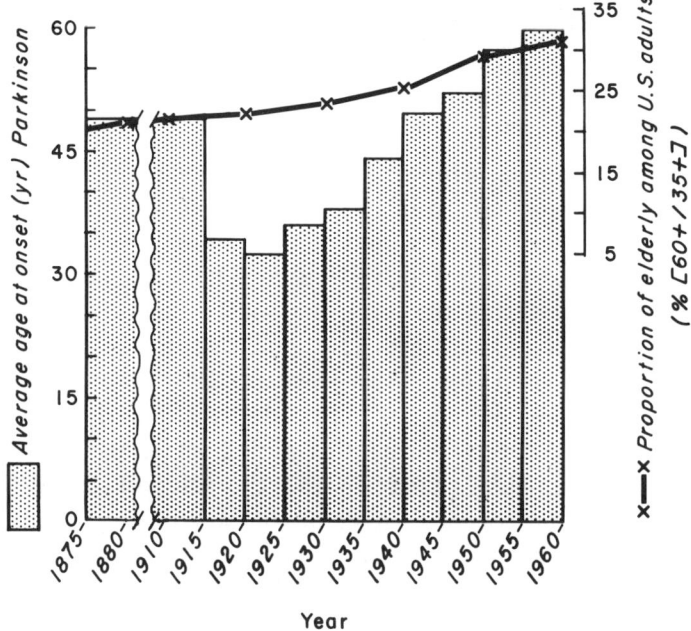

Figure 3.6 Mean age at onset for parkinsonian patients, according to calendar intervals when first seen at Massachusetts General Hospital, 1875–1960, compared with the proportion of elderly among United States white adults (Source: MGH data redrawn from Poskanzer and Schwab 1963.)

parkinsonism patients seen at the Massachusetts General Hospital increased steadily, almost on a year-to-year basis, after 1920. This accounted for their "cohort concept" in the encephalitis etiology of idiopathic parkinsonism. The mean age increased from about 40 years in 1935 to about 57 in 1958 (see Fig. 3.6). In contrast to this, the mean ages at onset of the parkinsonism patients in the Rochester population study during this same period showed no such cohort effect; the average age at onset was 63 for 1935-39 and 67 during 1955-59. Kurland and his associates (1969c) concluded that the shift in age distribution of parkinsonism patients at the Massachusetts General Hospital postulated by Poskanzer and Schwab (1963) was not necessarily caused by the cohort effect of common exposure to the encephalitis lethargica epidemic:

Such a shift can be explained equally well, and perhaps better, as a reflection of changes in medical practice and particularly specialty services, which have been sought by, and become available to, the elderly patient with increasing frequency in recent years. The specialty clinics in the United States are more and more attending to the chronic and progressive illnesses in elderly patients which previously had been largely the concern of the general practitioner.

This view is further supported by a study of parkinsonism among all Mayo Clinic patients from 1935 to 1967. During this period there were 11,320 patients for whom this diagnosis was made, and the mean age increased from about 51 years in 1935 to about 63 years in 1967. However, during the same period, the mean age of patients with other neurologic diseases also increased; for herpes zoster, for example, it increased from 48 to 56 years. This was interpreted as an indication that increased utilization by the elderly of specialty facilities was occurring during this period and not that there had been any appreciable change in the character of disease. It was further noted that for all patients at the Mayo Clinic from 1935 to 1965 (as well as at the Massachusetts General Hospital) the mean age had changed very little; at the Mayo Clinic the analysis was carried one step further and revealed that during the thirty-year interval the percentage distribution of patients had doubled for those under 10 years of age and for those over 65 years of age.

Poskanzer and Schwab (1963) also had reported:

Cases born after 1920 might be attributed to the reported occurrence of sporadic cases of encephalitis lethargica up to 1931. No case of Parkinson's syndrome born after 1931 and only one case born after 1930 occurred in this [the Massachusetts General Hospital] series.

Of 3,100 patients with parkinsonism observed at the Mayo Clinic from 1960 to 1967, 27 were less than 40 years of age. All 27 were born after 1925, and 7 were born after 1931.

As Poskanzer and Schwab pointed out, the cases from the Massachusetts General Hospital cannot be assigned to any population-based denominator. Further analysis of their data was made by Kurtzke (unpublished data), who compared their patients prior to 1915 and in each five-year interval thereafter with the proportion of elderly* in the United States in those same years. He noted that the mean ages of the parkinsonism patients corresponded well with this proportion before 1915 and after 1950. There was a significant difference during the years between 1915 and 1935, attributable to

---

*The percentage of those 60 years of age or more (in whom parkinsonism is most likely to occur) to those aged 35 or older (an age below which parkinsonism is essentially absent).

inclusion of the encephalitis cases. By 1935, the number of such cases (generally occurring at a much younger age than the idiopathic form of parkinsonism) was decreasing markedly and after 1940 there were few, if any, new postencephalitic cases. Further, where a special disease clinic exists, as at the Massachusetts General Hospital, one might expect that over time the increased numbers of registrants consequent thereto would more nearly represent the general population than the typically younger hospital series; from population studies, an average age at onset near age 65 seems likely for parkinsonism. This is supported by the Mayo Clinic data previously noted.

In other words, we have one illness of the elderly, that of paralysis agitans. This pool of cases was suddenly diluted with another illness, postencephalitic parkinsonism of the young. As the postencephalitics became older at onset—and especially fewer in number—their influence on the mean age at onset of all parkinsonian patients decreased and was essentially vestigial by the 1940s. Accordingly, the clinical separation of paralysis agitans from postencephalitic parkinsonism as two completely different entities appears to be upheld.

Familial Features

The role of heredity in parkinsonism is still to be determined. Unfortunately, most studies have dealt with selected patients or ill-defined family relationships. In the early study of Rochester, Minnesota, a history of a similar illness in an immediate member of the family was recorded in at least 16 percent of the cases of idiopathic parkinsonism (Kurland 1958*b*). Mjönes (1949), in Sweden, personally interviewed a large number of patients and obtained positive family histories from 41 percent of his idiopathic patients, 42 percent of his encephalitic patients, and 19 percent of his "arteriosclerosis" patients. (Family histories were considered to be least reliable in the last group.) In Iceland, Gudmundsson (1967*b*) recorded positive family histories for 20 percent of his idiopathic and arteriosclerotic patients and for 13 percent of his postencephalitic patients. Mjönes (1949), and Allan (1937) in the United States, compiled striking series of pedigrees in which parkinsonism was noted in members of several generations that had a pattern compatible with autosomal dominance with incomplete penetrance. In a series of patients in whom parkinsonistic features developed during therapy with phenothiazines, Myrianthopoulos and his associates

(1962) found a higher frequency of parkinsonism among their relatives than among those of a matched group of patients without this side reaction to the same drugs. Although this finding could have important genetic implications, it has yet to be confirmed.

Summary and Conclusions

The United States mortality statistics for 1959-61 compiled for the current effort were similar to the mortality statistics previously reported from the United States and from Canada a decade earlier. The data indicated a slightly higher mortality rate per 100,000 for parkinsonism as an underlying cause for males (1.8) than for females (1.5). Rates for whites were much higher than those for nonwhites (1.8 vs 0.4). Geographic variations were minimal, but the lowest rates were recorded for the southern United States. This probably represents underreporting rather than true differences. Death rates were essentially 0 for patients less than 40 years old and increased sharply to a peak of about 22 per 100,000 for those 75 through 84 years old. In the group 85 and older, the rate was 19 per 100,000.

International mortality comparisons showed wide variations, but available prevalence studies suggest that the variations may be more a reflection of reporting artifact than an indication of true geographic differences.

A number of prevalence studies for parkinsonism have been done, but only two seemed to approach complete ascertainment, those from Rochester, Minnesota, and from Iceland. For these two studies an annual incidence rate of nearly 20 per 100,000 and a prevalence rate of nearly 200 per 100,000 were recorded. Taking the annual mortality rate as nearly 2 per 100,000, we may infer a case-fatality rate of 10 percent (2 vs 20 per 100,000) and, with the prevalence rate, an average duration of about ten years (200 vs 20 per 100,000) for parkinsonism.

Age-specific prevalence rates increased with age from essentially 0 for persons less than 40 years old to a rate of 2.2 percent for those 85 or older. Age-specific incidence rates also increased from almost 0 for those under 40 to a peak at about 75 years of age, above which there appeared to be a decline. The mean age at onset was about 65. On the basis of these data, each year about 1 per 5,000 in the total population and about 1 per 1,000 of those 50 or older are newly affected. If we can project these findings to the entire country, then for the United States this represents the addition of about 40,000 new cases per year, and the existence at present of between 300,000 and 400,000 clinically identifiable cases of parkinsonism. Thus parkinsonism is one of the most numerous of the serious neurologic problems and one that, in the absence of effective treatment or prevention, will become more serious with the increasing life-span of our population.

Except for a few instances attributable to toxins or specific cerebral lesions, virtually all parkinsonism at present can be classed as idiopathic paralysis agitans. A separate category of parkinsonism with arteriosclerosis seems unnecessary in our view. The best available evidence indicates that new cases of parkinsonism which are a sequela of von Economo's type A encephalitis have essentially disappeared. From both morbidity and mortality data, the frequency of parkinsonism seems essentially stable in the recent decades of this century when age-specific rates are considered. The increasing numbers of cases reflect an aging population.

There appears to be an increased familial frequency for parkinsonism, and present information is compatible with its transmission as an autosomal dominant trait with reduced penetrance. However, further genetic studies are indicated before the relative roles of heredity and environment can be assessed.

4 / MULTIPLE SCLEROSIS

John F. Kurtzke
Leonard T. Kurland
Irving D. Goldberg
Nung Won Choi

The demyelinating diseases are a group of disorders so called because the most obvious pathologic change in the nervous system is the loss of the myelin sheath. The most frequently occurring disease of this group is multiple sclerosis (MS), which is generally considered to be a chronic, essentially progressive affliction characterized by multiple and disseminated lesions in the white matter of the central nervous system. Among young adults, MS is the most common primary disease of the nervous system in our western culture, and one in which the cause is unknown and the treatment unsatisfactory.

Multiple sclerosis is a condition in which the diagnosis is based on clinical criteria; no sign or group of signs is distinct. Some investigators contend that MS is not a single disease, but rather a syndrome of varied cause and course. As generally considered, MS is "a disease scattered in time and space," that is, one in which more than one lesion is present and in which continued or repeated evidence of disease activity is manifested by new or worsening symptoms, although at times there are intervening remissions and improvement. The most satisfactory set of diagnostic requirements probably is that of the Schumacher committee (1965). However, since these criteria cannot be applied to studies already completed, the comparisons must be based on the classifications which were usually employed—namely, "probable," "possible," or "unlikely" MS. The group of cases considered most likely to be MS on the basis of such a classification by different investigators does provide diagnostic criteria which appear similar to one another.

The geographic distribution of MS in particular has been the subject of extensive mortality analyses and intensive population surveys in recent decades, and efforts have been made to identify possible causative factors whose distribution would parallel that of the disease. It is but slight exaggeration to state that the investigation of MS has provided the foundation for modern neuroepidemiology.

The unique geographic distribution of MS remains a tantalizing clue to those concerned with the etiology of the disorder. This has been the subject of recent symposia (Hyllested and Kurland 1966; Alter and Kurtzke 1968) and an excellent review by Acheson (1965) and by others (Kurland et al. 1965; Poskanzer 1967). In his chapters on the epidemiology of MS, Acheson presented a critical and interpretive analysis of the reported distribution of the disease. He considered the possible importance of genetic factors, of climatic and meteorologic variations, of predisposing infections, and of dietary or trace-element deficiencies or excesses, but he had to conclude that no specific mechanism could be identified to explain the remarkable distribution of MS.

Mortality Data

The limitations of mortality data are especially pertinent to MS. A recent survey in Winnipeg, Canada, revealed that MS as a cause of death would not have been discovered in approximately 40 percent of the fatal cases during a ten-year period had the study been limited to a review of death certificates listing MS as the underlying cause of death; furthermore, the diagnosis of MS was erroneously reported in about 18 percent of the death certificates coded to MS as the underlying cause (Stazio et al. 1964). Nevertheless, the availability of death data for MS provides a broad overview geographically at minimal cost. Further, the omissions need not all be considered as errors because death from the disease is not its inevitable outcome. Thus mortality data particularly concern "severe MS," plus or minus errors of coding and diagnosis.

Data are available for only a few countries regarding the frequency with which MS was coded as a secondary cause of death (Table 4.1). In Norway for 1956-60 (Statistisk Sentralbyra 1961), in 23 percent of 350 death certificates on which MS was recorded, it was classified as a secondary cause of death. In the Netherlands (Central Bureau of Statistics 1961), the figure was about 15 percent of 1,909 deaths during 1953-57 and 1959-61 (data not available for 1958). In the United States (National Center for Health Statistics 1965) in 1955, MS was coded as a secondary cause in 28 percent of the death certificates on which the condition was listed.

International Mortality Data

Limburg (1950) demonstrated an inverse relation between crude mortality rates for MS in many countries and the mean annual

Table 4.1 Death certificates listing multiple sclerosis as primary or secondary cause of death, with percent listed as primary cause: selected countries, various years, 1953-61
(ISC code 345)

Country	Years	Total deaths	Percent primary
Norway[a]	1956-60	350	77
United States[b]	1955	1,943	72
Netherlands[c]	1953-60	1,681	85
Netherlands[d]	1961	228	81

[a] All secondary causes considered.

[b] Up to four secondary causes considered.

[c] Only one ("most important") secondary cause considered; excludes deaths for 1958 (not available).

[d] Up to three secondary causes considered.

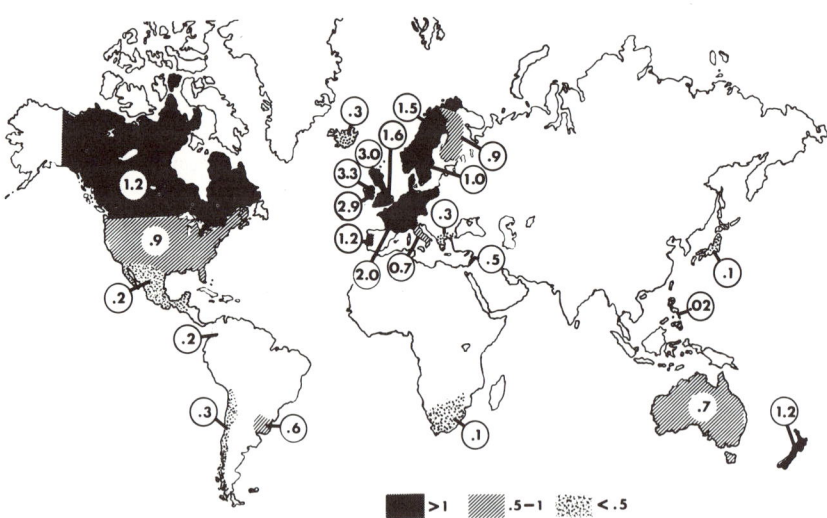

Figure 4.1 Average annual age-adjusted death rates per 100,000 population for multiple sclerosis: selected countries, various years, 1951–58 (Source: Modified from Kurland et al. 1965. By permission of the New York Academy of Sciences.)

temperature of the major city of each country. A more recent study also showed a relation between death rates and latitude in thirty-one countries, although the data for several, such as Iceland, Japan, and Portugal, deviate from this pattern (Goldberg and Kurland 1962) (Fig. 4.1 and Table A.4.1).

There is a lack of uniformity in many of the reporting sources. Thus we must look at mortality rates in areas that have reasonably comparable systems of medical-practice terminology and death coding. Table 4.2 is based on data from the United States and Canada (Goldberg and Kurland 1962) and on a study from selected British Commonwealth countries (Acheson 1961; 1965). The rates for Northern Ireland and Scotland were higher than for England and

Table 4.2 Age-adjusted[a] death rates per 100,000 population for multiple sclerosis: selected British Commonwealth countries and United States, various years, 1950-59
(ISC code 345)

Country and years	Range of approximate latitude	Rate
United Kingdom (1954-56)		1.8
Scotland	55° - 60° N	2.9
Northern Ireland	54° - 56° N	3.1
England and Wales	50° - 55° N	1.6
Australia (1950-59)		0.7
Tasmania	40° - 42° S	1.3
Victoria	34° - 39° S	1.0
New South Wales	29° - 37° S	0.7
Southern Australia	26° - 37° S	0.7
Queensland	10° - 29° S	0.8
Western Australia	13° - 35° S	0.4
New Zealand (1950-59)		1.2
South Island	41° - 47° S	1.3
North Island	34° - 41° S	1.0
Union of South Africa (1950-58)	22° - 35° S	0.1
Canada (1953-57)	42° - 69° N	1.2
United States (1953-57)	24° - 47° N	0.9

[a]Death rates are adjusted to the structure of the United States population in 1950. The figures for Australia, New Zealand, South Africa, and the United States are for the white population only. Commonwealth data from Acheson 1965; Canada and U.S. data from Goldberg and Kurland 1962.

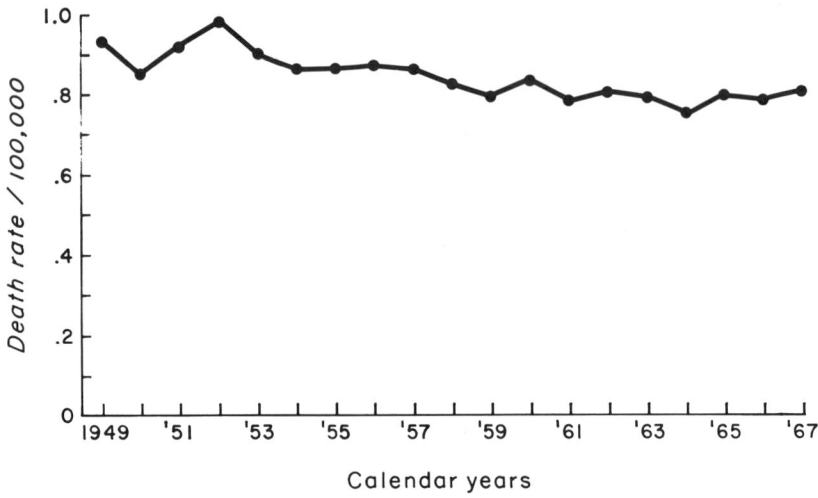

Figure 4.2 Crude death rates per 100,000 population for multiple sclerosis by year: United States, 1949–67

Wales, and these in turn were higher than for Canada, which exceeded the rate in the United States. In the English-speaking countries of the Southern Hemisphere, people of British descent generally had a lower mortality rate for MS than did people inhabiting the British Isles. The pattern also suggests that the rate increases as one proceeds south from the equator, at least in New Zealand and parts of Australia.

United States Mortality Data, Trend

Figure 4.2 shows crude death rates by year from 1949 to 1967 for deaths coded to MS as underlying cause in the United States. There was a slight decline over the entire interval, but most of the decline seems to have occurred before 1960; thereafter there appears to have been little change. The age-adjusted rates for the United States were 0.9 for 1949-51, 0.8 for 1959-61, and 0.8 for 1965-67. In Canada, the MS death rates (age adjusted) declined from 1.3 for 1949-51 to 1.0 for 1959-61 (Kurland et al. 1965).

The assumption of a noteworthy decline in MS death rates may reflect either a decline in MS incidence or an increase in MS survival, or both. The incidence rate for MS has not changed appreciably during the twenty years to 1959 in Winnipeg (Stazio et al. 1964) or New Orleans (Stazio et al. 1967). Reported average durations of MS were much shorter before World War II than those cited since. If the increased duration is valid, a declining death rate would be expected until the new survival rate has stabilized, and this may be the preferable explanation for the mortality trend. There is still another point. If more patients survive to old age, one would expect an increasing frequency of deaths unrelated to MS but associated with the infirmities of aging. In the Winnipeg study, the average age at death was 46 years when MS was cited as primary cause, and 51 years when MS was listed as a secondary cause of death (Stazio et al. 1964).

United States Mortality Data, 1959-61

Age, sex, and color. The 1959-61 average annual crude rate per 100,000 population for all ages combined was 0.8 (Table A.4.2). The rates for females of either color were slightly greater than the corresponding rates for males. The female preponderance was noted in all regions of the United States where numbers were sufficient for comparison (Table 4.3).

The age-specific death rates by sex and color are shown in Fig. 4.3 and Table A.4.2. The rates for both sexes and colors combined were

Table 4.3   Average annual age-adjusted death rates per 100,000 population for multiple sclerosis by sex: United States and census regions, 1959-61
(ISC code 345)

Region	Rate		M:F ratio
	Male	Female	
United States	0.7	0.8	0.9
New England	0.9*	1.1	0.8
Middle Atlantic	0.8	1.0	0.8
East North Central	0.8	1.0	0.8
West North Central	0.8*	1.0*	0.8
South Atlantic	0.5*	0.7	0.7
East South Central	0.4*	0.5*	0.8
West South Central	0.4*	0.4*	1.0
Mountain	0.8*	1.0*	0.8
Pacific	0.7*	0.8*	0.9

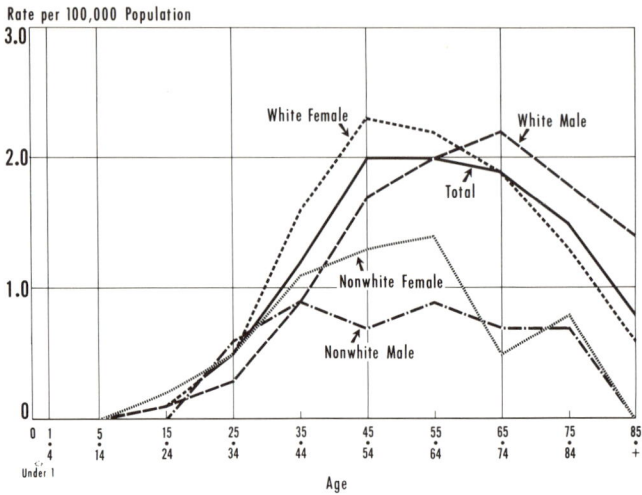

Figure 4.3 Average annual age-specific death rates per 100,000 population for multiple sclerosis by color and sex: United States, 1959-61

negligible prior to age 15, increased sharply and steadily to a plateau at age 45-74, and then decreased sharply.

The rates for females of either color who were under age 65 exceeded those for the males of corresponding age; at older ages among the whites, the rates for males were slightly greater.

For the whites, male rates appeared to lag behind those for females, so that at most ages the rate for males was about the same as that for females ten years younger (see Fig. 4.3). The rates for nonwhites were based on about 100 deaths per year, and the pattern irregularly followed that of whites but at a lower level for corresponding age groups.

Age-adjusted rates for whites were about 1.6 times those for nonwhites (Table 4.4). However, when the individual regions of the United States were considered, the ratios were close to unity for most of the regions. Only in the Mountain and Pacific regions (where there were only 1 and 9 nonwhite deaths, respectively) were the ratios appreciably larger. In regions where there were less than 10 nonwhite deaths during this three-year period, the ratios varied considerably (for example, New England 1.0, and Mountain 4.5).

Aside from general problems of diagnostic accuracy, the mortality data for nonwhites are open to question because of the population undercount (see Chapter 2). In addition, differential migration by

Table 4.4 Average annual age-adjusted death rates per 100,000 population for multiple sclerosis by color: United States and census regions, 1959-61

(ISC code 345)

Region	Rate		White:nonwhite ratio
	White	Nonwhite	
United States	0.8	0.5*	1.6
New England	1.0	1.0*	1.0
Middle Atlantic	0.9	0.8*	1.1
East North Central	1.0	0.5*	2.0
West North Central	0.9	0.6*	1.5
South Atlantic	0.6	0.5*	1.2
East South Central	0.5*	0.5*	1.0
West South Central	0.4*	0.4*	1.0
Mountain	0.9	0.2*	4.5
Pacific	0.8	0.2*	4.0

age and color from the rural South to other regions may influence these rates. For example, in Denver, Colorado, in the ten years prior to 1950, the nonwhite population increased by 112 percent, in contrast to a 27-percent increase among the whites (Kurland and Westlund 1954).

Accordingly, it seems best to reserve judgment on the importance of this color variation, except to state that for deaths resulting from MS recorded for the United States as a whole the mortality rate for nonwhites was two-thirds that for whites, but that for most of the individual regions of the United States the differences by color were much smaller. In one sense, the national ratio is an artifact, being a reflection of the preponderance of nonwhites in the South, together with the low death rates for MS in the South.

Geographic distribution. Age-adjusted death rates by state (Fig. 4.4), and by the nine geographic census regions (Table 4.3), both according to residence at death, showed the same geographic pattern of MS as that previously described. Rates by state of birth are shown in Table A.4.3. Generally, the death rates increase as one proceeds from south to north. The same south-to-north pattern was observed when the rates for those 65 or older were compared (Table A.4.4). When distribution of the rates for all ages by longitude was studied, no gradient was apparent either by states or by regions.

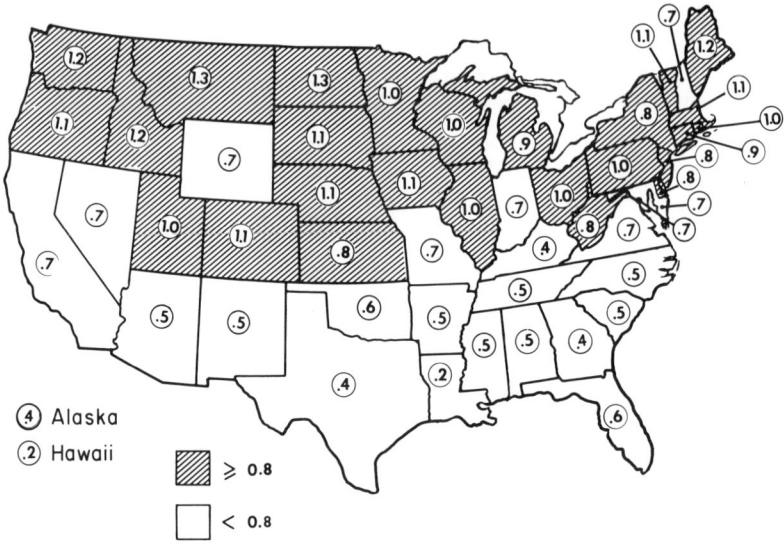

Figure 4.4 Average annual age-adjusted death rates per 100,000 population for multiple sclerosis by state of residence at death: United States, 1959–61 (Source: Kurtzke et al. 1971. By permission of Lancet Publications, Inc.)

Comparison by color had to be limited to the census regions because of small numbers of nonwhites. In Table 4.4, the north-south gradient was noted also for nonwhites, although the differences were smaller than those for whites. Further detail is provided in Table A.4.4.

Crude death rates were available for states and census regions according to residence at birth (regardless of residence at death). The rates for states of birth are displayed according to color in Table A.4.3 and summarized in Fig. 4.5. The demarcation between areas that had high and low rates was perhaps more definite when analyzed by place of birth than by residence at death. The major change was at about the 37 degree parallel of north latitude. The results for whites only were similar (Table A.4.3). Figure 4.6 shows the death rates by state for whites whose state of birth and state of residence at time of death were the same. The geographic differentiation between a northern (high) tier and a southern (low) tier is again observed, and although the gradient described in earlier studies is noted, a dichotomous pattern also seems to be a possibility. The shading in these

MULTIPLE SCLEROSIS / 73

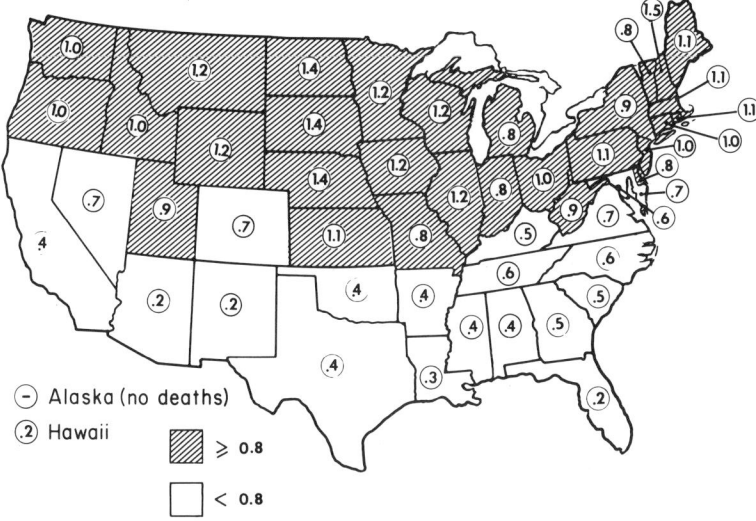

Figure 4.5 Average annual crude death rates per 100,000 population for multiple sclerosis among native born by state of birth: United States, 1959–61. Rates based on less than 20 deaths are indicated by an asterisk (*) in Table A.4.3. (Source: Kurtzke et al. 1971. By permission of Lancet Publications, Inc.)

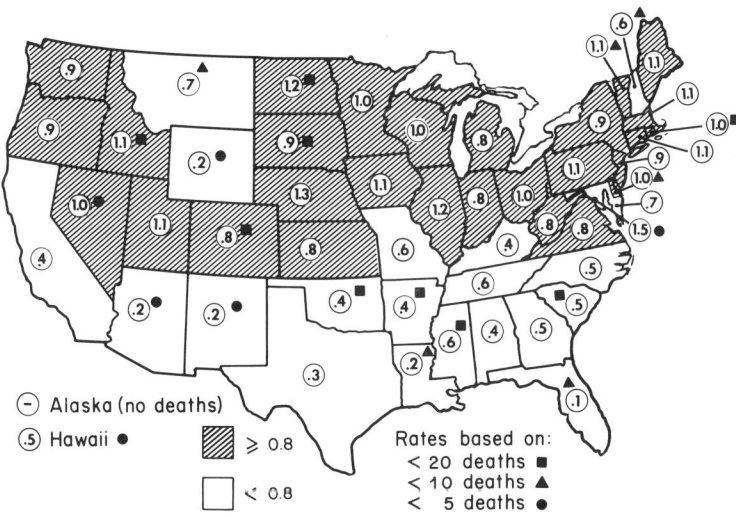

Figure 4.6 Average annual crude death rates per 100,000 population for multiple sclerosis, white persons whose state of birth was state of residence at death, by state: United States, 1959–61 (Source: Kurtzke et al. 1971. By permission of Lancet Publications, Inc.)

maps defines those areas which were at or above the national age-adjusted death rate of 0.8 per 100,000.

An investigation of migration between the high-risk northern states and the low-risk southern states would provide some clues as to the time at which a geographic-related risk factor might be operative. For example, if those born in the southern tier who died in the northern tier had a low risk, and if the opposite direction of migration were marked by a high risk, then the critical time would seem closely related to the period of birth.

Considering only place of birth or death for all MS patients combined could mask the effect of migration,* because those who changed tiers accounted for only a small proportion of all MS deaths. In order to investigate this problem, we need geographic areas larger than states, but areas in which we can still define a high-risk North versus a low-risk South. The census regions, which divide the United States into nine parts, closely follow such a division for the eastern two-thirds of the country, although the two western regions (Mountain and Pacific), which extend from Canada to Mexico, are not useful in such an analysis. The eastern portion is divided into a northern tier of four regions (New England, Middle Atlantic, East North Central, West North Central) and a southern tier of three regions (South Atlantic, East South Central, West South Central).

The interrelation of place of birth and place of death for MS among all nine census regions is displayed in Table A.4.5, where crude death rates for MS are listed according to region. These death rates are shown in Fig. 4.7 for the seven census regions that comprise the northern and southern tiers, for those persons for whom the region of birth and the region of death were the same. The two-to-one ratio for the northern tier versus the southern tier as seen by state in Fig. 4.6 is still apparent.

If we now analyze the mortality data for those who have migrated between regions at some time between birth and death, we note in Table A.4.6 the MS deaths in 1959-61 listed according to region of birth versus region at the time of death. Also shown in the table are the corresponding three-year population figures, based on the 1960 census.

*"Migration" is used here in the sense of differing census regions for residence at birth versus residence at death among the seven regions considered. It is of course impossible to determine from death data the age, duration, or frequency of any such changes. It is also obvious that of those who actually migrated between regions only that fraction will be identified whose region of birth and death differed. For example, should a migrant have returned to his region of birth a month before death, he would be identified as a "nonmigrant."

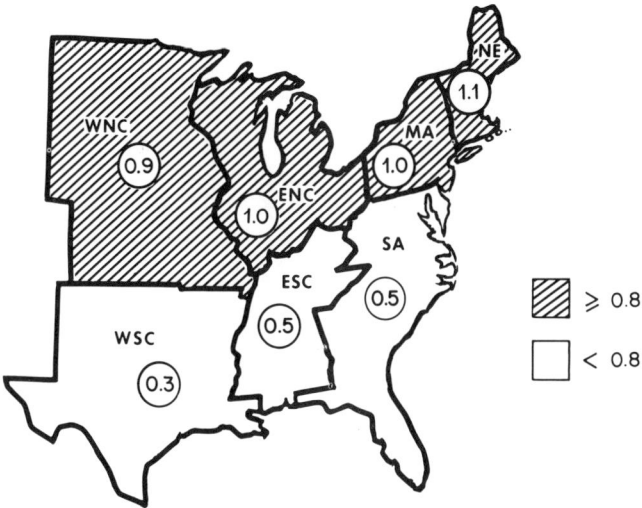

Figure 4.7 Average annual crude death rates per 100,000 population for multiple sclerosis, persons whose census region of birth was region of residence at death, by census region: census regions except Mountain and Pacific, United States, 1959-61 (Source: Kurtzke et al. 1971. By permission of Lancet Publications, Inc.)

What happened when movement was known to be between regions within the *same* northern or southern tier? Figure 4.8 shows death rates for MS according to region of death for all born in the same northern *or* the same southern tier. For example, a rate of 1.1 was cited for New England. This was the result of 293 deaths from MS in New England, comprising 265 such persons who were born and who died in New England, plus 28 who died in New England but who had been born in the Middle Atlantic (24), East North Central (3), and West North Central (1) regions. The population at risk was derived from the 1960 census multiplied by 3 to cover the same three years—1959-61. The estimated three-year total population residing in New England in 1960 who were born in New England was 23,962,000 plus 1,725,000 who had been born in the Middle Atlantic region but resided in New England, and so forth. If we exclude those who were born and died in the same region and limit attention only to the migrants from northern regions to other northern regions, the death rates by place of death were 1.2 for New England, 1.7 for Middle Atlantic, 1.2 for East North Central, and 1.7 for West North Central, or a rate of 1.4 for all northern migrants within the northern tier.

The southern tier in the same manner showed rates of 0.5 (South

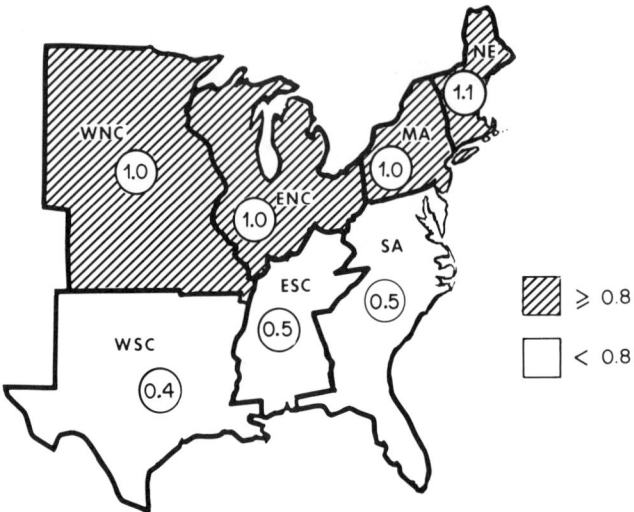

Figure 4.8 Average annual crude death rates per 100,000 population for multiple sclerosis, persons whose place of birth and residence at death were in same tier (northern or southern), by census region of death: census regions except Mountain and Pacific, United States, 1959-61 (Source: Kurtzke et al. 1971. By permission of Lancet Publications, Inc.)

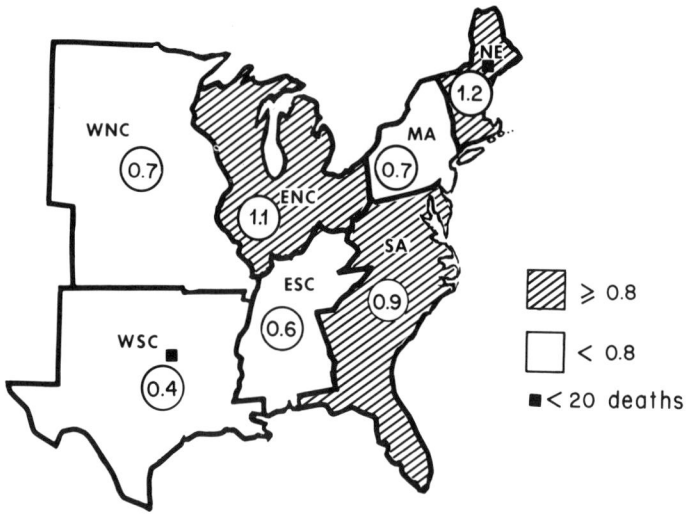

Figure 4.9 Average annual crude death rates per 100,000 population for multiple sclerosis, persons whose place of birth and residence at death were in *opposite* tiers (northern or southern), by census region of *birth:* census regions except Mountain and Pacific, United States, 1959-61 (Source: Kurtzke et al. 1971. By permission of Lancet Publications, Inc.)

Atlantic and East South Central) and 0.4 per 100,000 (West South Central) according to region of death. Again the rates for the southern migrants only within this tier were 0.5 (South Atlantic), 0.4 (East South Central), and 0.8 (West South Central), or a total rate of 0.6 for the southern migrants within the southern tier.

Accordingly, movement *within* the tier preserved the north-south differential in the risk of MS. What, then, is the effect of changing tiers? Figure 4.9 shows the rates for those who died in the opposite tier according to the individual region of birth. For example, the rate of 1.2 for New England was based on 15 persons who were born in New England and who died of MS in any of the three southern regions. The other northern rates were based on 33, 49, and 21 MS deaths in Middle Atlantic, East North Central, and West North Central regions, respectively. The southern rates were generated from 77 (South Atlantic), 44 (East South Central), and 14 (West South Central) deaths among MS patients who were born in the respective southern regions but who died in the northern tier.

Because the combination of regions will be different when region of death is specified, we note in Fig. 4.10 the similar migration

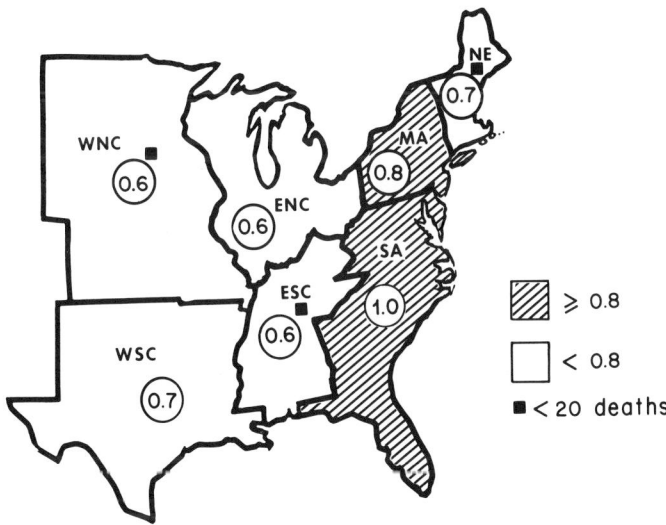

Figure 4.10 Average annual crude death rates per 100,000 population for multiple sclerosis, persons whose place of birth and residence at death were in *opposite* tiers (northern or southern), by census region of residence at *death:* census regions except Mountain and Pacific, United States, 1959-61 (Source: Kurtzke et al. 1971. By permission of Lancet Publications, Inc.)

patterns with rates expressed according to region of death for those who had been born in the opposite tier. The rate of 0.7 for New England refers to the 6 persons with MS who had been born in one of the three southern regions and who died in New England. Numbers underlying the other northern rates of 0.8, 0.6, and 0.6 were 46, 69, and 14, respectively, from east to west. In the southern tier, the respective numbers were 85, 9, and 24 for the rates of 1.0, 0.6, and 0.7.

Although some of these rates for migrants were based on small numbers, the resultant impression was that the striking north-south differential—seen for all MS deaths by place of birth, by place of death, for those where both states or regions were the same at birth and death, *or* for those who migrated within the tier—had disappeared when the tiers differed between birth and death. There was then a tendency for all the regional rates to approximate the mean death rate for the country as a whole. It seemed to make little difference whether one moved from the northern tier to the southern tier or vice versa; changing tiers reduced the north-south differential in the risk of MS.

This observation and conclusion is summarized in Table 4.5. There was a two-to-one ratio of the rates for those who were born and died in the northern tier versus those who were born and died in the southern tier (1.00 vs 0.46). There was no significant difference when the rate for those born in the northern tier who died in the southern tier was compared with the rate for those born in the southern tier who died in the northern tier (0.87 vs 0.68). Place of birth seemed to provide a stronger influence on MS risk than place of death, but the migration data would indicate that residence in the northern tier increased the risk of dying of MS.

Type of county. There was little difference in the age-adjusted death rates for MS between metropolitan and nonmetropolitan counties for either sex (Table A.4.7). The rates for either type of county generally followed the same geographic pattern by census region as previously noted.

Marital status. Age-adjusted death rates by marital status are shown in Table 4.6. In general, lower rates were noted among the married and widowed than among the single or divorced. By sex, divorced males and single females had the highest rates, but these differences between the sexes had largely disappeared among the elderly. It is

Table 4.5 Deaths and average annual death rates per 100,000 population for multiple sclerosis among native born by residence at birth and death: **nor**thern tier[a] and southern tier[b] of United States, 1959-61
(ISC code 345)

	Place of birth	
Place of death	Northern tier	Southern tier
	Rate ± SE rate	
Northern tier	1.00 ± 0.02	0.68 ± 0.06
Southern tier	0.87 ± 0.08	0.46 ± 0.02
	Deaths, 3-year totals	
Northern tier	2,356	135
Southern tier	118	662
	1960 census population x 3 (1,000's)	
Northern tier	236,330	19,709
Southern tier	13,641	142,528

[a] New England, Middle Atlantic, East North Central and West North Central census regions.

[b] South Atlantic, East South Central and West South Central census regions.

Table 4.6 Average annual age-adjusted death rates per 100,000 population for multiple sclerosis by age, sex and marital status: United States, 1959-61
(ISC code 345)

Age and sex	Single	Married	Widowed	Divorced
15 & over				
Total	2.3	0.9	1.3	2.4*
Male	1.9*	0.7	1.6*	3.1*
Female	2.8	1.0	1.3	1.9*
15-64				
Total	2.3	0.8	1.3	2.3
Male	1.9	0.6	1.5*	3.1*
Female	2.8	0.9	1.3	1.8*
65 & over				
Total	2.6*	1.9	1.5	2.9*
Male	2.5*	1.9	2.3	2.9*
Female	2.6*	1.7*	1.3	2.9*

likely that disease in the young female is a bar to marriage, and that the afflicted young male may suffer divorce when he is unable to care for his family. Among the married less than 65 years of age, there was a preponderance of females for all MS deaths. Why the rates for the widowed should have been higher among males—especially elderly males—is not clear.

Nativity. The age-adjusted death rates for MS among the white foreign-born population (Table 4.7) were somewhat less than those among the white native born. The relationship held for all ages and for the elderly alone, as well as for both sexes. However, there were notable differences according to country of birth (Fig. 4.11 and Table A.4.8). Rates were between 1 and 3 per 100,000 for immigrants from most of Europe, including the USSR, but those from Greece, Switzerland, the Netherlands, Hungary, and Yugoslavia were lower, although based on very small numbers. For immigrants from Mexico, the death rate was 0.5, and for the remainder of Central and South America, it was 0.1. All these rates were for whites. Among the 352 foreign born with known country of birth who died of MS in these three years, there were only 3 nonwhites, who were all from Central and South America. There were but 5 MS deaths among the Asian born, all of whites, providing a rate of 0.8. Absence of Orientals among the immigrant deaths should not be construed as

Table 4.7 Average annual age-adjusted death rates per 100,000 population for multiple sclerosis, white persons, by age, sex and nativity: United States, 1959-61 (ISC code 345)

Nativity and age	Rate			M:F ratio
	Total	Male	Female	
Native born				
All ages	0.8	0.7	0.9	0.8
65 & over	2.0	2.3	1.8	1.3
Foreign born				
All ages	0.6	0.6*	0.7*	0.9
65 & over	1.5	1.7*	1.4*	1.2

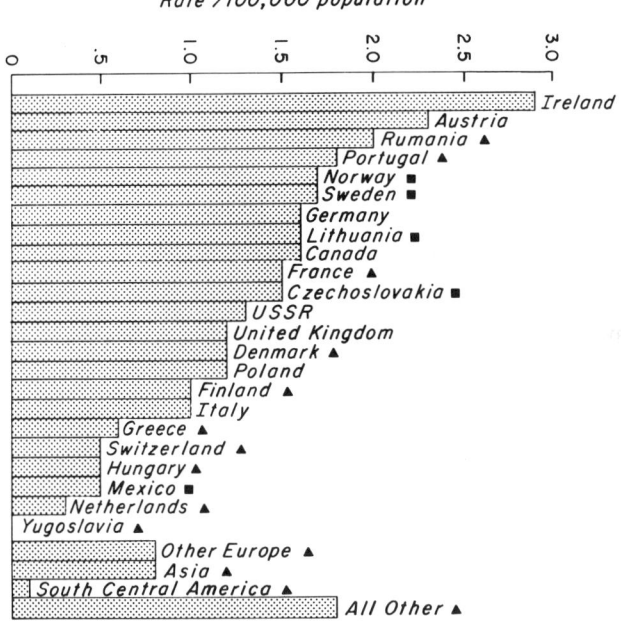

Figure 4.11 Average annual crude death rates per 100,000 population for multiple sclerosis among foreign-born white residents of the United States by country of birth: United States, 1959–61. Solid triangle (▲) represents rate based on less than 6 deaths and solid square (■) the rate based on less than 20 deaths.

meaning Oriental immunity, since the population at risk was small and the 95-percent confidence interval on the mortality rate for no deaths among the Oriental Asians would include 0.7 per 100,000 for males and 1.0 for females.

In order to compare death rates for immigrants with those for their native lands, only countries that provided more than 5 deaths in the three years in question were considered. This experience can be related to the international mortality rates for the 1950s, discussed in an earlier section, but using the crude rates for comparison instead of the age-adjusted rates of Table A.4.1. These crude rates are listed as "native rates" in Table 4.8 (Goldberg and Kurland, unpublished data). The agreement is surprisingly close, despite the uncertainties underlying both sets of data. If these data are valid, they suggest that migrants carry with them the MS risk of their homeland. Obviously, further inquiry into this possibility is in order.

Table 4.8   Average annual death rates per 100,000 population for multiple sclerosis among immigrants to the United States by birthplace and reported rates for residents of their native countries: United States, 1959-61, and specified countries, various years, 1952-58
(ISC code 345)

Country of origin	Immigrants to U.S.	Residents of native country
Ireland	2.9	2.8
Germany	1.6	2.3[a]
Czechoslovakia	1.5*	2.1
Austria	2.3	2.2
Norway	1.7*	1.7
Canada	1.6	1.0
Sweden	1.7*	1.2
Italy	1.0	0.7
Mexico	0.5*	0.1

Source of resident rates for native countries: Goldberg and Kurland, unpublished data.
[a] West Germany only.

Morbidity Data

Many studies have described the characteristics of MS in defined populations. Surveys of populations in different environments around the world and comparisons of subpopulations in the same environment have been the major sources of the statistics on incidence and prevalence of MS. These often provide a more accurate, albeit more localized, distribution pattern than do the mortality statistics.

The uncertainty of onset date, the often long time interval between onset and diagnosis, and the inaccuracies in diagnosis of early cases have led most investigators to limit comparisons to the larger and statistically more stable prevalence rates. However, prevalence rates also are subject to extraneous influences, including differences in the extent and intensity of case-finding and diagnostic procedures. The diagnostic classification of the individual investigator also affects the rates, although most investigators limit cases for inclusion to those that are generally considered "probable" or "highly likely" MS. Also, prevalence rates in different populations may be affected by a differential migration of patients and unaffected persons into or out of a community, or by differences in the rate of progression of illness and survival associated with the availability of supportive medical care.

Prevalence

In general accord with the mortality rates, prevalence of MS has been found to be high in the higher latitudes of western Europe and North America, with but little difference between the continents. More recent efforts also have resulted in some information from the Far East and the Southern Hemisphere.

General pattern of geographic distribution. In Table 4.9 are listed most of the recent prevalence studies of MS which have been conducted with reasonably comparable standards, though there still may be differences in case ascertainment. Our efforts shall be directed to determining from these studies whether or not there is a general pattern definable to geographic distribution.

A geographic gradient based on a few population studies was initially described in Europe. In these countries, however, variations in language and medical practice were annoying circumstances in the effort to develop comparable studies. Thus, population surveys were instituted about twenty years ago in parts of the large land mass of the United States and Canada where differences in classification and medical practice were appreciably reduced. The prevalence rates for many of these studies are shown in Table 4.9.

The first thorough morbidity survey of MS in the United States was that of MacLean and his co-workers (1950) for Rochester, Minnesota. The prevalence rate per 100,000 of 64 for all residents and 55 for those who were residents prior to onset was the highest reported anywhere up to that time. Intensive retrospective surveys carried out later (Siedler et al. 1958; White and Wheelan 1959; Kurland et al. 1965) in other communities of about the same latitude and size—Kingston, Ontario, and Missoula, Montana, both about 30,000 population—provided prevalence rates that were almost identical with Rochester's rate.

Further refinements led to comparative prevalence studies in different areas by the same teams of investigators to obviate

Table 4.9 Prevalence rates per 100,000 population for multiple sclerosis: specified localities, various years, 1950-68

Location (source)	Degrees latitude (approx.)	Year of report	Rate[a]
Orkney and Shetland, Scotland (Allison 1963)	60 N	1963	128
Vestfold, Norway (Oftedal 1966)	59 N	1963	80
Denmark (Hyllested 1956)	56 N	1956	64
Rochester, Minnesota, USA (MacLean et al. 1950)	44 N	1950	64
Missoula, Montana, USA (Kurland et al. 1965)	47 N	1958	59
Kingston, Ontario, Canada (Kurland et al. 1965)	44 N	1959	57
Hamburg, Germany (Behrend 1966)	54 N	1963	57
Northern Scotland (Sutherland 1956)	58 N	1956	55
Switzerland (Georgi and Hall 1960)	47 N	1960	51
Northumberland and Durham, England (Poskanzer et al. 1963a)	55 N	1963	50
Iceland (Gudmundsson and Gudmundsson 1962)	66 N	1962	44
Northern Ireland (Allison and Millar 1954)	55 N	1954	41
Boston, Massachusetts, USA (Kurland and Westlund 1954)	42 N	1954	41
Winnipeg, Manitoba, Canada (Westlund and Kurland 1953)	50 N	1953	40
Denver, Colorado, USA (Kurland and Westlund 1954)	40 N	1954	38
Western Norway (Presthus 1966)	64 N	1963	38
South Australia (Rischbieth 1966)	30 S	1966	35
Faroes, Denmark (Allison 1963)	56 N	1963	34
Halifax, Nova Scotia, Canada (Alter et al. 1960)	45 N	1960	32
Hobart, Tasmania (McCall et al. 1968)	40 S	1968	32
San Francisco, California, USA (Kurland and Westlund 1954)	38 N	1954	30
Perth, Western Australia (McCall et al. 1968)	32 S	1968	20
New Castle, Australia (McCall et al. 1968)	33 S	1968	20
Charleston, South Carolina, USA (Alter et al. 1960)	33 N	1960	14
Marseilles, France (Behrend 1966)	44 N	1963	14
Parma, Italy (Macchi et al. 1962)	45 N	1962	12
Southern Queensland, Australia (Sutherland et al. 1966)	25 S	1963	12
Republic of South Africa (white English-speaking) (Dean 1967)	30 S	1967	11
Houston, Texas, USA (Chipman 1966)	30 N	1959	7
Northern Queensland, Australia (Sutherland et al. 1966)	15 S	1963	7
New Orleans, Louisiana, USA (Westlund and Kurland 1953)	30 N	1953	6[b]
Israel (Alter et al. 1962)	32 N	1962	4
Niigata, Japan (Kuroiwa 1967)	38 N	1964	4
Republic of South Africa (white Afrikaners) (Dean 1967)	30 S	1967	3
Fukuoka, Japan (Kuroiwa 1967)	34 N	1964	2
Sapporo, Japan (Okinaka et al. 1960)	43 N	1960	2
Kumamoto, Japan (Okinaka et al. 1960)	33 N	1960	2

[a] Rate includes "possible MS" in some studies.
[b] The rate based on a study by Stazio et al. 1967 was 10 per 100,000 population.

disparities in diagnostic criteria: Winnipeg, Canada, and New Orleans, Louisiana, were compared (Westlund and Kurland 1953), as were Halifax, Nova Scotia, and Charleston, South Carolina (Alter et al. 1960). Both Winnipeg and New Orleans were later resurveyed by a single team and essentially the same prevalence rates were found as in the previous studies (Stazio et al. 1964; 1967).

In the European surveys of Hyllested in Denmark (1956) and of Georgi and Hall in Switzerland (1960), no attempt was made to provide for an independent examination of each patient by the investigators. However, this was done by several other investigators in Great Britain (Allison and Millar 1954; Sutherland 1956; Poskanzer et al. 1963a), Iceland (Gudmundsson and Gudmundsson 1962), and Italy (Macchi et al. 1962).

With the exception of the results in Vestfold, Norway (Oftedal, 1966), and Orkney-Shetland, Scotland (Allison 1963)—the latter having been chosen because a high rate had been noted there previously (Sutherland 1956)—the prevalence rates were similar in the Canadian and northern United States cities and in the northwestern European centers. This differed from the findings in the mortality analysis data, where the rates were generally higher in the northwestern European countries than in the United States and Canada; however, the morbidity data appear to be more reliable than the mortality data.

In northern Europe, the results of several of the recent studies provided prevalence rates which exceeded those reported previously (for example, Vestfold, Norway, and Orkney-Shetland, Scotland). Better case ascertainment, greater survival, and differential migration were factors that might cause this increase without any change in the incidence of the disease. The mortality rates seemed to have declined somewhat in North America, which could be a result of increased survival, decreased incidence, or both. On the basis of the studies in Rochester (Percy et al. 1968), Winnipeg (Stazio et al. 1964), and New Orleans (Stazio et al. 1967), there was no indication of a changing incidence.

Interpretation of geographic differences. Table 4.9 reveals that MS prevalence rates were about 30 to 80 per 100,000 population in northern Europe, southern Canada, and northern United States, whereas in southern Europe and southern United States, the rates were about 6 to 14 per 100,000. These data have been interpreted in two ways, by the "gradient" and the "zonal" theories.

The gradient concept holds that MS is rare in the indigenous population of the tropics, increases in the subtropics, and is of increasing frequency from the lower to the higher temperate regions. Prevalence rates for selected studies in the United States and Canada are so described in Fig. 4.12a (Kurland and Kurtzke 1972). A similar gradient has been offered for the Eastern Hemisphere from immigrants to Israel, as seen in Fig. 4.12b (Alter et al. 1962).

In the zonal theory, a band or zone of high-prevalence MS is delineated from a zone of medium prevalence (Kurtzke 1964; 1966b), which in turn is contiguous to a zone of low prevalence. High zones include southern Canada, northern United States, and northern Europe. Medium zones include southern United States and southern Europe. Africa and Asia comprise low zones. Southern New Zealand and southern Australia are in the high intermediate zone. The "dividing line" between high- and medium-prevalence zones is at about 46 degrees north latitude in Europe and at about 37 degrees in the United States. In the Northern Hemisphere, to the far north, there is little information on MS prevalence; what there is indicates a general decrease in prevalence north of about 55 degrees in North America and 65 degrees in Europe. In the surveys of the 1950s, prevalence rates were about 30 to 60 per 100,000 population in the high zone and 5 to 15 in the medium zone (Fig. 4.13a and b). Data from other northern Italian communities suggest that they were also in the medium zone for prevalence (Mapelli and Ramelli 1967; Caruso et al. 1968; Barlow 1969b).

Some support for the zonal concept was provided by Beebe and his associates (1967) in a matched control study of United States Army servicemen with MS in World War II. The MS case-control ratio showed a sharp change from low to high at about 38 degrees north latitude, according to place of birth (Fig. 4.14). Recently, Behrend (1969) has indicated that the prevalence of MS is markedly different among four small communities situated along the Rhone River in France, being high in the two northern communities of about 45 degrees and in the medium range in the two southern communities. These towns are separated by only a few miles.

Conversely, data from Australia suggest the possibility of a regular gradient. Queensland (Sutherland et al. 1966) had a lower rate than did Perth (McCall et al. 1968) or Newcastle (McCall et al. 1968); and Hobart, Tasmania (McCall et al. 1968), and South Australia (Rischbieth 1966) had higher rates of about 30 per 100,000.

Regardless of which theory is used, the distribution of MS in Asia

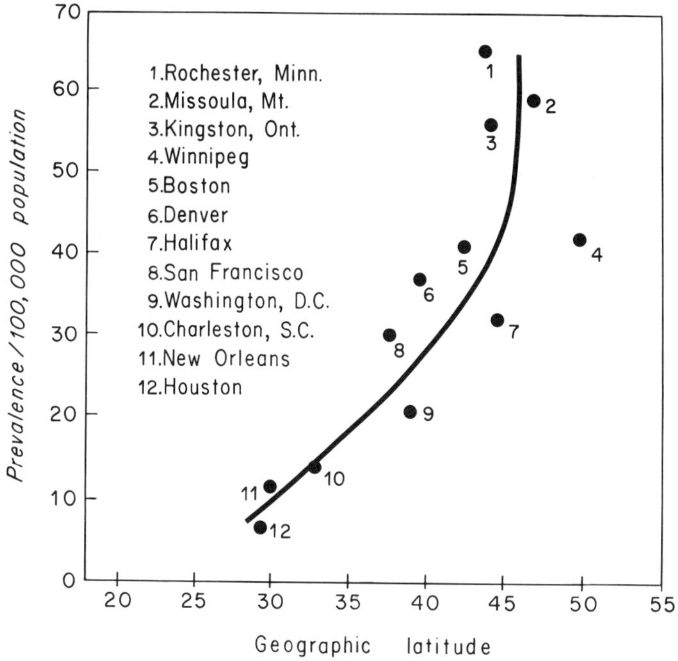

Figure 4.12 Prevalence rates per 100,000 population for multiple sclerosis. *a.* By geographic latitude, selected surveys, United States and Canada, various years, 1950–60 (Source: Kurland and Kurtzke 1972. By permission of McGraw-Hill Book Company, Inc.) *b.* By geographic latitude of birthplace for immigrants to Israel, 1960 (Source: Redrawn from Alter et al. 1962. By permission of the American Medical Association.)

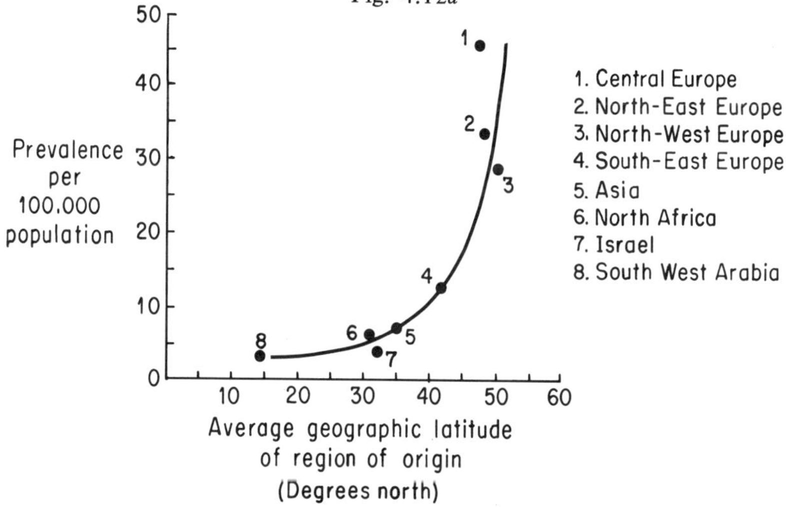

(insofar as it is known) does not conform to a regular pattern. Rates in Japan were low, whether north or south (Table 4.9). The prevalence rate in South Korea has been estimated at about 2 per 100,000 (Kurtzke et al. 1968*b*) and seems to be about 1 per 100,000 in South Vietnam (Thong 1965), based on the ratio of MS-to-ALS (amyotrophic lateral sclerosis) hospitalized patients. Data from hospital series collected by Barlow (1969*a* and *b*) imply low rates for China and Siberia. Admittedly none of this information is

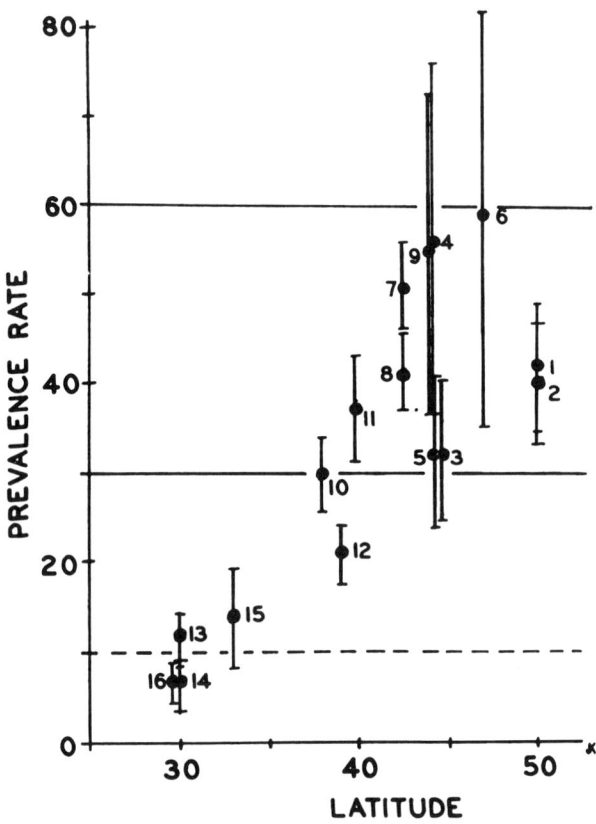

Fig. 4.13*a*

Figure 4.13 Prevalence rates per 100,000 population for multiple sclerosis by geographic latitude. The vertical ranges indicate the 95-percent confidence band for the given prevalence rate. *a*. Selected surveys: United States and Canada, various years, 1947–65. Numbers 1–5 are from Canada and 6–16 from the United States. *b*. Selected surveys: Europe, Australia, Asia, and Africa, various years, 1947–65. Numbers 17–36 are from Europe, 37–48 are from Australasia, and 49 from Africa. All studies are from the Northern Hemisphere except numbers 41, 42, and 49. (Source: Kurtzke 1966*b*. By permission of the American Medical Association.)

definitive. The only formal prevalence studies were those for Japan (Okinaka et al. 1960; Kuroiwa 1967), where clinical neurology is a new discipline and the populace may not yet be attuned to appropriate consultation for neurologic ills.

The prevalence rates from South America are unknown quantities. From hospital figures, Barlow (1969*b*) concluded that the prevalence of MS in South America was low. However, around Buenos Aires, Argentina, a region of major European immigration, the rate seemed higher; the origin of the patients was uncertain but many may have immigrated from Europe. Alter (1969) has found relatively few cases of MS among government employees and their families enrolled in a social medical system in Mexico City. Barlow (1969*b*) has cited reports to indicate that prevalence in Czechoslovakia, Poland, and northwestern Yugoslavia was relatively high, but southeastern Yugoslavia was of medium prevalence. Bulgaria had a prevalence of about 6 per 100,000 population, a rate that was in the low or medium range.

Several years ago, Grashchenkov and his colleagues (1960) reported that in the USSR, on the basis of relative frequency of hospital

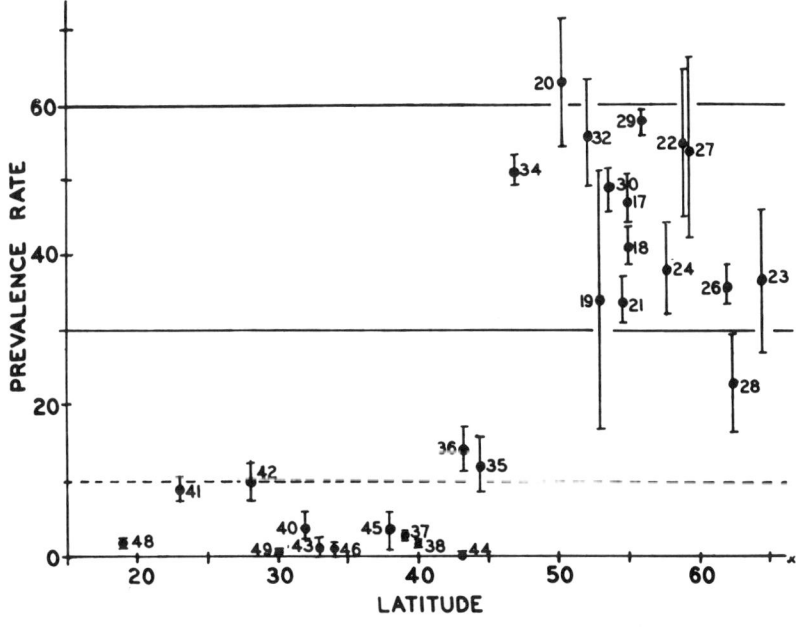

Fig. 4.13*b*

Figure 4.13 (*continued*)

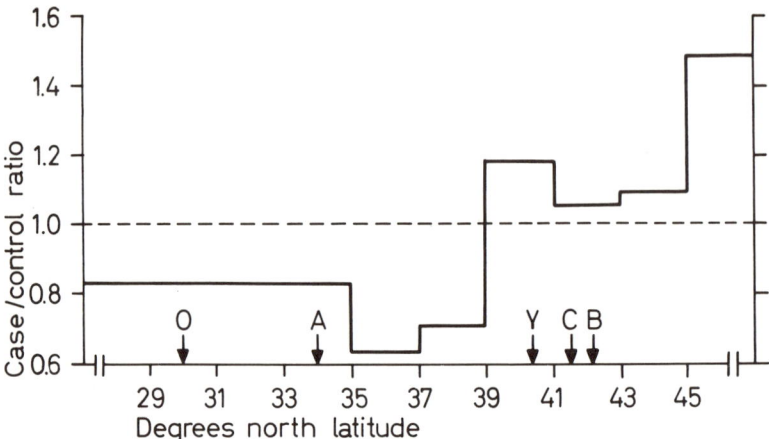

Figure 4.14 Case-control ratios for multiple sclerosis cases in United States Army males in World War II versus controls matched by age, sex, color, date of induction, and length of service, by latitude of place of birth. Five cities are spotted on the graph for reference: Los Angeles (A), Boston (B), Chicago (C), New Orleans (O), and New York (Y). (Source: Beebe et al. 1967. By permission of Lancet Publications, Inc.)

admissions, MS was more common in the northwest than in eastern or southern cities. Khodos (1960) reported that MS was rare in Irkutsk, Siberia, before 1933, but has been increasingly diagnosed since that time. Most of the increase was probably associated with immigration from western USSR, but the rate for Irkutsk was estimated still to be below that for western Europe. The data provided come from his personal experience during thirty-five years at Irkutsk, but they refer to hospital admissions rather than to a population base. He was unaware of any diagnosed cases in the population of Outer Mongolia. Khodos considered that the increase over time was caused by some local factor, because 85 percent of his patients had not been out of the area for at least ten years before onset.

Barlow (1967) also believed that MS was rarely diagnosed and reported in North Korea as well as in China and Siberia.

If we can accept these estimates, there would be not only a north-south differential in Europe but also an east-west change, with the differentiating longitude lying in the more eastern half of the USSR, so that all of Asia would be of low prevalence for MS. Validation of this distribution would be exceedingly important and appropriate study procedures to provide prevalence, incidence, and mortality rates referable to specified populations are highly desirable.

Foci of MS. Kurtzke (1966*b* and *c*) has stated that, within the high-risk zone of Europe, MS is distributed in clusters or foci in Switzerland, Denmark, northern Scotland, Norway, Sweden, and Finland. Such clusters were noted also when age-specific rates Kurtzke (1967*a*) and small administrative units (Kurtzke 1967*b*) were assessed. Kurtzke (1965*b*) found that the MS distributions did not correlate with those of medical facilities. He suggested that the pattern in the northern countries was such as to describe one single high-prevalence "Fennoscandian focus" (Kurtzke 1968*a*), comprising southern Norway, contiguous Sweden, and southwestern Finland (see Fig. 4.15).

Kurland (1970), among others, has expressed doubts as to the validity of these interpretations, pointing out exceptions to this focal pattern in the studies of Northern Ireland (Allison and Millar 1954), Iceland (Gudmundsson and Gudmundsson 1962), and the Northumberland-Durham counties in England (Poskanzer et al. 1963*a*). Recently, Allison (1969) has noted that the prevalence rate for MS was low in Belfast according to birthplace but that the rates elsewhere in Northern Ireland were rather homogeneous. As to Northumberland, the interpretation of homogeneity was made by the authors for residence at onset, but they noted that residence at birth was *not* uniform.

It is recognized that if a sufficient number of countries are divided into small units, in addition to chance variation, differences in diagnostic habits of physicians may also affect patterns of relative frequency or infrequency of the disease. Although such foci should continue to be sought, and if possible explained, "convincing proof of focalization must await the recognition of some meaningful pattern" (Kurland 1970), by which is meant the definition of factors responsible for the distribution noted. Among these are the combined effects of several factors, including chance fluctuation and quality in diagnostic practice that are not necessarily related to the number of physicians or hospitals in a community.

Incidence

Age-specific and sex-specific MS incidence rates were determined for several populations included in Table 4.9. In cities of the United

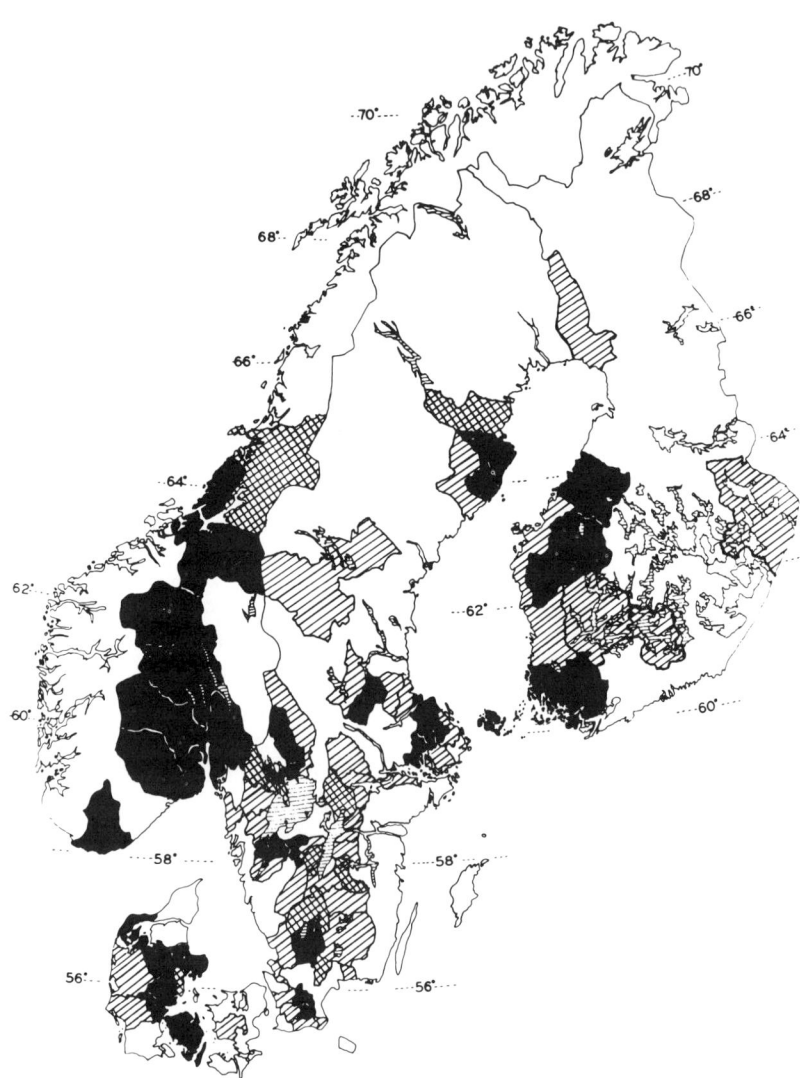

Figure 4.15 Prevalence rates per 100,000 population for multiple sclerosis: Norway and Denmark (counties), Finland (hospital districts), and Sweden (small administrative units), various years, 1925–64. Regions significantly high are solid black; those high but of dubious significance are cross hatched; those insignificantly above the mean are diagonal lined. The open or white areas are below the respective national mean prevalence rates. (Source: Kurtzke 1968a. By permission of Lancet Publications, Inc.)

States and Canada, the age-specific rates, which were 0 for early childhood, increased rapidly during late adolescence to reach a peak for persons about 30 years of age, followed by a steady decline, with few new cases occurring in persons 45 or older (Kurland and Westlund 1954). In Fig. 4.16, the age-specific and sex-specific rates were based on the large series of Hyllested (1956) in Denmark and an appropriate population base (Kurtzke 1968b). The maximal age-specific rates were for young adults, being about 7 to 9 per 100,000 for females and 6 to 7 per 100,000 for males. In adolescence and early adulthood, the rates for females were about twice those for males of the same age, but by age 40 the rates were about equal.

Multiple sclerosis rarely begins before age 10 and is unusual before age 15 (Kurtzke 1970). Reported onsets much after 45 are believed to be largely a reflection of the inability of the patient to recall early symptoms of the disease or of the physician to inquire about such symptoms. However, in some studies, such as those in Northumberland, onset after age 45 was more than occasionally reported; the

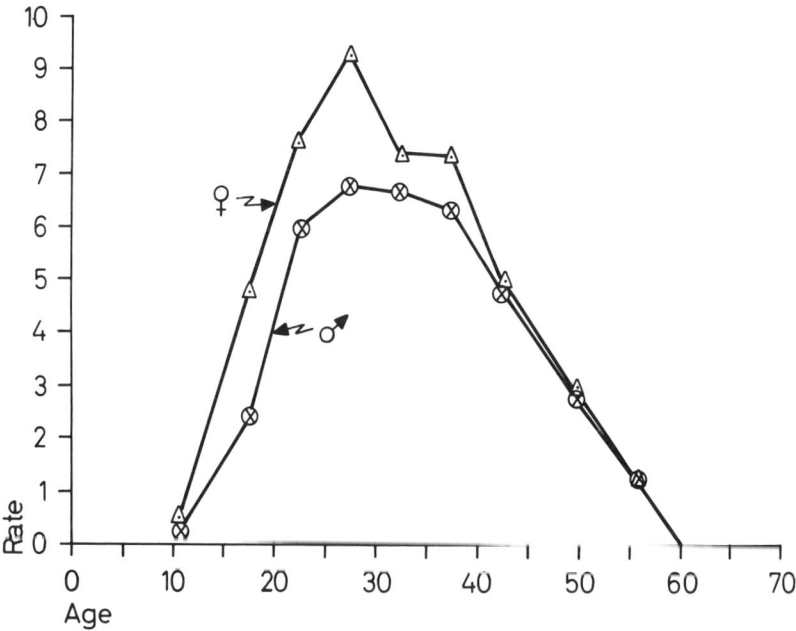

Figure 4.16 Average annual age-specific incidence rates per 100,000 population for multiple sclerosis by sex: Denmark, based on prevalence survey of 1949. Rates are based on population in 1938, the median year of onset. (Source: Modified from Kurtzke 1968b. By permission of Lancet Publications, Inc.)

authors of that report (Poskanzer et al. 1963*a*) believed that physicians were discouraged from making the diagnosis of MS even when all other evidence favored it because of the prevailing view that MS did not begin after age 45.

The overall annual incidence rate in high-risk MS areas is probably close to 2 per 100,000 general population. The incidence of MS has been unchanged in Winnipeg, Canada (MacLean et al. 1950), and in New Orleans, Louisiana (Stazio et al. 1967), during the twenty years through 1959. Information available for the population of Rochester, Minnesota, from 1905 to 1965 does not support the view that the incidence of MS has been increasing appreciably (Percy et al. 1968). Allison's cohort analysis (1969) revealed that for more than thirty years the annual incidence rates for MS in Northern Ireland were stable. Thus the increasing prevalence and decreasing mortality rates discussed previously are best explained by increasing survival rather than by a change in incidence rates.

Other Characteristics of MS

Duration

Early estimates of survival in MS were based on historical data of nonsurvivors of hospital series, and the figure was about ten years. The mean survival was found to be at least twenty years after clinical onset in population studies of the early 1950s (Kurland and Westlund 1954).

Life table methods were used to calculate survival rates for the MS patients who were residents of Rochester, Minnesota (Percy et al. 1968). This was also done for United States Army male MS patients hospitalized in World War II and included in a follow-up study (Kurtzke et al. 1970*a*). The Army patients were divided into two groups: one being those (A) who had the onset in a bout separate from that for which they had been hospitalized in the Army, and the other being those (B) so hospitalized for their initial bout. Figure 4.17 gives the survival rates for the Rochester patients and the Army groups (Kurtzke 1970). In all instances, about three-fourths of the MS patients had survived twenty years of illness and about two-thirds had survived at least twenty-five years. The average duration of illness, or median survival, was estimated at about thirty-five years (Kurtzke 1970; Kurtzke et al. 1970*a*). After twenty years of illness, the survival rate was about three-fourths of normal (expected)

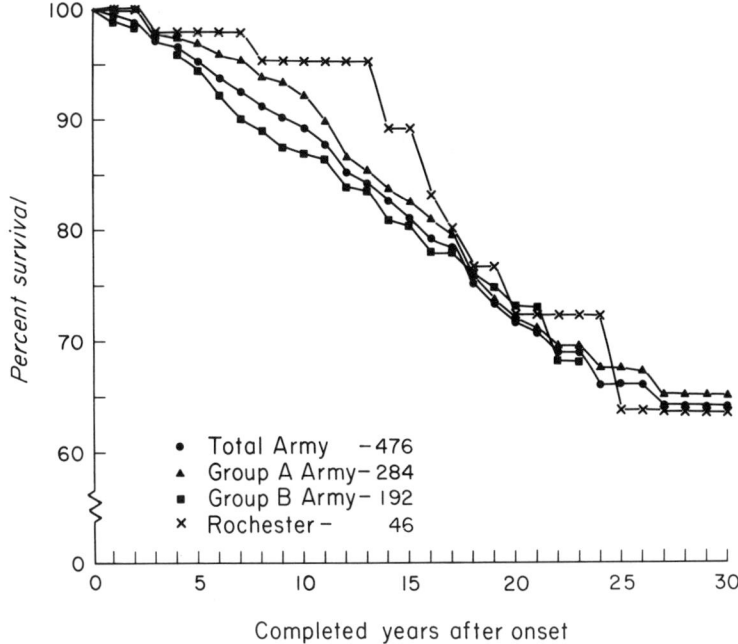

Figure 4.17 Percent survival among patients with multiple sclerosis by years after onset: Rochester, Minnesota, and United States Army males (Source: Kurtzke 1970.)

survival for both subgroups of the Army series *and* for the Rochester patients. Among the latter, half the survivors were still ambulatory after about twenty years of disease. Although the Rochester experience might suggest that the extensive case-finding procedures in that study assured discovery of mild cases as well as the more seriously affected, the Army results were similar for the group B with severe initial bout (Kurtzke et al. 1968*a*). Accordingly, these estimates may be reasonable for all MS occurring in a circumscribed population.

Familial Features

Numerous studies have shown that familial aggregation is excessive in MS. In Sutherland's series (1956), 7 of 545 siblings (1.3 percent) of the 127 patients also had MS, whereas in Hyllested's experience (1956), 44 of 11,924 siblings (0.4 percent) were affected. A "positive family history" of MS was reported in 3.8 percent of probable cases in the recent Winnipeg survey (Stazio et al. 1967), although in the previous studies in Winnipeg and New Orleans, familial aggregation seemed to be uncommon. The 3.8 percent was considered to be a minimal figure, based only on the number of cases personally ascertained; it did, however, include not only siblings and parents but also more distant relatives. For all known relatives, the familial incidence reported by Pratt and his colleagues (1951) in England was 6.5 percent, while in the highly inbred Orkney, Shetland, and Faroe Islands, it was reported to be as high as 12 percent (Allison 1963).

These findings, however, do not take into account the size of the "families," and if cousins are included, the numbers at risk may be substantial and the relative risk to family members may be difficult to ascertain. Also, familial aggregation, if present, does not differentiate between the effects of an environmental exposure common to members of the same family and the role of genetic predisposition. However, Mackay and Myrianthopoulos (1966), as a result of their study and follow-up of twins, contended that MS is "an autosomal recessive trait with reduced [43 percent] penetrance." Schapira and his colleagues (1963) in northeastern England found a second case in 5.8 percent of the families investigated, but concluded that there was inadequate evidence for a simple genetic basis for familial aggregation of MS. They preferred to consider a possible infectious mechanism in the disease. Kurtzke (1965a) also concluded that the increased familial frequency probably was not on a genetic basis.

A further argument against a purely hereditary basis for MS is that concordance with respect to MS in identical twins has been low (Müller 1953; Kurtzke 1970). The lack of any proved selection by race or nationality independent of geography is also a potent argument against simple genetic predisposition to which might be added some exogenous precipitating factor. The rarity of the disease in Japan and presumably in Asians in general does not necessarily favor either viewpoint.

Migration and "Latency"

Migration of groups to or from different risk areas offers unique opportunties for investigating geographic influence on MS. First Rozanski (1952) and later Alter and his co-workers (1962; 1968) took advantage of the unusual population composition of Israel to study this question. A large segment of the Jewish population in Israel has been exposed to the influence of diverse climatologic and geographic conditions. They have gathered as one population in

Israel where immigration is not limited by medical restrictions, where the doctor-patient ratio is among the highest in the world, and where political isolation practically ensures that patients are treated within the country. The prevalence rate for immigrants from northern Europe was five to ten times higher than that for immigrants from Asia and Africa or for the native-born population of Israel, even if the parents of the native born came from Europe. Prevalence rates calculated for each national group of immigrants matched those expected for their native lands (see Fig. 4.12a). The lower prevalence rates previously reported among native-born Israelis have been questioned recently (Leibowitz et al. 1972), but the different rates between European and Afro-Asian immigrants still appear valid.

Dean (1967) in the Republic of South Africa also found that migrants from a high- to a low-prevalence area carried with them their risk for MS. The prevalence rate for white Afrikaans-speaking natives was 3 per 100,000 and for the white English-speaking natives was 11 per 100,000. For immigrants from Great Britain and northern or central Europe, the prevalence rate was about 48 per 100,000. Upon further assessment (Dean and Kurtzke 1970), sharp transition in the risk among these northern European immigrants according to age at immigration has been found: for those less than 15 years old at immigration, the prevalence rate was estimated at about 13 per 100,000, while for those aged 15 to 19 at immigration, the prevalence rate was more than 60 per 100,000. The rates for age groups older than this at immigration (with one exception) were close to 50 per 100,000. Thus immigrants older than 15 at immigration retained the risk of their birthplace, whereas immigrants who entered South Africa under the age of 15 apparently acquired the risk of their new homeland (Kurtzke et al. 1970b). The implications of this study are wide-ranging, and confirmatory evidence is greatly needed.

In Israel, Alter and co-workers (1966) related a similar pronounced difference in MS risk for immigrants who migrated before they were 15 years old compared with those who migrated after they were 15, but risk by age subgroups could not be estimated.

In Australia, rates for immigrants have generally been higher than those for native-born Australians. McCall (1968) noted a rate of 32 per 100,000 for European immigrants and 20 for native born (a difference which was not statistically significant). Sutherland and his associates (1966) found little difference in the area of Queensland, where the rate per 100,000 was 12 for immigrants and 9 for the native born. However, support for the concept of higher rates among immigrants was afforded by Saint and Sadka (1962) in Western Australia. In Australia, age at immigration could not be assessed, and there was probably some selection against immigration for those already affected. In other studies pertaining to migration, Khodos (1960) implied a higher risk for western Soviet immigrants to Irkutsk than for the natives, and Moffie (1966) noted a much higher rate among immigrants than natives in the Dutch Antilles.

In essence then, almost all migrant studies indicated that the adult subject brought with him the MS risk of his homeland. This was also suggested by the death rates for United States immigrants discussed previously. Further, two studies demonstrated that this carrying of risk is age dependent: immigration before age 15 from a high- to a low-risk area apparently subjugates the risk.

The MS death rates for native born in the United States also provided evidence that some period *between* birth and death was critical for the increased risk of development of MS by residence at some time in the high-risk northern tier of states. This period can be narrowed to that between birth and perhaps age 20, from the data of Beebe's group (1967). In this matched control study, residence at birth or at induction into the Army showed the same north-south differential in the risk of MS previously noted. However, in this case-control comparison, military residence after induction but *before* clinical onset, or an equivalent date in controls, showed no significant deviation from unity for each of the three geographic tiers (northern, middle, southern).

Until these studies, the concept of a latent or "incubation" period in MS was largely speculative, but these works suggest that the pathologic mechanism for MS may develop in late childhood, even though the clinical features may not be apparent until much later. Alter and his associates (1966) noted that the average minimal interval was about nine years for subjects in whom MS developed after emigration to Israel from northern or central Europe; in Dean's study (1967), the interval to onset of MS for all patients combined averaged about thirteen years after emigration to South Africa from Europe or after the return to South Africa from a visit to Europe. The age at onset and the interval from immigration to onset, though, were both influenced by the age at immigration. The average age at onset in these immigrants with MS was 33, and the *first* immigration age group showing a high risk of MS was the one aged 15-19. Thus the incubation period theoretically would be about fourteen to eighteen years for this group.

After evaluating familial aggregations of MS cases, Schapira and his fellow-workers (1963) concluded that exposure to an environmental factor might be critical for the development of MS and computed latent periods on the assumption of common exposure during the period of common habitation of affected members of the same family. The calculated incubation period for siblings was twenty-one years. Because the mean age at onset in their study was 35, it was "tenuously concluded" that common exposure might have occurred about the age of 14 (range: 3 to 23 years). Kurtzke (1965c) considered the age at which the geographic concentration of cases was maximal in several series, as well as other factors including the Northumberland sibling study of the Schapira group (1963), and concluded that MS may begin in the pathologic sense at about age 10 to 15 among residents of high-risk areas, with an interval averaging about twenty years before symptoms develop.

Some Differential Features of MS Patients

Many investigators have attempted to determine whether some condition(s) related to geography might be identified as etiologic risk factors in MS. Acheson and his colleagues (1960) studied men who were discharged for MS from Veterans Administration hospitals between 1954 and 1958, according to their residences at birth and on admission to the hospital. By multiple regression analyses of *place* of birth of MS patients, the highest correlations found were negative ones with annual hours of sunshine and December solar radiation. However, the case-control study for birthplace and residence at induction for *patients* with MS conducted by Beebe and his associates (1967) showed no significant relation to sunshine or solar radiation.

Barlow (1960) has indicated that the known distribution of MS throughout the world showed a higher correlation with geomagnetic latitude than with geographic latitude, particularly with reference to the low rate in Japan. One possible explanation he offered is that cosmic radiation, which is affected by geomagnetic latitude, might have an etiologic role in MS. He later suggested that perhaps periodic solar flares also might be of importance, because cosmic radiation is largely filtered out by the atmosphere (Barlow 1966). The geomagnetic concept does not fit the pattern if the entirety of China and Siberia are considered low-frequency areas.

Dietary aberrations have been considered in MS, the most persistent of which has been the concept of Swank and his colleagues

(1952) that a high-fat diet is of etiologic importance in MS. This hypothesis is based in part on their survey of MS in Norway where it was claimed that prevalence was higher in inland dairy-farming areas than in the coastal villages. The published data, though, suggest that MS was most prevalent in the entire southeastern plains area of Norway but extended from coast to coast (see Fig. 4.15). There were pronounced differences in the regional distribution of MS in Denmark, although diet seemed to be uniformly high in fat (Kurtzke 1966c), and the western coastal (largely fishing) region of Finland was the high-risk area of that land (Kurtzke 1967a; 1968a). It is unlikely that the farming Afrikaners of South Africa eat less fat than do their more urban English-speaking peers, yet they may have less MS (Dean 1967). Dietary habits did not differ between patients and controls in Winnipeg (Westlund and Kurland 1953) or in Israel (Alter et al. 1968).

In view of the suggested relation between MS and swayback, a demyelinating disease that affects sheep and lambs, and the reports by Campbell and his colleagues (1950) on lead and MS, the effect of deficiencies and excesses of a number of trace elements such as copper and lead has been studied in relation to MS (Dean 1949). Warren and his associates (1967) have raised the possibility that lead in soil, which might be taken up by plants, could be associated with a broad pattern of MS, as well as with smaller foci. However, there is as yet no convincing evidence that these elements have a direct role in the etiology or pathogenesis of the disease. Several clinical series of patients and controls have been investigated because of these reports, and no alteration of trace elements has been discovered in serum or urine (Acheson 1965; Alter and Kurtzke 1968 .)

In an attempt to elucidate an etiologic factor, numerous characteristics of the Winnipeg patients prior to onset of MS were obtained retrospectively and compared with a matched sample of the general population of Winnipeg (Westlund and Kurland 1953). No statistically significant difference was found with regard to the limited areas of Europe from which the persons or their ancestors had migrated, or with regard to place of birth, birth order, education, occupation, urban or rural residence, source of water and types of food, exposure to farm and domestic animals, vaccinations and inoculations, previous illnesses, and prior head or back injuries. There was also no difference in the prevalence rates for persons of English, French, or Ukrainian descent.

A case-control comparison was also used by Poskanzer (1965;

1968) in a retrospective search for pre-illness features of etiologic value. The major finding was that patients had had tonsillectomy more often than their spouse or nearest sibling. This observation needs confirmation, as it is of potential importance in our understanding of the pathogenesis of MS.

An intensive comparison of patients and matched controls was accomplished in Israel (Antonovsky et al. 1967; Alter et al. 1968). By retrospective questionnaires, a large number of items of socioeconomic, dietary, and medical import were evaluated. Aside from simple geography, the only major differences were possible relations with sanitation and some features of urbanization, but most impressive was the predominance of negative results. In a study of MS in Minnesota, Alter and Speer (1968) found essentially no difference between 36 patients and 72 controls on a large number of historical items including infections, allergies, vaccinations, operations, trauma, toxins, and ownership of pets and other animals.

A significant methodologic advance was made by Beebe and his associates (1967) in the effort to elucidate *prior* to the onset of symptoms characteristics that might distinguish the multiple sclerotic from the unaffected. This involved a comparison of nearly four hundred MS patients and matched controls from the United States Army with respect to various geographic and biologic factors. Factors that were tested originated in data obtained routinely for cases and controls before MS was diagnosed in the Army.

Characteristics that significantly differentiated MS cases from controls were (*a*) geographic location at birth or induction but not geographic location while in military service, (*b*) degree of urbanization of residence at birth or induction, (*c*) socioeconomic status at induction, and (*d*) visual defects in the form of refractive errors at induction. There was also a lower risk for MS among Negroes.

The geographic differentiation in the United States was such that the highest risk of MS was in the northeastern part of the country and the lowest in the southwestern. The greatest difference was found between the northern and middle tiers of states. There was a preponderance of MS cases in the metropolitan or urban areas and least in the rural regions. The risk of MS was directly proportional to the educational level, the induction intelligence-test score, and the census scale for occupational status.

Defective vision at induction, which was correctable to the same degree in cases and controls, was found in significant excess among the MS cases. A similar finding had been noted previously in a separate study of optic neuropathy in which MS later developed (Kurland et al. 1966).

The risk of MS for nonwhites was about half the expectation based on Army-wide racial distributions, even when the rates were corrected for place of residence or birth (Beebe et al. 1967). However, no further analysis of this feature was possible in this study.

Beebe and his colleagues concluded:

> In general, this study provided further evidence that the cause or causes of MS will be found in certain environmental factors and that a genetic predisposition could assume significance only in association with some exogenous influence. Perhaps the most striking finding was that all the characteristics which served to differentiate MS cases invariably pertained to events that antedated military service, even in those with clinical onset after induction. This indicated, therefore, that the determinative events in the acquisition of MS may well occur in the early years of life. Although the environmental factors identified here were quite nonspecific, their value may best lie in channeling our attention to features which distinguished culturally advantaged children in urban communities from the disadvantaged in rural areas during the first half of this century.

In the past twenty years, a large body of literature has grown out of attempts to relate MS to experimental allergic encephalomyelitis, and thus to consider the human disease an autoimmune disorder. Although this has been discussed extensively (Kurland and Westlund 1954; Allison 1963; Acheson 1965; Alter and Kurtzke 1968), no relationship has been established. If there is an immune mechanism in MS, it would appear to be a part perhaps of the immediate pathogenesis but would not explain the epidemiologic characteristics.

Is There an Infectious Origin to MS?

Multiple sclerosis has not been regarded as a disease transmitted from man to man because of the low incidence of conjugal cases and the relatively low rate in siblings. However, the risk in siblings, although low, is several times greater than the risk in unrelated persons (Allison 1969), and if we accept that the disease may be acquired in childhood, an increase in conjugal rate would not be expected.

MS is not considered a disease that can be transmitted from animals to man by some insect vector, because a vector considered to be geographically appropriate has not been recognized. With respect to diseases transmitted directly from animals to man, there is none that appears to have a similar geographic pattern, although scrapie has been the subject of much recent study. Scrapie is a disease of sheep, generally manifested by its effect on the nervous system. It can be transmitted experimentally by inoculation or by exposure of susceptible sheep to various tissues from affected animals or even to the grazing areas of affected animals. It also has been transmitted by inoculation to goats and mice. Symptoms begin only after a prolonged incubation period. The agent is considered one of the class called "slow viruses." Infectivity of the brain inoculum apparently persists even after a brief period of boiling or exposure to formalin. Under natural conditions transmission requires a genetic factor, since susceptibility varies appreciably with the species of the sheep.

Field and his colleagues (1962) described a patient who died after an acute illness apparently heralded by an attack of viral encephalitis; the diagnosis was MS. This case presented some unusual histologic features—specifically, rod-like structures enclosed within vacuoles in large glial cells. In Iceland, intracerebral inoculation of material from the patient's brain into sheep produced a disorder histologically indistinguishable from scrapie. However, this work has not been confirmed through independent efforts to passage the presumed agent to sheep elsewhere. Campbell and his co-workers (1963) have described a case of subacute encephalitis that was somewhat similar to subacute sclerosing panencephalitis and associated with extensive destruction of myelinated fibers in the spinal cord. Material from the spinal cord and brain of the patient injected intracerebrally into Icelandic sheep was also followed, after an interval of two to three years, by a severe neurologic illness and pathologic changes characteristic of scrapie. Whether typical MS can be transmitted to these sheep is still under active investigation.

Poskanzer and colleagues (1963b) have presented their hypothesis that "multiple sclerosis represents the occasional neurological manifestation of a widespread enteric infection ... just as paralytic poliomyelitis is a rare manifestation of infection with the virus of poliomyelitis." The analogy is developed on the basis of the geographic variation in prevalence of the two diseases, the similarity in urban and rural attack rates with a higher age at onset in the rural population, a similar proportion of family members who are affected, a shift toward the upper social class in the distribution of the disease, an increase in risk with pregnancy, the localizing effects of trauma, and the incidence rates of the diseases themselves. This is an intriguing hypothesis, but it does seem appropriate to review and add to the authors' own critical evaluation, as well as to provide some additional comments on the analogy that they presented.

(1) They interpreted the lower rates for both disorders in the tropics on the basis of lower socioeconomic conditions that lead to early exposure and immunity; whereas in temperate zones, later exposure and higher socioeconomic settings were associated with a greater probability of clinical disease. It should be noted, however, that the MS rate was low among the "Europeans" in South Africa, northern Australia, and the Israeli population—peoples whose standard of living is equivalent to that found in much of Canada and Great Britain.

(2) The risk for paralytic poliomyelitis was higher for those traveling from a high-incidence region for paralytic disease (such as the United States) to endemic infectious regions of low paralytic incidence. Although the MS rate for European immigrants to South Africa and to Israel was higher than for the native-born population, it did not exceed that of the areas from which the immigrants had come.

(3) The authors reported a similarity in the overall incidence and familial aggregation for MS and paralytic poliomyelitis, which may be but an interesting coincidence for a few areas from which data are available. They also described the increased association of both diseases with pregnancy, trauma, and vaccination, although other carefully documented studies comparing MS patients with the "general" population failed to show such associations (Westlund and Kurland 1953; Antonovsky et al. 1967; Alter et al. 1968; Alter and Speer 1968).

(4) Although they noted no significant difference in MS prevalence rates between urban and rural areas and although the ages at onset overlapped considerably, the reported mean age at onset in the rural areas was greater than that in the urban areas, as was true for paralytic poliomyelitis. Their report was one of the few instances wherein adequate data were available for comparison. It may be recalled that in MS, urbanization was one of the risk factors found in the Army study (Beebe et al. 1967). If Kurtzke's concept of "foci" in Europe is accepted, this aspect would need additional amplification. Also, there was no correlation in geographic distribution between MS and polio in Scandinavia and Switzerland (Kurtzke 1966a).

(5) The authors pointed out that several known facts about MS may be inconsistent with a hypothesis that implicates infection. These include the apparent absence of seasonal and year-to-year variation, although the uncertainty of onset in many cases could well

"mask seasonal and annual fluctuations." The age distribution, as the authors noted, although it differed from that in paralytic poliomyelitis, cannot be considered as inconsistent with an infectious etiology, particularly if the concept of a long "latent period" is correct.

(6) In interpreting the South African immigrant data, Dean (Dean and Kurtzke 1971) came to the same conclusion, also with the polio analogy, that the childhood immigrants are "protected" and the older ones are "susceptible." However, Kurtzke (Dean and Kurtzke 1971) interpreted the same data as indicating that MS was more likely "caught" near the age of 15 in the high-risk areas of northern Europe and became clinically manifested after a lengthy incubation period, even though the patient migrated to South Africa before clinical onset. The pathogenetic inferences from the opposing viewpoints would differ markedly. The question of etiology is even more at variance: Does one seek the cause of MS where the disease flourishes or where it is absent?

There are said to be similarities in the distributions of acute upper respiratory infections (Duff 1953) or of rheumatic fever (Ziegler 1959) to that of MS in the United States. The former can be questioned, and the latter was not found in the European comparisons (Kurtzke 1966a). Other possible relationships have been discussed elsewhere (Acheson 1965; Alter and Kurtzke 1968).

A number of workers have reported elevated levels of measles antibody in the serum of MS patients (Adams and Imagawa 1962; Reed et al. 1964; Sibley and Foley 1965; Sever and Zeman 1968). The significance of this finding remains to be determined. The relation of measles and other myxoviruses to disease of the nervous system (including MS) was the topic of a recent symposium on measles virus and subacute sclerosing panencephalitis (SSPE) (Sever and Zeman 1968).

Perhaps the greatest evidence for an infectious origin in MS has nothing to do with MS, and that is the concept of slow and latent virus diseases in human neurologic ills, including SSPE and measles (Sever and Zeman 1968), kuru (Gajdusek et al. 1967), progressive multifocal leukoencephalopathy (Zu Rhein and Chou 1968), and Jakob-Creutzfeldt disease (Gibbs and Gajdusek 1969).

A remote specific event, perhaps infectious, may be the agent in question that accounts for the unique geographic distribution of MS, but the precipitating factor for the development of symptoms may be immunologic (Soll 1968). Serum and cerebrospinal fluid from MS patients are cytotoxic for certain cell lines, according to Bornstein and Crain (1965), although the changes produced are *not* unique for MS fluids. At the moment, an immune mechanism need not be postulated for MS any more than for tuberculosis or syphilis. The geographic differentiations and the migration studies suggest that the best model for MS would be an infectious disease of prolonged latency, but the proof of this concept is awaited and is likely to come from the laboratory rather than from the epidemiologist.

Comment

The distribution of MS from the mortality and prevalence data does not conform to any readily apparent pattern; for every etiologic hypothesis that has been proposed, some exceptions can be found. Poor experimental design in some instances may account for these discrepancies; in others, problems of case ascertainment particularly related to diagnostic criteria and classification continue to cloud the emerging picture of population selection associated with the disease. In spite of the differences, there has been considerable agreement as to the acceptable results, and to a lesser extent as to their interpretation.

Multiple sclerosis is a disease that is clinically recognizable in the prime of reproductive life, but in which pathologic onset probably occurs at an appreciably younger age than the onset of clinical manifestations. There may be several relatively common abortive forms of this disease, such as retrobulbar neuritis, which in most instances does not develop into MS (Kurland et al. 1966; Kurtzke 1970). Although MS reportedly has occurred about equally in both sexes, the rate now appears to be slightly higher in females. The prognosis for life is generally good and is far better than was thought from earlier hospital experience.

There is no valid evidence that the incidence rate in a given locale has changed during this century. Increasing prevalence rates and slightly declining mortality rates probably reflect longer survival. The observation of a remarkable geographic distribution continues to persist, as additional studies have indicated that the disease is indeed much more common in the temperate zone than in the subtropics and tropics. The validity of the existence of foci or clusters of MS, however, requires reasonable biologic interpretation before it can be accepted.

Most of the studies indicate that persons who emigrate from high- to low-incidence areas carry with them the MS risk of their original native land. In two studies the immigrants retained the prevalence of their birthplace if immigration took place after the age of 15, while they acquired the low risk of their newly adopted country if they arrived before the age of 15.

The clinical characteristics and course of MS appear to be the same regardless of geography, once the disease has developed. This, together with the susceptibility of some MS patients to aggravation of symptoms with increased environmental temperatures, would suggest that movement of those already affected to a warmer climate may not be beneficial even though the latter is a low-risk area.

A genetic factor does not appear to be determinative in MS, despite the contention of Berry (1969), who in an excellent review of the disease concluded not only that such a role does exist, but also that "an inborn error of fatty acid metabolism can be envisaged as predisposing towards development of clinical multiple sclerosis." Most of the current epidemiologic evidence suggests that continued intensive laboratory efforts to transmit the disease would seem to be the most promising lead in order to define the etiology of this enigmatic disorder.

5 / AMYOTROPHIC LATERAL SCLEROSIS AND OTHER MOTOR NEURON DISEASES

Leonard T. Kurland
John F. Kurtzke
Irving D. Goldberg
Nung Won Choi

About a century ago Charcot described amyotrophic lateral sclerosis (ALS), which is characterized by a progressive and fatal motor paralysis occurring in adults. The clinical features are attributable to degeneration of the motor nuclei at the spinal or brain-stem levels, or at both levels, usually with involvement of the Betz cells of the cortex and demyelination of corticobulbar and corticospinal (pyramidal) tracts.

When the clinical involvement is characterized by anterior-horn-cell involvement alone, the state is called progressive (myelopathic) muscular atrophy (PMMA) or progressive bulbar palsy (PBP), depending on the level of involvement. Together, they are now denoted as progressive muscular atrophy (PMA). These clinical differentiations are indistinct, and it is common to class them all (ALS, PMMA, PBP) as variants of one disorder, motor neuron disease.

In this chapter we shall use for convenience the term ALS or motor neuron disease (MND) when referring to PMMA or PBP or those instances of combined anterior-horn-cell and lateral-column dysfunction, which meet the literal translation of the term amyotrophic lateral sclerosis (amyotrophy-muscle wasting, lateral sclerosis-gliosis of pyramidal tracts).

This neuronal degeneration results in skeletal muscular wasting and weakness that may affect all skeletal and lower bulbar levels before respiration or swallowing becomes so impaired that death intervenes. The disease is progressive and the duration averages three to four years, although it may be as brief as one year or as long as ten years. Upper motor neuron disease in the form of spasticity and increased or pathologic reflexes is likely to be present during the course of the illness, even in the presence of muscular wasting. Whether upper motor neuron disease is recognized clinically or not, demyelination of the corticospinal tracts with degeneration of Betz cells is usually found at autopsy. Systems other than the motor system (for example, the cerebellar or sensory) are rarely affected, but when they are they may provide points of differentiation in the classification of ALS that is to be presented later in this chapter.

Although the ISC classification of the motor neuron diseases includes the "idiopathic" pyramidal tract involvement of primary lateral sclerosis (PLS), this is not included in our interpretation of ALS. Primary lateral sclerosis is a syndrome that may be a consequence of cervical spondylosis or may develop in the course of familial spastic paraplegia, multiple sclerosis, or other disorders. However, it is believed that PLS accounts for only a small fraction of all deaths included in the MND category.

Although ALS is not difficult to diagnose in its late clinical course, it poses some difficulties in the early stages, particularly when PMMA is the prominent form. On such occasions the clinician need be concerned with ruling out the diagnosis of polymyositis, which is associated with a better prognosis than is PMMA. There is also a clinical impression that the duration of illness from onset of symptoms to death may differ in PMMA from that in PBP or the complete ALS picture.

Mortality Statistics

Before 1949, MND was not retrievable from death data because the disorder was not separately coded. The Sixth and Seventh Revisions of the ISC provided for code 356 as "motor-neurone disease and muscular atrophy." There were optional subcategories: 356.0 was PMMA and PBP; 356.1 was ALS (but it also included PLS); 356.2 was primarily for relatively rare but distinct forms of presumably hereditary progressive muscular atrophy of infants (Werdnig-Hoffmann disease) and of young adults with peroneal atrophy (Charcot-Marie-Tooth disease); and 356.3 was for "other and unspecified manifestations." As of 1969, the Eighth Revision of the ISC has been in effect, and now these disorders recognized as being hereditary are coded separately. The MND code is 348, ALS (and PLS) is 348.0, PBP is 348.1, PMMA is 348.2, and 348.9 is "other and unspecified." As previously stated, PLS is a minor addition to the ALS category, but would be more appropriately assigned to an independent subcategory. Data in this chapter are limited to code 356 of the Sixth and Seven Revisions for the years 1949-68.

When a death is attributed to ALS, it is our impression that this is likely to be a correct diagnosis; but of course there is no way from the mortality data alone to retrieve the undiagnosed cases. When MND was certified as a cause of death, it was listed as the underlying cause in about 80 to 90 percent of the certificates according to data from Norway, the Netherlands, and the United States. This is shown in Table 5.1.

International Mortality Data

Deaths from MND (all of ISC code 356) occurred in all countries for which mortality statistics were available; in western Europe and North America, as well as in Australia, New Zealand, and Japan, it accounted for about 1 per 1,000 of all adult deaths. The age-adjusted death rates for most of the developed countries range from about 0.5 to 1.2 per 100,000 population per year, according to data for the 1950s, as calculated by Goldberg and Kurland (1962) and shown in Fig. 5.1. There was a consistent preponderance for males, the sex ratio averaging about 1.6 to 1 (Table A.5.1).

Table 5.1 Death certificates listing motor neuron disease (MND) and amyotrophic lateral sclerosis (ALS) as primary or secondary causes of death, with percent listed as primary cause: selected countries, various years, 1953-61

(ISC codes 356 and 356.1)

Country and years	MND (356)		ALS (356.1)	
	Total deaths	Percent primary	Total deaths	Percent primary
Norway (1956-60)[a]	235	93	---	---
United States (1955)[b]	1,309	76	859	84
Netherlands (1953-60)[c]	1,084	83	---	---
Netherlands (1961)[d]	125	89	---	---

[a] All secondary causes considered.

[b] As many as four secondary causes considered.

[c] Only one ("most important") secondary cause considered; excludes deaths for 1958 (not available).

[d] As many as three secondary causes considered.

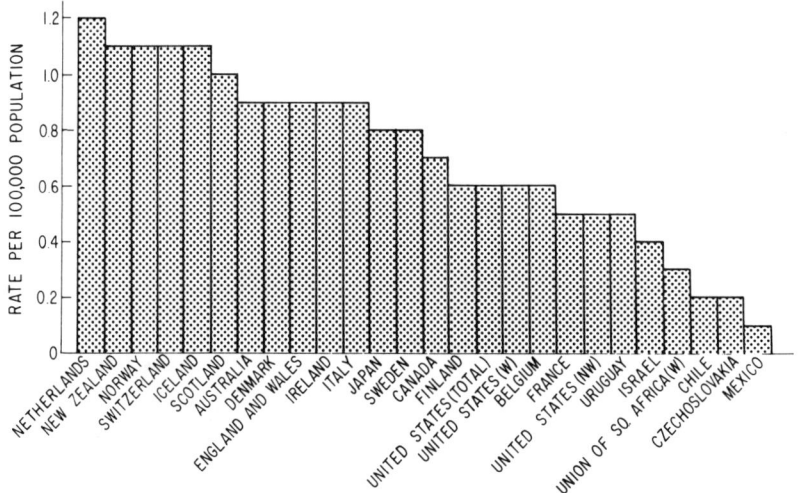

Figure 5.1 Average annual age-adjusted death rates per 100,000 population for motor neuron disease: selected countries, various years, 1951-58 (Source: Goldberg and Kurland 1962. By permission of Lancet Publications, Inc.)

United States Mortality Data, Trend

The major components of the MND category are ALS (356.1) and PMA (356.0). For the entire MND category 356, the crude death rates in the United States have remained essentially constant at about 0.7 per 100,000 for 1949-64 (see Fig. 5.2). While the rate for ALS increased from 0.4 per 100,000 in 1949 to 0.6 by 1959, the rate for PMA went from 0.2 to 0.1 per 100,000 population. This would be consistent with change in diagnostic custom—in other words, with more frequent usage of ALS in preference to PMA. From 1949 to 1964, the components of the MND code changed; ALS went from about 60 to 85 percent and PMA from 35 to 10 percent of MND deaths (Table A.5.2).

United States Mortality Data, 1959-61

In 1959-61, 83 percent as the MND deaths were coded as ALS (356.1) and 13 percent of PMA (PMMA + PBP) (356.0), with the remaining 4 percent divided as 3 percent familial (356.2) and 1 percent "other" (356.3). The detailed analysis of the United States

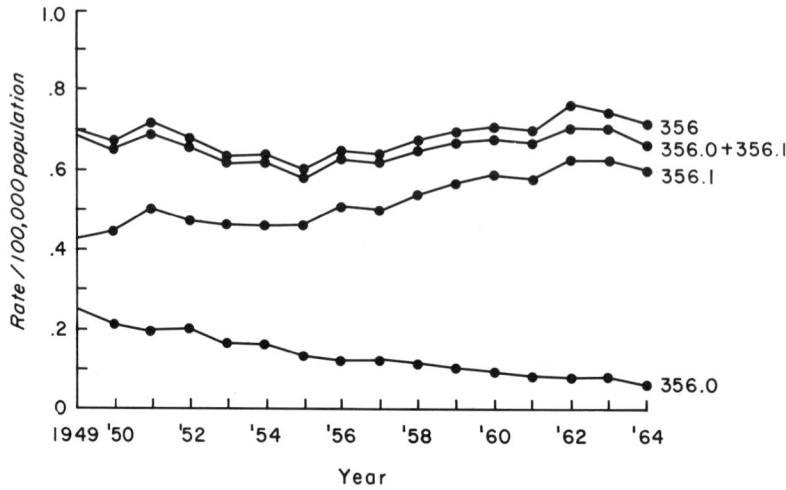

Figure 5.2 Crude death rates per 100,000 population for amyotrophic lateral sclerosis (code 356.1), progressive muscular atrophy (356.0), and motor neuron disease (356) by year: United States, 1949–64

mortality experience in this chapter will be concerned primarily with ALS (356.1) coded as the underlying cause of death for these three years.

Age. Age-specific death rates for ALS in the United States, 1959-61, are depicted in Fig. 5.3 and Table A.5.3. Of 3,149 certificates listing ALS as the primary cause of death, 98 percent were for persons between 35 and 84 years old. Only 8 percent of the deaths occurred in persons under 45, and 73 percent occurred in those over 54. The rates were highest at about age 70 and then decreased sharply.

The median age at death for the ALS decedents in the United States was approximately 62 years, and the mean age was 61.1 years. If we assume a four-year duration from clinical onset to death, the mean age at onset would be about 57, or five years older than reported in the clinical series by Mulder (1957) and by Friedman and Freedman (1950). The mean age at death was about twelve years greater than for the ALS decedents on Guam, where a form of this disease is a major cause of death (Reed et al. 1966).

Sex and color. The death rates for ALS were about 1.8 times as high for males as for females (Table 5.2); this was true for whites as

ALS AND OTHER MOTOR NEURON DISEASES / 113

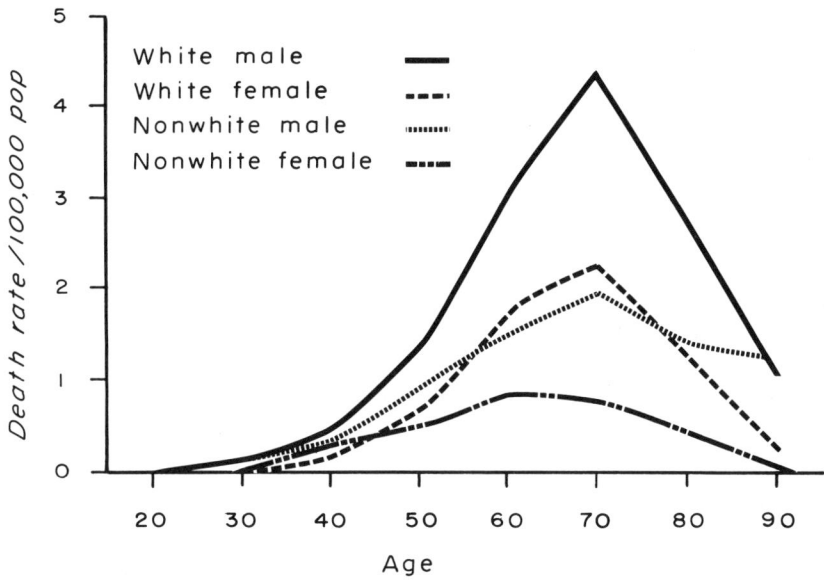

Figure 5.3 Average annual age-specific death rates per 100,000 population for amyotrophic lateral sclerosis by color and sex: United States, 1959-61 (Source: Kurland et al. 1969a. By permission of Grune & Stratton, Inc.)

Table 5.2 Average annual age-adjusted death rates per 100,000 population for amyotrophic lateral sclerosis by race, age and sex: United States, 1959-61
(ISC code 356.1)

Age and sex	All races	White	Nonwhite				
			Total	Negro	Indian	Japanese	Other
All ages							
Total	0.5	0.5	0.3*	0.3*	0.2*	0.9*	0.7*
Male	0.7	0.7	0.4*	0.4*	-	1.4*	1.0*
Female	0.4*	0.4*	0.2*	0.2*	0.5*	0.4*	-
Under 15							
Total	0.0*	0.0*	-	-	-	-	-
Male	-	-	-	-	-	-	-
Female	0.0*	0.0*	-	-	-	-	-
65 & over							
Total	2.6	2.7	1.2*	1.1*	-	6.0*	-
Male	3.7	3.7	1.7*	1.6*	-	8.9*	-
Female	1.8	1.9	0.6*	0.6*	-	2.5*	-

well as for nonwhites. The excess among males was noted for all regions in the United States (Table 5.3), suggesting that the unidentified factor responsible for selection for males is ubiquitous. The white-nonwhite ratios of the age-adjusted rates varied in the nine geographic regions (Table 5.4). Lower ratios were noted in the East North Central (1.2 to 1) and Middle Atlantic (1.3 to 1) regions, and the highest ratios were recorded from the southern areas. However, as may be seen in Table 5.4, the nonwhite rates by region are based on too few deaths to provide reliable regional comparisons with respect to the white-nonwhite ratios. Among the nonwhites nationwide, male Japanese-Americans had a rate of 1.4 per 100,000, twice as high as that for white males, but this rate was based on fewer than 15 deaths in three years (Table 5.2).

Geographic distribution. The age-adjusted death rates for ALS showed little variation by census region (Tables 5.3 and 5.4). Figure 5.4 shows the rates by individual state. There was a somewhat wider range than by region, as might be expected, but it was only from 0.3 to 1.0 per 100,000 population. All but six of the states had rates within the range of 0.4 to 0.7 per 100,000. The rates by state are provided in Table A.5.4 for all ages, as well as for those 65 or older. In this last age grouping, however, comparisons were of limited value because the age-specific rates were based on so few deaths.

Although more rates in the northern states were above the total

Table 5.3 Deaths and average annual age-adjusted death rates per 100,000 population for amyotrophic lateral sclerosis by sex, with male-female ratio of adjusted rates: United States and census regions, 1959-61 (ISC code 356.1)

Region	Male		Female		M:F ratio
	Deaths	Rate	Deaths	Rate	
United States	2,007	0.7	1,142	0.4*	1.8
New England	121	0.7*	83	0.4*	1.8
Middle Atlantic	419	0.7	240	0.3	2.3
East North Central	440	0.7	265	0.4	1.8
West North Central	234	0.9	129	0.5*	1.8
South Atlantic	228	0.6	116	0.3*	2.0
East South Central	104	0.6*	50	0.3*	2.0
West South Central	134	0.5*	92	0.3*	1.7
Mountain	77	0.8*	34	0.4*	2.0
Pacific	250	0.7	133	0.4*	1.8

Table 5.4 Deaths and average annual age-adjusted death rates per 100,000 population for amyotrophic lateral sclerosis by color, with white-nonwhite ratio of adjusted rates: United States and census regions, 1959-61
(ISC code 356.1)

Region	White		Nonwhite		White: nonwhite ratio
	Deaths	Rate	Deaths	Rate	
United States	2,987	0.5	162	0.3*	1.7
New England	204	0.5*	-	-	-
Middle Atlantic	629	0.5*	30	0.4*	1.3
East North Central	668	0.6*	37	0.5*	1.2
West North Central	356	0.7*	7	0.4*	1.8
South Atlantic	306	0.5*	38	0.3*	1.7
East South Central	140	0.5*	14	0.2*	2.5
West South Central	208	0.5*	18	0.2*	2.5
Mountain	109	0.6*	2	0.3*	2.0
Pacific	367	0.6*	16	0.4*	1.5

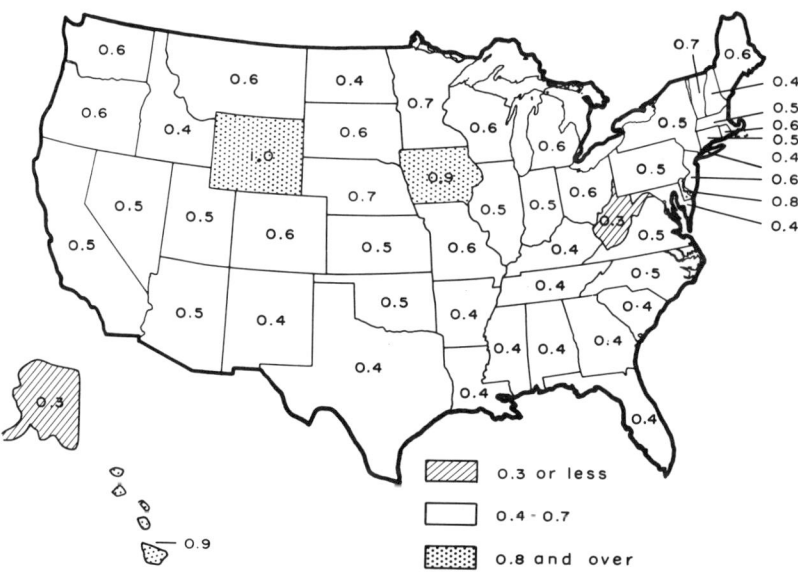

Figure 5.4 Average annual age-adjusted death rates per 100,000 population for amyotrophic lateral sclerosis by state: United States, 1959–61. None of the rates meets the standard of reliability or precision as defined in Notes on Tables and Figures. (Source: Kurland et al. 1969a. By permission of Grune & Stratton, Inc.)

rate for the United States of 0.5 per 100,000, what is striking is the small number of states that recorded high or low rates (that is, above 0.7 or below 0.4): Delaware (0.8), Iowa (0.9), Hawaii (0.9), and Wyoming (1.0); West Virginia (0.3) and Alaska (0.3). The numbers of deaths in these states were few, and the distribution by state must be considered homogeneous. (In Denmark also, the distribution of ALS was essentially uniform among the various regions of the country; see Kurtzke 1969a.)

Type of county. Age-adjusted mortality rates by metropolitan and nonmetropolitan counties are shown in Table 5.5. For both whites and nonwhites, by sex, and for the nine regions, there was little difference between metropolitan and nonmetropolitan rates, and no consistent deviations—again supporting the homogeneity of these rates.

Marital status. In general, the rates for males were nearly twice as high as those for females in each of the four marital categories; this held for those aged 15-64 years, as well as those 65 or older (Table 5.6). As previously mentioned, a similar pattern prevailed throughout each of the nine census regions. Thus the mortality from ALS does

Table 5.5 Average annual age-adjusted death rates per 100,000 population for amyotrophic lateral sclerosis by color, sex and type of county: United States and census regions, 1959-61 (ISC code 356.1)

Region and color	Metropolitan counties			Nonmetropolitan counties		
	Total	Male	Female	Total	Male	Female
United States	0.5	0.7*	0.4*	0.5*	0.7*	0.3*
Region						
New England	0.5*	0.6*	0.4*	0.6*	0.9*	0.3*
Middle Atlantic	0.5*	0.7*	0.4*	0.5*	0.7*	0.3*
East North Central	0.6*	0.7*	0.4*	0.6*	0.8*	0.4*
West North Central	0.6*	0.8*	0.5*	0.7*	0.9*	0.4*
South Atlantic	0.4*	0.6*	0.3*	0.4*	0.6*	0.2*
East South Central	0.4*	0.6*	0.2*	0.4*	0.6*	0.3*
West South Central	0.5*	0.7*	0.4*	0.4*	0.4*	0.3*
Mountain	0.6*	0.8*	0.4*	0.5*	0.7*	0.3*
Pacific	0.6*	0.8*	0.4*	0.5*	0.6*	0.3*
Color						
White	0.5	0.7*	0.4*	0.5*	0.7*	0.3*
Nonwhite	0.3*	0.5*	0.2*	0.3*	0.3*	0.2*

Table 5.6 Average annual age-adjusted death rates per 100,000 population for amyotrophic lateral sclerosis by age, sex and marital status: United States, 1959-61
(ISC code 356.1)

Age and sex	Single	Married	Widowed	Divorced
15 & over				
Total	0.7*	0.7	0.6*	0.7*
Male	1.0*	0.9	0.9*	1.1*
Female	0.5*	0.5*	0.5*	0.5*
15-64				
Total	0.6*	0.5	0.4*	0.6*
Male	0.8*	0.6	0.6*	0.9*
Female	0.3*	0.3	0.4*	0.4*
65 & over				
Total	2.5*	3.0	2.1	2.2*
Male	2.8*	3.8	3.5	3.2*
Female	2.3*	1.8*	1.8	1.2*

not appear to have any association with marital status—perhaps because this fatal disease is of short duration and the age at onset is usually past middle age.

Nativity. The age-adjusted death rates for the foreign born were similar to those for the native born, as shown in Table 5.7. The preponderance of males in these rates (nearly 2 to 1) was seen in

Table 5.7 Average annual age-adjusted death rates per 100,000 population for amyotrophic lateral sclerosis, white persons, by sex and nativity: United States and census regions, 1959-61
(ISC code 356.1)

Region	Native born			Foreign born		
	Total	Male	Female	Total	Male	Female
United States	0.5	0.7	0.4*	0.5*	0.7*	0.4*
New England	0.5*	0.7*	0.3*	0.5*	0.5*	0.5*
Middle Atlantic	0.5*	0.7*	0.4*	0.6*	0.8*	0.4*
East North Central	0.6*	0.8*	0.4*	0.5*	0.6*	0.4*
West North Central	0.7*	0.9*	0.5*	0.6*	1.0*	0.2*
South Atlantic	0.5*	0.7*	0.3*	0.3*	0.6*	0.1*
East South Central	0.5*	0.7*	0.3*	0.4*	0.8*	-
West South Central	0.5*	0.6*	0.4*	0.4*	0.5*	0.2*
Mountain	0.6*	0.8*	0.3*	0.3*	0.5*	0.1*
Pacific	0.6*	0.8*	0.4*	0.5*	0.5*	0.5*

both groups for the United States as a whole and by region of the country, although there was some fluctuation in the latter, probably related to the few deaths among the foreign born.

Death rates among foreign born by country of origin were obtained for the total MND category (356) rather than for ALS alone (356.1). When classified according to country of origin, the crude death rates for motor neuron disease among foreign-born United States residents seemed to vary appreciably (Table A.5.5). However, for many countries the number of deaths and the population at risk were small, and it is doubtful that any significance can be attached to deviations in the rates. Although most of these crude rates were high, compared to those of the total United States population, the foreign born were older on the average. Age adjustment for whites only (data not shown) brought the total rate of 1.8 among foreign-born whites (2.4 males and 1.2 females) down to a rate of 0.6 (0.8 male and 0.5 female) which is similar to that for native-born whites of 0.6 (0.9 male and 0.4 female) for the entire MND category. Age-adjusted rates among whites for ALS alone are compared in Table 5.7.

Morbidity Data in ALS

Based on the average annual mortality rate of about 1 per 100,000 population for ALS and an expected duration of approximately four years, a prevalence of about 4 per 100,000 population might be expected if all deaths were ascertained. There are, however, only three population surveys that permit a direct estimation of incidence and prevalence.

Rochester, Minnesota

In an early study, the average annual incidence of ALS from 1945 to 1954 was reported as about 1.7 per 100,000 among the resident population of Rochester, Minnesota (Kurland 1958*a*). This survey has now been extended to cover 1925-64 (Kurland et al. 1969*a*).

During these forty years, there were 17 acceptable cases of ALS (8 males and 9 females). There was a tendency for the crude rates to increase in succeeding decades, but this upward trend was not statistically significant and was less marked when the rates for each decade were age and sex adjusted as in Table 5.8. The average annual incidence rate, age adjusted to the 1950 United States population, was about 1.3 per 100,000 population for the entire forty-year period.

Table 5.8 Number of cases and average annual incidence rates per 100,000 population for motor neuron disease among residents: Rochester, Minnesota, 1925-64

Period	Population [a]	Number of cases			Rate, both sexes	
		Total	Male	Female	Crude	Adjusted[b]
Total	29,885[c]	17	8	9	1.4	1.3[d]
1925-34	20,621	2	1	1	1.0	1.1
1935-44	26,312	2	2	0	0.8	1.0
1945-54	29,885	5	2	3	1.7	1.5
1955-64	40,663	8	3	5	2.0	1.8

[a] Decennial census 1930, 1940, 1950, and 1960.

[b] Adjusted for age and sex to United States white population 1950.

[c] 1950 population used for crude rate (1925-64).

[d] Male-female ratio of age-adjusted rates is 1.6 to 1.

In all four decades the general population of females outnumbered that of males in Rochester, especially in the older age groups. Therefore, although the number of ALS cases involving females exceeded those involving males, the rates by sex, when adjusted to a standard population, actually showed a higher rate for males, with a male-female ratio of 1.6 to 1.

All the patients were white; their national origins varied, as did those of the community, and included Scandinavian, English, German, and Irish. In this small series there was no obvious selection of cases by occupation or social status or any indication that the onset occurred in a particular season.

The age distribution in the Rochester cases was similar for males and females. The mean age at onset for all persons was 64 years, which was clearly older than that in the series reported by Mulder (1957) for Mayo Clinic patients or by Friedman and Freedman (1950) in their own series and in the other series that they reviewed, or in the series by Norris and Engel (1965). It is possible that the usual hospital or clinic series are biased in favor of younger patients who travel to the better-known neurologic centers from which many such statistics are derived. The mean age of the Rochester patients was much greater than that reported in series of familial cases (Kurland and Mulder 1955) and on Guam (Kurland and Mulder 1954; Reed et al. 1966). The possibility that the small Rochester series is aberrant with respect to age at onset cannot be ruled out.

Sixteen of the 17 patients in the Rochester series have died and, in every case, ALS was reported on the death certificate as the underlying cause. The duration from onset to death was essentially the same for both sexes, about two and a half years. In the 9 cases in which autopsies were performed, the diagnosis of ALS was confirmed.

Carlisle, England

Brewis and colleagues (1966) surveyed this city of 71,000 population in 1961 and obtained data on the incidence and prevalence of various neurologic diseases for 1955-61. Based on the 5 patients discovered in this period, the average minimal incidence for ALS in Carlisle was 1.0 per 100,000 population. The prevalence rate was 7 per 100,000, as all 5 patients were alive and resident in Carlisle on prevalence day in 1961.

Iceland

Gudmundsson (1968b; 1969) has provided valuable data on the population characteristics of neurologic disorders in the country of Iceland, where he was the only neurologist. For the ten years 1954-63, he discovered 24 cases in that country, with a male-female ratio of 2.0 to 1. The average annual incidence rate was 0.8 per 100,000, and the mortality rate was 0.7 per 100,000. Duration averaged 7.7 years, largely because of 4 patients with onset at ages 21-33 who were alive more than eight years after onset, two of whom died after ten and twelve years of illness. With these cases of long duration included, the prevalence rate was 6.4 per 100,000 population from the 12 patients alive in 1963. Median age at onset was in the age range 51-60 years. There was a familial frequency of 8 percent, 2 of the 24 patients being related.

The prevalence rates based on small numbers were estimated at about 6 per 100,000 in the three population studies. If these were valid, then either the national mortality rates were underestimates or the duration was longer than our clinical evidence generally indicates. For this fatal disorder each incidence rate noted herein was somewhat higher than the appropriate mortality rate, which would support the concept of incomplete retrieval of ALS deaths.

Classification of ALS

We agree with Espinosa and his associates (1962) that currently it is reasonable to classify ALS (or MND in general) into three types: the classic and usually sporadic form, the familial and presumably hereditary form as seen in the United States and other countries, and the Mariana Islands form as seen among the Chamorros and perhaps others who have lived in the western Pacific islands (see Table 5.9). Although the major pathologic and clinical features of the three groups appear to be similar, the underlying pathogenesis may be dissimilar if the distinguishing features referred to are real.

Classic or Sporadic Form

About 90 to 95 percent of the cases observed in the United States occurred sporadically and had the classic features of progressive lower motor neuron disease usually accompanied by evidence of upper motor neuron involvement. The sites of initial wasting and weakness varied, but in most series about 40 percent of the sites were in the upper extremities, 25 percent were in the head (bulbar), 25 percent were in the lower extremities, and about 10 percent were in mixed sites (Mulder 1957).

The possibility that sporadic cases of ALS reflect some biochemical defect which might be genetically determined was considered in an earlier paper (Kurland 1957b). Dermal changes, which include increased mucopolysaccharide concentrations, connective tissue disorientation, elastosis, and disorganization of collagen structure, are believed to reflect such a biochemical defect. They were noted in about 50 percent of the sporadic cases in the United States and in the same proportion of cases on Guam (Fullmer et al. 1960). Unfortunately, no later information is available on this aspect of the disease.

Familial Form

Prior to the studies on Guam, almost all neurologists considered ALS to be nonfamilial and nonhereditary. Because of the familial aggregations of ALS observed on Guam, the question was appraised in a series of patients seen at the Mayo Clinic. It was concluded that the disease was familial in about 5 to 10 percent of these cases, and closer study revealed an autosomal dominant pattern of inheritance with high penetrance (Kurland and Mulder 1955; Mulder 1957).

Table 5.9 Selected clinical and pathologic features of amyotrophic lateral sclerosis

Features	Sporadic cases	Familial cases	Marianas cases
Approximate mean age at onset, years (usual range)	57 (25-75)	47 (25-65)	49 (25-65)
Sex ratio, M:F	1.6:1	1:1	2:1
Approximate mean duration, years (usual range)	3-4 (1-8)	3-4 (1-10)	3-4 (1-8)
Clinical features:			
Initial symptoms, lower extremities	20-25 percent	40-50 percent	20-25 percent
Initial symptoms of spasticity as in primary lateral sclerosis	Rare	Rare	About 10 percent
Extrapyramidal symptoms	Rare	Occasional	Frequent (if cases with both AlS and P-D are included)
Dementia present	Rare	Occasional	Infrequent in AlS alone; frequent in AlS/P-D
Sensory changes	Not detected	Not detected	Not detected
Histochemical changes in skin (collagen)	About 50 percent	Infrequent (?)	About 50 percent
Pathology in central nervous system:			
Posterior column demyelination and column of Clarke changes	Rare	About 50 percent	Rare
Neurofibrillary changes before age 60 years	Rare	Rare	Common
Granulovacuolar bodies	Rare	Rare	Occasional
Amorphous inclusions in anterior horn cells	Apparently absent	Present in some	Apparently absent

Although individual cases of familial ALS showed no distinctive findings on clinical examination, it appeared that a high proportion began with weakness and wasting in the lower extremities and had a relatively rapid rate of progression. Hirano and his associates (1967) described the pathologic features in several such cases. There was clinically silent involvement of the posterior columns and the spinocerebellar tracts, with loss of cells in the column of Clarke. Hyalin-like material was present within the cytoplasm of affected anterior horn cells. Occasionally a more deeply stained central core, which resembled Lewy's inclusions, was also observed in the affected neurons. In one case an accumulation of amorphous material was observed between the Purkinje cell layer and the granular cell layer of the cerebellum in the region of the culmen, the nature of which is unknown.

Thus there appeared to be at least one distinct form within the group of familial ALS cases; other familial cases, particularly when there was early cervical or bulbar involvement, seemed identical in all respects to the sporadic cases. Perhaps the group described by Hirano and his associates (1967) is a transitional type in a genetic spectrum that encompasses the hereditary ataxias and ALS.

The familial cases showed a one-to-one sex ratio, in contrast to the observed preponderance of males in the classic and Mariana Islands forms. The range of age at onset and the duration (approximately three to four years) were similar to those in sporadic cases, although the mean age at onset in the series reported by Kurland and Mulder (1955) was about 47. Histochemical changes observed in the skin in cases of the classic and Marianas forms have not yet been noted in the few familial cases that have been studied (Fullmer et al. 1960).

Mariana Islands Form

In about 1950 a form of ALS that was believed to be identical in its clinical and pathologic features to the classic form of the disease was observed on Guam and in other Mariana Islands in the western Pacific. Among the indigenous Chamorro population, it was about a hundred times more prevalent than in the population of the United States (Mulder and Kurland 1954; Mulder et al. 1954). About 1 percent of the adult Chamorros were found to be affected at any given time, and for an adult Chamorro, the lifetime risk of dying from ALS was about 10 percent. Although the original data suggested a genetic basis for this focus of disease, the more recent developments enumerated below have led to a renewed search for an exogenous factor:

(1) The recognition that another disease referred to as parkinsonism-dementia complex (P-D) is highly prevalent among the Chamorros (Kurland et al. 1961). Pathologically, neurofibrillary changes and granulovacuolar bodies are common in P-D, as Hirano and his associates (1969) have reported, but in areas of the brain not ordinarily affected in ALS. The same type of unusual neuronal changes were belatedly recognized in the Mariana Islands cases of ALS—again, most often in nonmotor neuron areas and tracts (Hirano et al. 1961).

(2) The observation that the small non-Chamorro population of nearby Saipan and Tinian, and possibly the non-Chamorro long-term residents on Guam, had more ALS than was usual among other populations (Elizan et al. 1966a).

(3) The reporting of a new focus of ALS in another area of the western Pacific, namely, the Kii Peninsula of Japan (Kimura et al. 1963). At least one of these patients at autopsy also had the unusual pathologic changes observed in the Marianas cases (Shiraki 1969).

(4) The frequent occurrence of muscular atrophy in the hands of adolescents and young adults and several cases of motor neuron disease in one other possible focus, Kepi (a small remote village near the southern coast of western New Guinea) (Gajdusek 1963). This disorder possibly is ALS, but pathologic confirmation is required.

(5) The prevalence of diaphysial aclasis (multiple exostosis), hyperuricemia, and perhaps hyperglycemia in the Chamorros and Carolinians of the Marianas (Krooth et al. 1961; Burch et al. 1966). Although the association of these disorders with the neurologic disease is uncertain, the possiblity of a common toxic factor must be considered.

The male-female sex ratio in the Marianas form of ALS was about two to one. Although the range of ages was similar, the mean age at onset of ALS in the islands was appreciably lower than in the sporadic cases of the United States. The mean duration of the disease was about three to four years, and there were no differences in the major pathologic features of anterior-horn-cell degeneration and demyelination of the long motor tracts (Elizan et al. 1966b). However, neurofibrillary changes and granulovacuolar bodies were common in the Marianas form of the disease but were infrequent in other cases. The histochemical changes observed in the skin in the sporadic cases were also noted in the cases in the Marianas but not, to date, in the few non-Guamanian familial cases studied. Terminally, about 10 percent of the Marianas patients with ALS had evidence of either extrapyramidal or intellectual deficits. This association of motor-neuronal, extrapyramidal, and mental effects, which is not uncommon in the Marianas cases, seemed to occur infrequently in either the sporadic or the familial cases of ALS. There have been occasional reports from Europe and the United States, some apparently stimulated by the studies on Guam, in which parkinsonism or dementia or both have been noted in patients with ALS (Robertson 1953; Van Bogaert and Radermecker 1954; Bonduelle et al. 1959; Poser, personal communication).

Comment and Conclusions

Motor neuron disease occurred in all countries for which mortality statistics were obtained and, where data seemed reliable, it accounted for about 1 per 1,000 adult deaths. The sex ratio was about 1.6 males to 1 female. Average annual age-adjusted death rates for the United States by region and for Canada, Australia, England and Wales, and several other western European countries were within the range 0.7 to 1.2 per 100,000 population. When variability in medical training, diagnostic facilities, and reporting and coding practices is considered, these rates appear remarkably similar.

In the United States there was no appreciable selectivity for ALS death rates by region, by metropolitan or nonmetropolitan counties, by marital status, or by native versus foreign birth. Although the reported death rate was higher for whites than for nonwhites (1.7 to 1), it is uncertain whether this reflects a true difference in mortality or whether it is related to the availability and utilization of diagnostic services. In Rochester, Minnesota, there has been a slight, but not statistically significant, upward trend in incidence during the past four decades, in which the annual incidence rate has averaged about 1.3 per 100,000 population age adjusted to the 1950 white United States population.

Despite the hazards of generalizing from the available data, on these bases it is estimated that in the United States there are nearly 3,000 new cases of MND annually and about 10,000 persons affected at any given time.

The mean age at death for ALS in the United States was about 61 for both males and females. Since the mean duration from onset to death seems to be three to four years, this suggests that the previously held concept of 52 as the mean age at onset (derived from clinical series) may be incorrect. The mean age at onset of the small series of Rochester cases was about 64 years.

Three forms of ALS have been described and referred to as the sporadic or classic form, the familial and presumably hereditary form, and the Mariana Islands form, perhaps more appropriately now called the "western Pacific islands" form. Although the major pathologic and clinical features of the three groups appear to be similar, the underlying pathogenic mechanisms may be dissimilar if the distinguishing features referred to are real. The opportunity afforded on Guam and the other western Pacific islands to examine so many patients within a relatively brief period offers us a rare view of the full spectrum of this disease entity, only segments of which are generally recognized elsewhere.

No single concept of the cause or pathogenesis of ALS has been widely accepted; and it is not unreasonable to consider that ALS may be more than a single disease entity. Case series have been described which suggest that the causative mechanism or agent may have been trauma; heavy metal or organic intoxicants; metabolic, vascular, or nutritional processes; prior poliomyelitis; or other infectious agents (the last-mentioned cause being associated with prior encephalitis). However, small numbers of cases, selection bias, and other methodologic explanations argue against the role of most of these concepts in the etiology of ALS.

Norris and Engel (1965) have described an association of ALS and malignancy in 10 percent of a series of 130 patients, but the absence of an appropriate "expected" value of malignancy in a population of similar age, sex, and duration of follow-up raises some doubt about the significance of this association. In the Rochester series of 17 patients, 2 had prior malignancies, both apparently treated successfully prior to onset of symptoms of ALS.

Among the Chamorros, ALS has been considered as familial for decades and perhaps for more than a century, but no simple pattern of inheritance has been recognized and no exogenous agent has yet been identified. Because the disease is no longer believed to be endemic among the Chamorros alone and because it is highly unlikely that the foci in Japan, the Marianas, and possibly New Guinea result from a single genetic identity of these peoples, there has been a renewal of efforts to find some exogenous factor common to these regions. The combination of prevalent neurologic disease, the collagen changes in the skin of such patients, and the multiple exostosis observed on Guam has led to intensive efforts to find some local food with lathyrogenic properties.

One source of toxin that has aroused considerable interest has been the nut of *Cycas circinalis* (cycad), which apparently has been an important source of starch on the island for more than a century (Proceedings 1964). In its natural form, cycad may contain a small quantity of lathyrogenic substance (Bell 1966), which could conceivably affect motor and other neurons. However, cycad also contains a remarkable water-soluble hepatotoxic and carcinogenic agent, the aglycone of cycasin (methylazoxymethanol), which can be removed by thorough elution. Several species of animals have been tested with the aglycone, which chemically resembles dimethylnitrosoamine (Proceedings 1964). Recent reports indicate that neurologic changes have occurred in a few animals (Mikelson 1970). It was also previously noted that cattle in Australia and Santo Domingo fed on cycad plants developed some disturbance of gait and demyelination of the posterior and lateral columns, particularly in the spinal cord (Innes 1966).

The possible roles of other nutritional agents, of heavy metals such as manganese, and of an infectious mechanism are still being explored. As to this last, several reports from the USSR have indicated that ALS may be transmitted to monkeys by intracerebral inoculation of human ALS central nervous system tissues (Zil'ber et al. 1961; Bunina 1962). This work has not been confirmed in the United States (Gibbs 1969; Johnson 1969), and following a review (Johnson 1969) of the pathologic tissues of the presumably affected monkeys by veterinary pathologists in the United States, the original report has been seriously questioned.

Thus the search for genetic and exogenous factors must still be continued. In the non-Pacific familial form of ALS, heredity as a dominant trait seems the most likely explanation. In the Mariana Islands form, it will be necessary to rule out a toxic etiologic agent. The sporadic cases are the major group and may represent more than one specific disease entity, in which especially the relative roles of heredity and environment remain to be explained. At the present time, aid from scientists in other disciplines seems necessary to help clarify the leads resulting from recent epidemiologic and genetic studies.

6 / MUSCULAR DYSTROPHY AND OTHER MYOPATHIES

Leonard T. Kurland
John F. Kurtzke
Irving D. Goldberg
Nung Won Choi

The myopathies include the muscular dystrophies in which heredity has a major etiologic role and the acquired myopathies in which the roles of heredity and environment are still to be clarified. Among the acquired myopathies the principal category is that of polymyositis. The population characteristics are available to a limited extent for some dystrophies and a few myopathies. Muscle disorders have been the subject of several recent volumes: Adams and associates (1960; 1962) and Walton (1969). Categorization of the dystrophies with emphasis on their genetic features is discussed in some detail by Pratt (1967).

Muscular Dystrophy

Muscular dystrophy (MD) refers to a group of syndromes, usually hereditary, that are manifested by weakness of striated muscles, with characteristic anatomic distribution. "In the majority of the cases, the significant pathological findings are confined to the muscles. There may be a few degenerative changes in the ventral horn cells or a slight reduction in their number, but as a rule the peripheral and central nervous systems are normal" (Merritt 1967).

Many classifications have been proposed, but the one advanced by Walton (1963; 1964), which was modified from a previous classification by Walton and Nattrass (1954), seems most reasonable. He divided his cases into three major groups: Duchenne type, facioscapulohumeral type, and limb-girdle type (Walton 1963). Myotonic dystrophy is separately classified. In addition, there are a number of other dystrophies, among them distal myopathy, ocular myopathy, congenital muscular dystrophy, dystrophy with true hypertrophy, and several nonprogressive dystrophies. Classifications are made on clinical, genetic, and even pathologic bases.

Duchenne Type

This variety is characterized by being found almost entirely in males; by onset generally within the first four years of life; and by a malignant course in which the children are generally nonambulatory by their teens, at which time they usually die from intercurrent infections. This disorder is transmitted as a sex-linked recessive trait, but perhaps half the recognized cases are sporadic, representing new mutants (Gardner-Medwin 1970). A high mutation rate of 1 in 10,000 pregnancies has been calculated (Tyler and Stephens 1951; Gardner-Medwin 1970). It is this type of dystrophy in which pseudohypertrophy of muscle is prominent.

A variant of the Duchenne type, but clinically similar to it, is that of x-linked recessive pseudohypertrophic dystrophy, as described by Becker (1962). In this variant the age at onset may be in the third decade of life and, most importantly, the course is benign and compatible with a normal life-span. Fortunately, fertility is notably reduced.

Whether there is truly an autosomal-recessive form of pseudohypertrophic dystrophy is conjectural. Pratt (1967) seems to have accepted its existence, but Gardner-Medwin (1970) believes that some of the patients actually have benign spinal muscular atrophy and that they never have the typical electrocardiographic changes of the Duchenne type of dystrophy, nor do their parents have the elevated creatine kinase levels by which the carriers are detected.

Facioscapulohumeral Type

This dystrophy is characterized by onset from late childhood to adult life in both sexes, with occurrence of abortive cases and transmission usually as an autosomal dominant trait (Walton 1963), possibly occasionally as a recessive one (Pratt 1967). Tyler and Stephens (1950) reported 58 cases of a kindred showing a typical mendelian dominant pattern of inheritance with complete penetrance and variable expressivity. They noted that the disease progressed more rapidly if the dystrophy began at an early age.

Limb-Girdle Type

Occurring in either sex, this variety has its onset usually within the first three decades of life, but occasionally later, and is generally transmitted "as an autosomal recessive character, but in rare instances as an autosomal dominant; many appear to be sporadic" (Walton 1963).

Mortality Data

Muscular dystrophy is included with amyotonia congenita (a disease of muscle and motor neurons present at birth) and myotonia in code 744.1 under the heading "inborn defect of muscle" in the Sixth and Seventh Revisions of the ISC coding.* Obviously, then, these deaths will be an admixture of all the aforementioned entities. In Canada, where the death rate from inborn defect of muscle was similar to that of the United States (0.2 per 100,000 in 1950-51), an analysis was made of death certificates allocated to this code in 1951 (Kurland 1958a). Of the 20 cases coded as underlying cause of death to 744.1, 16 were attributed to dystrophy, 4 to amyotonia congenita, and none to myotonia congenita. At the same time, there were an additional 7 deaths in which dystrophy was cited as a contributory cause of death. Although these numbers are small and based on a single year's experience, if the same proportion of deletions (amyotonia) and additions (muscular dystrophy coded as contributory cause of death) held for the United States, the annual death rate of persons who died of muscular dystrophy in this country would be roughly the same as (or perhaps only slightly higher than) the rate reported for ISC code 744.1.

International Mortality Data

Goldberg and Kurland (unpublished data) obtained data on deaths coded to 744.1 from nine countries for various years 1951-58. The crude death rates varied from 0.1 to 0.4 per 100,000 population, as shown in Table 6.1. Because most rates were based on but few deaths, the rates should not be assumed to differ appreciably; notably, the highest (0.4) and lowest (0.1) rates were found in the neighboring countries of Norway and Sweden.

*The Seventh Revision of the ISC is the basis for coding the mortality data utilized in this monograph. As noted, rubric 744.1 includes several distinct disease entities in addition to the major component, muscle dystrophies. Fortunately the Eighth Revision, to be used in future mortality studies, and the ICDA (National Center for Health Statistics 1962) for hospital data have distinct codes for muscular dystrophy, amyotonia congenita, myotonic dystrophy, myotonia congenita, and "other" forms of muscle disease.

Table 6.1 Average annual crude death rates per 100,000 population for inborn defect of muscle: selected countries, various years, 1951-58
(ISC code 744.1)

Country	Years	Rate
Canada[a]	1953-57	0.3
Iceland	1951-55	0.4
Ireland	1954-58	0.1
Israel[b]	1956-58	0.2
Italy	1955-57	0.1
New Zealand[c]	1952-56	0.2
Norway	1953-57	0.4
Sweden	1954-57	0.1
United States	1953-57	0.3
White	1953-57	0.2
Nonwhite	1953-57	0.3

[a] Yukon and Northwest Territories were included in 1956 and 1957 only.
[b] Jewish population only.
[c] Excludes Maori population.

United States Mortality Data

Trend. For each year 1949-51, the first three years in which this group of conditions was separately coded under the Sixth Revision of the ISC, the crude death rate in the United States was 0.2 per 100,000 for code 744.1. In 1952 the rate was 0.3, and it remained almost unchanged at that level for each succeeding year through 1967, the most recent year for which published statistics are available. It is likely that there has been no real change in the death rates from 1949 to 1967, and the variations noted reflect artifacts of coding or reporting or the effect of chance fluctuation or rounding off.

Age. Age-specific death rates revealed a trimodal distribution for whites and nonwhites, with the highest rate noted for those less than

Table 6.2 Deaths and average annual death rates per 100,000 population for inborn defect of muscle by age, color, and sex: United States, 1959-61 (ISC code 744.1)

Age	Total			White			Nonwhite		
	Total	Male	Female	Total	Male	Female	Total	Male	Female
Number of deaths									
All ages	1,697	1,183	514	1,587	1,106	481	110	77	33
Under 1	317	181	136	305	172	133	12	9	3
1-4	94	36	58	85	34	51	9	2	7
5-14	191	132	59	181	124	57	10	8	2
15-24	439	420	19	416	399	17	23	21	2
25-34	102	78	24	90	71	19	12	7	5
35-44	95	51	44	85	46	39	10	5	5
45-54	136	82	54	119	69	50	17	13	4
55-64	155	99	56	143	91	52	12	8	4
65-74	110	66	44	105	62	43	5	4	1
75-84	52	34	18	52	34	18	-	-	-
85 & over	6	4	2	6	4	2	-	-	-
Crude death rate									
All ages	0.3	0.4	0.2	0.3	0.5	0.2	0.2	0.3	0.1
Under 1	2.6	2.9	2.2	2.9	3.2	2.6	0.7*	1.0*	0.3*
1-4	0.2	0.1	0.2	0.2	0.2	0.3	0.1*	0.1*	0.2*
5-14	0.2	0.2	0.1	0.2	0.3	0.1	0.1*	0.1*	0.0*
15-24	0.6	1.2	0.1*	0.7	1.3	0.1*	0.3	0.5	0.0*
25-34	0.1	0.2	0.1	0.1	0.2	0.1*	0.1*	0.2*	0.1*
35-44	0.1	0.1	0.1	0.1	0.1	0.1	0.1*	0.1*	0.1*
45-54	0.2	0.3	0.2	0.2	0.3	0.2	0.3*	0.4*	0.1*
55-64	0.3	0.4	0.2	0.3	0.4	0.2	0.3*	0.4*	0.2*
65-74	0.3	0.4	0.2	0.3	0.4	0.3	0.2*	0.3*	0.1*
75-84	0.4	0.6	0.2*	0.4	0.6	0.2*	-	-	-
85 & over	0.2*	0.4*	0.1*	0.2*	0.4*	0.1*	-	-	-
Age-adjusted death rate									
All ages	0.3	0.4	0.2	0.3	0.5	0.2	0.2*	0.3*	0.1*
Under 15	0.3	0.3	0.2	0.4	0.4	0.3	0.1*	0.2*	0.1*
65 & over	0.3	0.5	0.2*	0.3	0.5	0.3*	0.1*	0.2*	0.1*

1 year of age. A peak at ages 15-24 was also apparent, and there was an additional, though less marked, peak for those 75-84 years old (Table 6.2 and Fig. 6.1).

The trimodal distribution of age-specific death rates suggests that at least three entities are involved in the code 744.1. The disease in infants would include amyotonia congenita and muscular dystrophy not otherwise specified. The peak at ages 15-24 was likely a result of muscular dystrophy of the Duchenne type, and the late peak was caused by the addition of both the facioscapulohumeral and the limb-girdle types, but especially of the myotonic dystrophies.

Almost all of those aged 15-24 with lesions classified as inborn muscle defects were males, which again indicates that these cases are likely to be the Duchenne type of muscular dystrophy (Fig. 6.1). The reason for the slight preponderance of males over females in the

MUSCULAR DYSTROPHY AND OTHER MYOPATHIES / 133

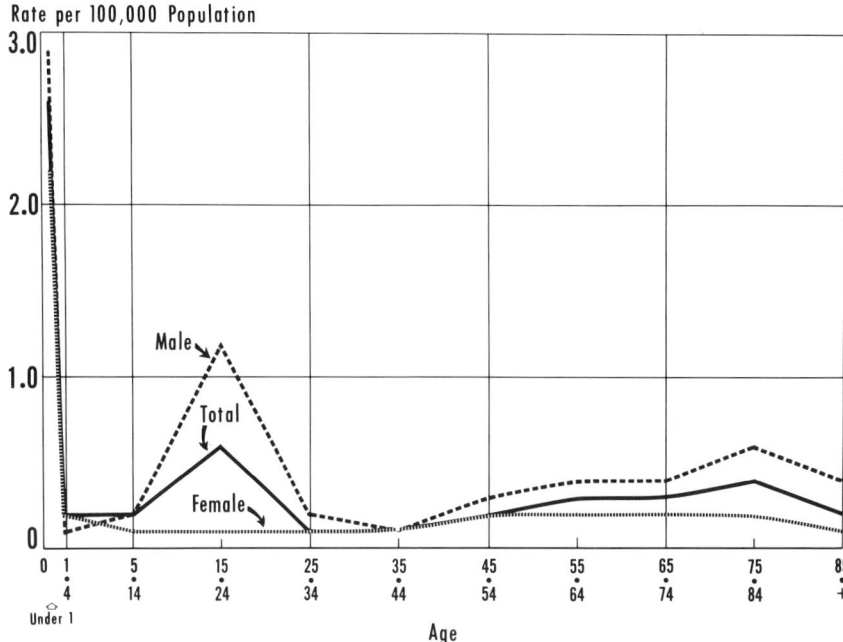

Figure 6.1 Average annual age-specific death rates per 100,000 population for inborn defect of muscle by sex: United States, 1959–61

group under 1 year of age is unclear, since amyotonia congenita and infantile muscular dystrophy not otherwise specified tended to occur in infants equally in both sexes (Thomasen 1948; Brandt 1950). This male preponderance is offset in the age group 1 to 4 years old by a comparable female excess; taken together, the number of deaths by sex in the group under 5 years old was approximately equal.

The elderly also manifested a definite male preponderance, which was not expected on the assumption that both limb-girdle and facioscapulohumeral types occur equally in both sexes. However, progressive muscular atrophy and amyotrophic lateral sclerosis (see Chapter 5), which are more common than muscular dystrophy and do occur selectively in males, also affect muscle (though secondarily to neuronal degeneration); the misclassification of these conditions as muscular dystrophy is sometimes made and possibly accounts for some of the male preponderance for dystrophy in older age groups. A contribution to the male excess is probably also made by the Becker type of pseudohypertrophic dystrophy, but the frequency of this variant is not known.

Table 6.3 Average annual age-adjusted death rates and death rates under age 1 per 100,000 population for inborn defect of muscle by sex: United States and census regions, 1959-61 (ISC code 744.1)

Region	All ages			Under age 1		
	Rate		M:F ratio	Rate		M:F ratio
	Male	Female		Male	Female	
United States	0.4	0.2	2.0	2.9	2.2	1.3
New England	0.4*	0.2*	2.0	3.1*	2.4*	1.3
Middle Atlantic	0.5*	0.2*	2.5	3.6	2.2	1.6
East North Central	0.5*	0.2*	2.5	2.5	2.8	0.9
West North Central	0.5*	0.2*	2.5	2.4*	1.7*	1.4
South Atlantic	0.4*	0.1*	4.0	2.0*	2.3	0.9
East South Central	0.6*	0.2*	3.0	3.7*	2.8*	1.3
West South Central	0.4*	0.1*	4.0	2.5*	1.0*	2.5
Mountain	0.4*	0.2*	2.0	3.6*	1.9*	1.9
Pacific	0.4*	0.2*	2.0	3.4	2.4*	1.4

Sex. The mortality rates, both crude and age adjusted, for males were about twice those for females (Tables 6.2 and 6.3). As previously suggested, some of the male excess at older ages may result from possible misclassification of muscular atrophy as dystrophy. The male-female pattern was fairly consistent by census region (Table 6.3), considering the small numbers at hand. The sex difference for deaths under 1 year of age was notably less than for all ages, although male deaths still predominated.

Color. While the rates for whites were higher than for nonwhites in most age groups, the greatest difference was for those less than 1 year old (Table 6.2). The crude and age-adjusted rates for all ages were 0.3 for whites, with 0.5 male and 0.2 female, versus 0.2 for nonwhites, with 0.3 male and 0.1 female. It is not certain whether this represents a real difference by color or whether it is a result of underreporting of deaths for nonwhites. Herndon (1954) reported a significantly higher prevalence rate for muscular dystrophy among the white population in his surveys in North Carolina (5.4 per 100,000 population for whites vs. 3.5 for nonwhites). He also commented that the difference in rates might be caused by gene frequency, but could be an artifact in case-finding efficiency.

Geographic distribution. There appeared to be no appreciable differences in the age-adjusted death rates by region, although there

Table 6.4 Average annual age-adjusted death rates per 100,000 population for inborn defect of muscle by color and age: United States and census regions, 1959-61
(ISC code 744.1)

Region	White			Nonwhite		
	All ages	Under 15	65 & over	All ages	Under 15	65 & over
United States	0.3	0.4	0.3	0.2*	0.1*	0.1*
New England	0.3*	0.3*	0.4*	0.1*	-	-
Middle Atlantic	0.3*	0.4	0.3*	0.1*	0.1*	-
East North Central	0.4	0.4	0.3*	0.2*	0.1*	-
West North Central	0.4*	0.3*	0.4*	0.2*	0.1*	-
South Atlantic	0.3*	0.4	0.3*	0.2*	0.1*	0.2*
East South Central	0.4*	0.5*	0.4*	0.4*	0.1*	0.1*
West South Central	0.3*	0.3*	0.3*	0.2*	0.2*	0.1*
Mountain	0.3*	0.3*	0.3*	0.1*	0.3*	-
Pacific	0.3*	0.3	0.5*	0.1*	0.1*	0.4*

was a slightly greater variation in the death rates for nonwhites than for whites (Table 6-4.). This can be explained by the few deaths upon which the rates were based among nonwhites in the various regions.

Type of county. There was little difference in the age-adjusted death rates for all ages between metropolitan residents and nonmetropolitan residents in each of the geographic regions (Table 6.5). The ratio of whites to nonwhites was essentially the same by type of county, and there were no appreciable differences in the rates for nonwhites by type of county (Table 6.6). Therefore, there is no indication of a rural environmental effect.

Marital status. Age-adjusted death rates for inborn muscle defect by age, sex, and marital status are shown in Table 6.7. Among those 15 or older, the highest rates were noted for single persons of either sex. The rate for single males was more than three times as high as that for single females. When comparison was restricted to those 65 or older, there was little difference in the rates by marital status. It is more likely that young and middle-aged adults affected with the disease remained single because of their ill health rather than that the single marital status predisposed to disease occurrence. The death rates for married and widowed persons were similar for each age group (Fig. 6.2), but for those 45 through 64 years old, the rates for

Table 6.5 Average annual age-adjusted death rates per 100,000 population for inborn defect of muscle by sex and type of county: United States and census regions, 1959-61
(ISC code 744.1)

Region	Metropolitan counties			Nonmetropolitan counties		
	Total	Male	Female	Total	Male	Female
United States	0.3	0.4	0.2	0.3	0.5	0.2*
New England	0.3*	0.4*	0.2*	0.3*	0.5*	0.1*
Middle Atlantic	0.3*	0.5*	0.1*	0.3*	0.4*	0.2*
East North Central	0.4*	0.6*	0.2*	0.3*	0.5*	0.1*
West North Central	0.3*	0.5*	0.1*	0.4*	0.6*	0.2*
South Atlantic	0.2*	0.4*	0.1*	0.3*	0.5*	0.2*
East South Central	0.3*	0.4*	0.2*	0.4*	0.6*	0.2*
West South Central	0.3*	0.4*	0.1*	0.3*	0.5*	0.2*
Mountain	0.2*	0.3*	0.1*	0.3*	0.4*	0.2*
Pacific	0.3*	0.4*	0.2*	0.4*	0.6*	0.1*

Table 6.6 Average annual age-adjusted death rates per 100,000 population for inborn defect of muscle by age, color, sex and type of county: United States, 1959-61
(ISC code 744.1)

Color & sex	Metropolitan counties			Nonmetropolitan counties		
	All ages	Under 15	65 & over	All ages	Under 15	65 & over
Total						
Total	0.3	0.3	0.3	0.3	0.3	0.4
Male	0.4	0.3	0.5	0.5	0.4	0.5*
Female	0.2	0.2	0.2	0.2*	0.3	0.3*
White						
Total	0.3	0.3	0.3	0.3	0.4	0.4
Male	0.5	0.3	0.5	0.5	0.4	0.5*
Female	0.2	0.3	0.3	0.2*	0.4	0.3*
Nonwhite						
Total	0.2*	0.1*	0.1*	0.3*	0.1*	0.2*
Male	0.3*	0.2*	0.1*	0.3*	0.1*	0.4*
Female	0.1*	0.1*	0.1*	0.1*	0.1*	-

Table 6.7 Average annual age-adjusted death rates per 100,000 population for inborn defect of muscle by age, sex and marital status: United States, 1959-61
(ISC code 744.1)

Age and sex	Single	Married	Widowed	Divorced
15 & over				
Total	0.9	0.1*	0.1*	0.2*
Male	1.3*	0.1*	0.3*	0.2*
Female	0.4*	0.1*	0.1*	0.2*
15-64				
Total	0.9*	0.1*	0.1*	0.2*
Male	1.3*	0.1*	0.3*	0.3*
Female	0.4*	0.1*	0.0*	0.1*
65 & over				
Total	0.4*	0.4*	0.3*	0.3*
Male	0.6*	0.5*	0.7*	0.2*
Female	0.2*	0.3*	0.2*	0.3*

divorced persons were much higher than for married and widowed persons, again a likely reflection of the diseased state.

Nativity. Average annual age-adjusted death rates for both native-born whites and foreign-born whites by age and sex are shown in Table 6.8. Lower rates for all ages were noted among foreign-born whites. The number of deaths among the foreign born was relatively small, and little discussion of the differences seems warranted. It is of some interest that there is no male preponderance for the foreign born as was noted for the native-born groups. Presumably the Duchenne type of dystrophy, occurring in childhood and adolescence, would militate against immigration to the United States and result in a lower death rate in the young foreign born, particularly among the males.

Morbidity Data

The major population studies available are summarized in Table 6.9. Herndon (1954), using many sources of medical and orthopedic information in North Carolina, located 133 index cases (and 6 other

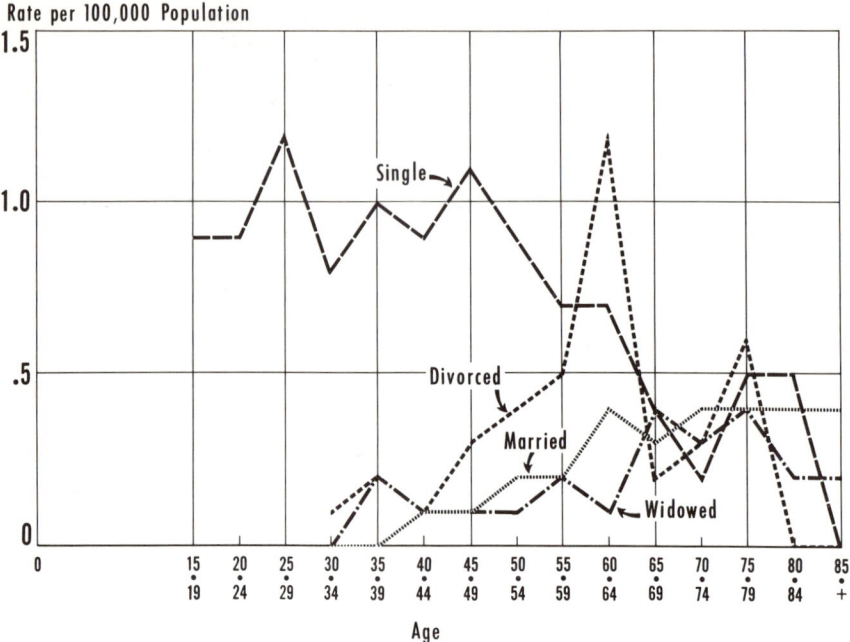

Figure 6.2 Average annual age-specific death rates per 100,000 population for inborn defect of muscle, persons age 15 and over, by marital status: United States, 1959-61

Table 6.8   Average annual age-adjusted death rates per 100,000 population for inborn defect of muscle, white persons, by age, sex and nativity: United States, 1959-61
(ISC code 744.1)

Nativity & age	Rate			M:F ratio
	Total	Male	Female	
Native born				
All ages	0.3	0.5	0.2	2.5
Under 15	0.4	0.5	0.3	1.7
65 & over	0.4	0.6	0.3*	2.0
Foreign born[a]				
All ages	0.2*	0.2*	0.2*	1.0
Under 15	0.3*	0.1*	0.5*	0.2
65 & over	0.3*	0.3*	0.3*	1.0

[a] Based on 51 deaths (30 male, 21 female).

Table 6.9 Cases and prevalence rates per 100,000 population for muscular dystrophy: selected surveys, various years, about 1950-63

Survey area (source)	Year	Cases	Rate
North Carolina (Herndon 1954)	c.1950	133	4
Northumberland-Durham, England (Walton and Nattrass 1954)	c.1952	84	4
Iceland (Gudmundsson 1968b)	1963	17	9
Carlisle, England (Brewis et al. 1966)	1961	5	7
Rochester, Minnesota (Kurland 1958a)	1955	2	6

cases in their families) in a population of about 3,500,000. He estimated that the minimal prevalence rate for North Carolina was 4 per 100,000 population.

Walton and Nattrass (1954) studied Northumberland and Durham counties in England, and in a population of about 2,262,000 found 84 cases of muscular dystrophy, for a prevalence rate of about 4 per 100,000 population. Of the 84 cases, 48 were of the Duchenne type, 18 of the facioscapulohumeral type, and 18 of the limb-girdle type. In addition, these authors observed two cases of distal myopathy and one of ocular myopathy.

With 5 patients, a prevalence rate of 7 per 100,000 population was described in Carlisle, England (Brewis et al. 1966). The four males were children with the Duchenne type; the only woman had adult limb-girdle dystrophy. In Iceland, Gudmundsson (1968b) recorded a prevalence rate of 9 per 100,000 population, with 17 living patients; 2 others had died before prevalence day. Eleven had the Duchenne type, 1 the facioscapulohumeral type, and 7 the limb-girdle type.

In Rochester, Minnesota, 1945-54, there were 4 diagnosed cases (1 Duchenne and 3 facioscapulohumeral type) in the 30,000 local population (Kurland 1958a). On the day prevalence was determined, 2 patients with the facioscapulohumeral type were living in Rochester (prevalence rate about 6 per 100,000 population).

The incidence of Duchenne muscular dystrophy was calculated at 33 per 100,000 males who survived to age 5 in northeastern England, or a rate of 17 per 100,000 for both sexes (Gardner-Medwin 1970). Morton and Chung (1959), by combining data from several series in the United States and England, estimated an incidence of 14 per 100,000 live births for the Duchenne type, 7 per 100,000 for the limb-girdle type, and 0.4 per 100,000 for the facioscapulohumeral type. In their own series, however, the rate for the Duchenne type was 28 per 100,000.

Myotonic Dystrophy

National mortality data for myotonic dystrophy are not available.

In Gudmundsson's survey (1968b), 18 (from 5 families) who were affected with the disorder were alive on the day prevalence was estimated in Iceland, for a rate of 10 per 100,000 population (Table 6.10). The Northumberland study indicated a prevalence rate of 1 per 100,000 population, based on 15 cases in the same community (Walton and Nattrass 1954). There were also 6 cases of myotonia congenita. In Carlisle (Brewis et al. 1966), the prevalence rate was 3 per 100,000 population, based on 2 cases. The same rate was recorded for Rochester, Minnesota (Kurland 1958a), with 1 case.

Table 6.10 Cases and prevalence rates per 100,000 population for myotonic dystrophy: selected surveys, various years, about 1952-67

Survey area (source)	Year	Cases	Rate
Rochester, Minnesota (Kurland 1958a)	1955	1	3
Northumberland-Durham, England (Walton and Nattrass 1954)	c.1952	15	1
Carlisle, England (Brewis et al. 1966)	1961	2	3
Iceland (Gudmundsson 1968b)	1963	18	10
Guam (Chamorros) (Chen et al. 1968)	1967	29	76

A recent study of the indigenous (Chamorro) population of Guam (Chen et al. 1968) disclosed a remarkable concentration of 29 patients in 4 apparently unrelated families, as of January 1, 1967. The pedigrees were compatible with that of an autosomal dominant trait. The prevalence rate of 76 per 100,000 population was the highest yet reported anywhere. There was no obvious relation between these cases and the amyotrophic lateral sclerosis, which was also prevalent on the island; the observation of myotonic dystrophy in the small population of the Kii Peninsula of Japan where ALS likewise was unduly prevalent is also unexplained, but could be more than coincidence.

In large populations, a rate of 1 to 3 per 100,000 population might be expected on the basis of the results of the English and Rochester surveys, but the possibility remains that the general prevalence rate may be appreciably higher. Both the Guam and Iceland surveys were conducted for neurologic diseases in general, without prior suspicion that the prevalence rate for any specific disease (other than ALS on Guam) was unusually high. The question arises then whether island populations in particular somehow carry a higher risk for the disease, or whether by chance the populations of the two islands studied happened to be extraordinary with respect to this disease. The populations of Iceland and Guam contain more males than females and are relatively inbred. Inbreeding per se does not influence the gene frequency if the trait is transmitted as a dominant; however, if the gene had been introduced when the population was small, it could by now account for a relatively large portion of the gene pool.

Inheritance is uniformly of an autosomal dominant nature (Thomasen 1948; Pratt 1967), even though there is a clinical impression that it is found more often in males (Merritt 1967). Perhaps the testicular atrophy that is characteristic leads to recognition of more cases of milder disease in the male.

Polymyositis

There are few estimates as to the incidence of polymyositis. This is a group of disorders classified according to Barwick and Walton (1963) as idiopathic (group 1), associated with mild collagen disease (group 2), associated with severe collagen disease (group 3), and associated with malignancy (group 4). Patients in group 1 may have acute polymyositis with myoglobulinuria, or—as in the other groups—the patients may have a subacute or chronic form.

The clinical characteristics of polymyositis are weakness and atrophy of striated muscle, most often of the limb-girdles, with the upper more involved than the lower. Fasciculations and atrophy are sometimes observed and fibrillation potentials may be detected in the electromyogram (EMG). Pain and tenderness of the muscle are common in the acute disease, and in the most florid cases systemic symptoms such as fever and malaise may occur. Pathologically, the muscles show degeneration and regeneration with round cell infiltrations. The erythrocyte sedimentation rate and serum enzyme levels are often elevated.

The diagnosis of polymyositis may be difficult. The differentiation must be made from limb-girdle dystrophy, "mixed" dystrophy, progressive myelopathic muscular atrophy, acute anterior poliomyelitis, and thyrotoxic myopathy.

The age at onset in the idiopathic variety of polymyositis may be from infancy to the senium, but the incidence is maximal in mid-adult life. In clinical series (Barwick and Walton 1963; Logan et al. 1966; Rose and Walton 1966) there was a female preponderance with a male-female case ratio of 0.5 to 1. Cases have been reported from all continents, and all races have been affected.

In Newcastle-on-Tyne, Barwick and Walton (1963) encountered 52 cases in the five years 1958-62. Of these, about one-third were considered idiopathic and about one-eighth were associated with malignancy. The remainder were associated with various collagen diseases.

The case series of Barwick and Walton (1963) has been enlarged to cover 1954-65 and includes 89 cases in the Northumberland population of about 2,300,000, from which Rose and Walton (1966) have estimated an average annual incidence rate of about 0.3 per 100,000 population. Pearson (1966) has collected a large series of cases and has estimated that the incidence rate was about 0.1 per 100,000 population in the United States. He found no genetic basis for the rare familial cases encountered. In Rochester, Minnesota, the average annual incidence rate for polymyositis was 0.6 per 100,000 population, and the prevalence rate was 6.3 (Kurland et al. 1969*b*). As the disorder becomes better recognized, all of these rates probably will be considered underestimates.

Other Myopathies

There is a group of glycogenoses, periodic paralyses, and other myopathies (such as thyrotoxic) that are classed as metabolic myopathies (McArdle 1963). Specific acute infectious myopathies would include trichinosis. Myopathies associated with sarcoidosis are also encountered. All our information on these rare entities comes from hospital series. In long-standing myasthenia gravis (see Chapter 7), a true myopathy occurs occasionally. In addition, new clinical entities are still being described and their position in the scheme of neuromuscular diseases remains to be clarified.

7 / MYASTHENIA GRAVIS

Leonard T. Kurland
Nung Won Choi
Irving D. Goldberg
John F. Kurtzke

Myasthenia gravis (MG), described by Thomas Willis in 1672, is a clinical entity of unknown cause that is characterized by striated muscle weakness and fatiguability. The clinical manifestations apparently are caused by a defect in the transmission of the nerve impulse at the myoneural junction (Merritt 1967). The disease may remain localized (for example, limited to the extraocular muscles) or it may become generalized. If the disease is generalized, the prognosis may be serious; if death occurs, it is then generally the result of ventilatory insufficiency. Drugs such as physostigmine or other anticholinesterases are important as diagnostic aids as well as in treatment. There are no consistent pathologic findings by light microscopy. The significance of changes seen at the motor end-plate region under the electron microscope is still uncertain.

Recent emphasis on autoimmune mechanisms of disease has led some to include MG in this category, a decision based largely on the clinical effect of thymectomy in some myasthenics and the finding (by fluorescent staining techniques) of antimuscle antibodies on the muscle fiber in some but not all patients. The significance of this last has been questioned because the antibodies are not at the site of the presumed lesion, the myoneural junction.

Recently, Goldstein and Hofmann (1969) elaborated on Goldstein's concept (1966) which, if substantiated, might explain the pathophysiology of this disorder. In their view, myasthenia gravis may be an autoimmune disease, but to thymus and not to muscle, since the thymus normally contains muscle-like cells. These investigators produced in guinea pigs and rats an autoimmune thymitis and what seemed to be a myasthenic syndrome, as indicated by nerve conduction studies and electromyography. The miniature end-plate potentials were believed to be reduced, as they are in human MG (but measurement of these potentials is difficult). The antigen, with a molecular weight of about 1,500, was called by these authors "thymine" and is also found in lesser amounts in normal thymus. Their interpretation of these findings was that perhaps "myasthenia gravis is thymotoxicosis." Future development of this concept will be followed with great interest. At the moment, though, the etiology of MG is unknown.

Mortality Data

International Mortality Comparisons

Because of the very low mortality from myasthenia gravis, the death rates for this disorder are presented in this chapter on a population base of 1,000,000 rather than the conventional 100,000 base used elsewhere in this monograph. This should be borne in mind when comparisons are made with the other rates.

The average annual mortality rate for myasthenia gravis as a primary cause of death in the United States was about 1.4 per 1,000,000 during the years 1950-54. In Canada, in 1951, the rate was 1.3 per 1,000,000 population for MG deaths coded to the underlying cause. However, by including the deaths listed as "contributory" or "complication," the rate became 2.2, which must be interpreted as that for persons dying *with* myasthenia gravis. In Norway and New Zealand, with 10 and 7 deaths respectively for the year 1951-54, the annual death rates for MG as an underlying cause were about 0.6 and 0.8 per 1,000,000 (Kurland and Alter 1961).

In Finland for 1957-66, Hokkanen (1969) reported for MG as the underlying cause of death an annual mortality rate of 0.9 per 1,000,000 population (0.7 among cases that he was able to confirm). Of the 48 deaths from his clinical series, 35 had MG coded as the underlying cause of death and 4 had it mentioned as a contributory cause; in 9 cases, there was no mention of MG on the death certificate.

Myasthenia gravis is coded as 744.0 in the Sixth and Seventh Revisions of the ISC, but deaths from causes coded to four digits are not routinely tabulated separately by most countries. However, Goldberg and Kurland (unpublished data) were able to determine the approximate death rates for myasthenia gravis in the following nine countries for different periods from 1951 to 1958: Canada (1953-57), Iceland (1951-55), Ireland (1954-58), Israel (1956-58), Italy (1955-57), New Zealand (1952-56), Norway (1953-57), Sweden (1954-57), and the United States (1953-57). For most of these countries, the crude rates were approximately 1 per 1,000,000 population (exceptions were Iceland with no deaths and Ireland with a rate of about 0.3 per 1,000,000). These data, along with those previously cited, indicate little if any material difference in the MG death rates among the countries considered, particularly in view of the few deaths involved.

United States Mortality Data, Trend

The crude death rates per 1,000,000 population for MG in the United States varied little between 1950 (1.5) and 1961 (1.3), and more recent data from the vital statistics reports of the United States show that the rate continued essentially unchanged each subsequent year through 1967, when the rate was 1.3 per 1,000,000. Although the highest rates were observed in 1950-52, this may be related to the fact that these were the first few years when MG was separately coded as an underlying cause of death according to the International Statistical Classification (Sixth Revision), and hence may represent artifacts of coding or reporting. In this regard, it is interesting to note that for inborn defect of muscle, ISC code 744.1 (see Chapter 6), the reverse was true: the death rate during 1949-51 was *lower* than in the subsequent sixteen years. In any event, during this entire eighteen-year period the MG death rate centered at about 1.3 per 1,000,000, ranging only from 1.1 to 1.6, without any discernible trend. Although a differential reporting of MG as underlying or secondary cause of death when the condition is known to exist at the time of death may have occurred during the period, there is no way to determine how this could have influenced the annual death rates over time.

United States Mortality Data, 1959-61

Age, sex, and color. Of 675 death certificates listing MG as the primary cause of death during 1959-61, more than 95 percent were for persons 15 years of age or older. This would indicate that "juvenile" MG accounted for only a small fraction of all MG deaths (Table A.7.1). The annual age-specific rates were less than 1 per 1,000,000 below age 15. The rate reached 1 at the 35-44 year age group and increased steadily to a maximum of about 6 at the 75-84 year group. The small numbers do not facilitate comparison by age, but females had a higher rate than males at each age group from 5 through 64 years of age, after which there was little difference by sex. For the nonwhites, among whom there were 108 deaths in these years, the rate reached 1 per 1,000,000 in the age group 15-24 years,

Table 7.1 Average annual crude and age-adjusted death rates per 1,000,000 population for myasthenia gravis by age, color and sex: United States, 1959-61[a] (ISC code 744.0)

Color and sex	Crude rate All ages	Age-adjusted rate		
		All ages	Under 15	65 & over
Total				
Total	1.3	1.2	0.2*	5.3
Male	1.0	0.9*	0.1*	5.8
Female	1.5	1.4	0.2*	5.0
White				
Total	1.2	1.0	0.1*	5.5
Male	1.0	0.9*	0.1*	6.0
Female	1.4	1.2	0.1*	5.1
Nonwhite				
Total	1.8	2.0*	0.4*	2.8*
Male	1.2	1.4*	0.1*	2.7*
Female	2.3	2.6*	0.6*	2.9*

[a] Detail in Table A.7.1.

and beyond that age it varied between 2 and 4 until the group age 85 or older, when it was 9.3 based on only 2 deaths. However, in all these age groups, the rates were subject to appreciable chance fluctuations. The age-adjusted rate, all ages combined, was greater for females than for males of either color group (Table 7.1). The age-adjusted rate for nonwhites was twice that for whites, with the excess mortality in the former limited to those under age 65 (Table A.7.1). Because Negroes accounted for 103 of the 108 nonwhite deaths, no assessment of racial variations among nonwhites is feasible.

Geographic distribution. The average annual age-adjusted death rates, all ages combined, varied only slightly for the nine geographic regions (Table 7.2). When the rates for whites only were considered, the findings were the same. Kurland and Alter (1961) reported a relatively even distribution of mortality rates among the same nine census regions of the United States for 1950-54.

The age-adjusted death rates for nonwhites varied by region, the highest being 4.8 per 1,000,000 population for New England and the

Table 7.2 Average annual age-adjusted death rates per 1,000,000 population for myasthenia gravis by color and sex: United States and census regions, 1959-61 (ISC code 744.0)

Region	Total			White			Nonwhite		
	Total	M	F	Total	M	F	Total	M	F
United States	1.2	0.9*	1.4	1.0	0.9*	1.2	2.0*	1.4*	2.6*
New England	1.2*	1.0*	1.3*	1.1*	1.0*	1.2*	4.8*	2.6*	6.8*
Middle Atlantic	1.2*	0.7*	1.5*	1.1*	0.7*	1.5*	2.2*	0.6*	3.6*
East North Central	1.2*	1.0*	1.7*	1.1*	1.0*	1.2*	2.9*	2.0*	3.8*
West North Central	1.2*	1.1*	1.2*	1.1*	1.0*	1.2*	1.7*	2.4*	1.1*
South Atlantic	1.1*	1.0*	1.2*	1.0*	1.0*	1.0*	1.4*	1.0*	1.7*
East South Central	1.3*	1.1*	1.4*	1.1*	0.9*	1.2*	2.0*	1.8*	2.2*
West South Central	1.2*	0.9*	1.5*	1.0*	0.8*	1.3*	2.0*	1.4*	2.6*
Mountain	0.7*	0.5*	1.0*	0.8*	0.5*	1.0*	-	-	-
Pacific	1.1*	0.9*	1.3*	0.9*	0.7*	1.1*	2.4*	2.0*	3.0*

lowest the Mountain region (with no deaths in its small nonwhite population) and 1.4 for the South Atlantic region, as shown in Table 7.2. Inasmuch as the rates for nonwhites were based on few deaths, the differences by geographic region may reflect chance variations or possible differences in diagnosis and reporting. The rates for nonwhites exceeded those for whites in eight of the nine regions. If there is a true color difference, the differences should be at least as great where medical facilities are above average as where they are below average. And indeed this was true; the most discrepant regions by color included the New England, East North Central, and Pacific regions, and the least difference was found in the South Atlantic region.

Type of county. There was no recognizable pattern to the distribution of MG age-adjusted death rates when the regions were subdivided into metropolitan and nonmetropolitan counties (Table A.7.2). Comparison of the rates per 1,000,000 for those 65 or older revealed that metropolitan death rates were 4.7 for whites and 3.7 for nonwhites, and those for nonmetropolitan areas were 6.9 and 1.5 respectively (Table A.7.3). There were, in all, only 11 deaths among nonwhites age 65 or older. Characterization of the individual geographic regions as to the type of county for MG deaths of the elderly probably was not reliable and showed no clear-cut pattern.

Table 7.3 Average annual age-adjusted death rates per 1,000,000 population for myasthenia gravis, white persons, by sex and nativity: United States and census regions, 1959-61

(ISC code 744.0)

Region	Native born			Foreign born		
	Total	Male	Female	Total	Male	Female
United States	1.1	0.9*	1.3	0.9*	1.0*	0.9*
New England	1.1*	1.0*	1.2*	0.6*	0.6*	0.7*
Middle Atlantic	1.1*	0.7*	1.5*	1.4*	0.8*	1.8*
East North Central	1.1*	0.9*	1.2*	1.0*	1.6*	0.4*
West North Central	1.2*	1.1*	1.2*	0.3*	0.1*	0.5*
South Atlantic	1.0*	1.0*	1.1*	1.1*	2.5*	-
East South Central	1.1*	0.9*	1.2*	-	-	-
West South Central	1.1*	0.8*	1.3*	0.9*	-	1.8*
Mountain	0.8*	0.6*	1.0*	0.4*	-	0.8*
Pacific	1.0*	0.7*	1.2*	0.6*	0.9*	0.3*

Nativity. Age-adjusted death rates for the foreign born differed little from those for the native born: 0.9 versus 1.1 per 1,000,000 for all ages. There were no noteworthy deviations by region for native and foreign born when the small number of cases, particularly among foreign born, was considered (Table 7.3).

Morbidity Data

Clinical series on MG are numerous, and these have been reviewed by Storm-Mathisen (1961; 1966). There are but few morbidity series with a population-based denominator (Table 7.4).

Incidence and prevalence rates for MG were presented by Kurland and Alter (1961) from surveys of Rochester, Minnesota (Kurland 1958a), and of Charleston County, South Carolina, and Halifax County, Nova Scotia (Alter and Talbert, unpublished data). Similar survey methods were used, incorporating a review of hospital records for the ten-year period 1945-54. In the Rochester study, records of the Mayo Clinic and affiliated hospitals in Rochester were taken as representing all major diagnosed illnesses in the community; in the other regions, practicing physicians also were canvassed for cases.

Prevalence

The MG prevalence rates per 1,000,000 population were 33 in Rochester, 26 in Charleston, and 5 in Halifax (Table 7.4). However, the rates are based on so few cases that no conclusions regarding possible differences can be drawn.

Garland and Clark (1956) reviewed their personal series of MG patients and estimated the prevalence rate in Leeds, England, in 1955 as 26 per 1,000,000, with 13 cases.

Storm-Mathisen (1961; 1966), who believed she would know of practically all suspected cases of MG in Norway through her clinic in

Table 7.4 Cases and average annual incidence rates and point prevalence rates per 1,000,000 population for myasthenia gravis from population surveys: selected areas, various years, 1941-65

Survey area and years (source)	Incidence		Prevalence[a]	
	Cases	Rate	Cases	Rate
Rochester, Minnesota (1945-54) (Kurland 1958a)	1	3	1	33
Charleston, South Carolina (1945-54) (Alter and Talbert, unpublished data)	11	5	6	26
Halifax, Canada (1945-54) (Alter and Talbert, unpublished data)	3	2	1	5
Leeds, England (1955) (Garland and Clark 1956)	---	---	13	26
Merseyside, England (1948-58) (Pennington and Wilson 1961)	33	2	32	23
Norway (1941-50) (Storm-Mathisen 1961)	(?)	2	70	22
Iceland (1954-63) (Gudmundsson 1968b)	14	4	12	64
Rochester, Minnesota (1960) (Kurland and Choi, unpublished data)	---	---	2	43
Finland (1956-65) (Hokkanen 1969)	102	2	117	25
Helsinki Central Hospital District (1956-65) (Hokkanen 1969)	31	4	40	42

[a]Prevalence day was at the end of the period cited except for the last two rates (Hokkanen) which were in 1968.

Oslo, provided a detailed description of a series in excess of 300 cases. As of 1950, the prevalence rate was calculated at 22 per 1,000,000 from 70 cases.

A more recent estimate of the prevalence rate for MG in Rochester, Minnesota, was 43 per 1,000,000, based on 2 cases (Kurland and Choi, unpublished data); 95-percent confidence limits on this rate are about 5 and 155. Again, no conclusion regarding any geographic pattern can be drawn.

The Merseyside conurbation, which includes Liverpool, is a well-defined region of the Lancashire-Cheshire plain of England. The prevalence rate for MG in 1958 was 23 per 1,000,000, with 32 living patients, according to the study of Pennington and Wilson (1961). In this study, as well as that of Storm-Mathisen (1961), the highest rates were noted for females 15-24 years old.

Gudmundsson (1968b) delineated the population characteristics of neurologic disease in Iceland. In 1963 the prevalence rate for MG, based on 12 living patients, was 64 per 1,000,000 population.

Recently, Finland was surveyed by Hokkanen (1969). The prevalence rate in 1968 was 25 per 1,000,000 population, with 117 cases. When the 40 cases from the Helsinki Central Hospital District alone were considered, a prevalence rate of 42 per 1,000,000 was calculated. Of the 117 cases, 32 were males and 85 females (populations by sex were not provided). Age at onset was somewhat concentrated between 11 and 50 years but ranged from the neonatal period to age 75.

Incidence

In the studies cited above the average annual incidence rates per 1,000,000 for MG were 3 in Rochester, 5 in Charleston, and 2 in Halifax, for 1945-54 (Table 7.4). In Merseyside, England, an incidence rate of 2 was noted in the 1948-58 period. The rate was also 2 in Norway for 1941-50 and was 4 in Iceland for the ten years 1954-63.

The annual incidence rate in Finland for 1956-65 was 2.3 per 1,000,000 population, with 102 cases. In the Helsinki Central Hospital District, the rate was 3.5 for the 31 cases, and in the city of Helsinki, it was 3.4 for the 17 cases.

Thus annual incidence rates per 1,000,000 for MG were about 3 or 4 and prevalence rates about 30 or 40 per 1,000,000 population—or about ten times the incidence rates.

Familial Features

The relative importance of genetic and environmental factors must still be clarified. The reported familial aggregations and twin cases of MG, extensively reviewed by Kurland and Alter (1961), did not seem to constitute sufficient evidence to suggest that genetic factors have an obvious role in the etiology of MG.

More recently, familial aggregation has been reported by Herrmann (1966), who suggested that exposure to a common factor in early childhood was one explanation for the familial cases. When the bias in case reports (one does not ordinarily report nonfamilial MG) and the sometimes difficult differential diagnosis from the myopathies are taken into account, it is not feasible to draw any conclusions regarding the relative importance of genetic and environmental factors in the etiology of MG.

Comment

Myasthenia gravis is a rare disease. The average annual death rates for MG as underlying cause were about 1 per 1,000,000 population in most of the countries for which data were available. The death rate for nonwhites in the United States was about 2 per 1,000,000 versus 1 for whites.

For both color groups, death rates for females with MG were higher than those for males until about age 65, after which the rates tended to be about the same. Overall, the rate for females was about 1.5 times that for males. There was no notable variation by region in the United States or by nativity.

From several population surveys, the average annual incidence rate of MG seemed to be about 3 or 4 per 1,000,000 and the prevalence rate about 30 to 40 per 1,000,000.

Although familial cases of MG have been recorded, no genetic patterns were discernible and the relative etiologic roles of heredity and environment are still to be established. The geographic uniformity and the rarity of the illness, however, do not suggest the existence of any particular environmental cause or precipitant, despite differences by sex and perhaps by color. The present epidemiologic studies have contributed little to direct etiologic studies. Metabolic, endocrine, or immune mechanisms would seem appropriate routes of etiologic investigation.

8 / DOWN'S SYNDROME

John F. Kurtzke
Irving D. Goldberg
Leonard T. Kurland

In Down's syndrome, mental retardation is associated with typical physical appearance: brachycephalic skull, epicanthal folds, narrowed palpebral fissures, depression of the bridge of the nose, large tongue, deformed earlobes, and changes in hands and feet with a simian palmar crease and a crease between hallux and second toe. Other neural and somatic anomalies may coexist (Merritt 1967). The term formerly used for this entity was mongolism (ISC Seventh Revision, code 325.4, and ICDA Eighth Revision, code 759.3). For obvious reasons, however, Down's syndrome is the preferred—albeit unofficial—designation, at least insofar as the Seventh Revision of the ISC is concerned.

A chromosomal aberration has been described in this disorder. Trisomy for chromosomes 21 (Denver system) caused by nondisjunction is found in the most common type of Down's syndrome, and this is the type that is associated with increased maternal age. A less common type with no relation to the age of the mother is that with translocation, usually for chromosomes 13-15. According to Penrose and Smith (1966), the translocation types are present in 2 to 3 percent of the cases, and a third type called mosaic mongolism (an admixture of cells with both normal and abnormal chromosomes) comprises perhaps another 2 percent of the cases of Down's syndrome.

A thorough review of the epidemiology of mongolism has been provided by Lilienfeld and Benesch (1969). They stressed the importance of separating the types of mongolism in epidemiologic inquiries and offered some estimates as to how this might influence various characteristics of such patients. However, except for selected series, the actual chromosomal analyses on which these differentiations currently rest are unavailable. In this chapter, therefore, Down's syndrome will be considered as a unit.

Mortality Data

For this disorder, mortality data based only on the primary (underlying) cause of death are likely to understate greatly the numbers affected. For the United States in 1955, only 87 deaths were attributed to Down's syndrome as the underlying cause among an estimated 1,516 deaths in which the condition was listed on the death certificate (National Center for Health Statistics 1965). To anticipate data to be presented, Down's syndrome as underlying cause of death under 1 year of age occurred at a rate of 4.3 per 100,000 in 1959-61, and this age group accounted for about three-fifths of all deaths coded to Down's in those years. From these figures, we may estimate that 7 per 100,000 eventually die with this cause listed as underlying on the death certificate. Multiplying this rate by 17.43, the ratio of total deaths with Down's syndrome to those where it was cited as underlying cause in 1955, we would predict from the total deaths an incidence rate of about 122 per 100,000 live births. As also will be seen, this last figure closely approximates the actual reported incidence of 1.2 per 1,000 live births for Down's. It is conceivable, therefore, that virtually all deaths referable to this condition would be retrievable if secondary causes of death were available. For the present, though, as in the remainder of this work, we are able to assess only those deaths coded as primary cause—and for Down's syndrome, only for the United States.

United States, Trend

Data are unavailable from the international comparisons for the 1950s as used in the other chapters because the status of Down's syndrome as a four-digit code in the ISC rendered it irretrievable from routine mortality statistics.

In the United States, deaths coded to Down's syndrome as an underlying cause were recorded for 1958-67. The rate per 100,000 population, all ages, varied between 0.1 and 0.2 with no consistent deviations. Accordingly, for this short period, there is no evidence of changing frequency in mortality from Down's syndrome.

Lilienfeld and Benesch (1969) reviewed the mortality experience reported in several series of patients with Down's syndrome. Studies through the 1950s revealed that less than half of the patients survived to the age of 10 years, with the greatest loss in the first years of life. A much more favorable experience was recorded by Forssman and Åkesson (1965) from Sweden, based on deaths in hospitals for the retarded. It is clear, though, that early infantile deaths were excluded from this series. It may be that the age-specific mortality rates to be reported next for the United States in 1959-61 may have changed their pattern, as supportive care and antibiotics became available, to one less pronounced in infancy than in earlier years. However, death rates are still maximal at the earliest ages.

United States, 1959-61

Age. There were 871 deaths coded to Down's syndrome as underlying cause of death in 1959-61. The average annual death rates by sex and color are summarized in Table 8.1, with supportive data provided in Table A.8.1. The crude rate, all ages, was 0.2 per 100,000 population, age adjusted to 0.1. About 60 percent of all

Table 8.1 Average annual death rates per 100,000 population for Down's syndrome by age, color and sex: United States, 1959-61[a]

(ISC code 325.4)

Color and sex	Crude rate					Age-adjusted rate	
	All ages	Under 1	Under 5	Under 15	15 & over	All ages	Under 15
Total							
Total	0.2	4.3	1.2	0.5	0.0	0.1	0.4
Male	0.2	4.3	1.2	0.5	0.0	0.1*	0.4
Female	0.2	4.2	1.1	0.4	0.0	0.1*	0.4
White							
Total	0.2	4.6	1.2	0.5	0.0	0.1*	0.4
Male	0.2	4.6	1.2	0.5	0.0	0.1*	0.4
Female	0.2	4.5	1.2	0.5	0.0	0.1*	0.4
Nonwhite							
Total	0.1	2.6	0.7	0.3	0.0*	0.1*	0.2*
Male	0.1	2.7	0.8	0.3	0.0*	0.1*	0.2*
Female	0.1	2.5	0.6	0.3	0.0*	0.1*	0.2*

[a] Detail in Table A.8.1.

deaths occurred under 1 year of age, providing an age-specific rate of 4.3 per 100,000 under 1 year. Age-specific rates declined rapidly to 0.4 for ages 1-4 and to 0.1 for ages 5-14. For age 15 and above, all the rates were less than 0.05 per 100,000; there were only 102 deaths, or less than 12 percent of the total number, at or over age 15 years.

Sex. At each age the death rates for Down's syndrome were equivalent for males and females, whether white or nonwhite (Table 8.1). The minor variations between the sexes by geographic region or by type of county are without any consistent pattern, and generally are within the bounds of chance fluctuation (Tables 8.2 and 8.3).

Color. Death rates for whites with this disorder were almost twice those for nonwhites, regardless of age or sex (Table 8.1). This was found also for residents of both metropolitan and nonmetropolitan counties. Although assessment of color within the nine census regions is affected by the small number of nonwhite deaths, there being but 70 in the United States during 1959-61 for both sexes combined, the pattern of higher mortality among whites persists in all regions. The consistency of the difference at each age group (and for residence in each type of county) suggests that this two-to-one difference by color may have validity. However, the questions raised in prior chapters as to death data for nonwhites are especially pertinent here because of the small numbers of deaths, particularly since these deaths as underlying cause account for only a small proportion of deaths *with* Down's syndrome.

Geographic distribution. The rates for deaths under 1 year of age provide perhaps the best measure of comparison for this disorder. In Table 8.2, these rates are distributed according to census region and by sex and color. Owing to small numbers, rates for nonwhites must be considered too unstable for assessment. Even for whites, the numbers in several regions are not large (Table A.8.2). The rates by region are rather homogeneous. There is no discernible north-south difference when the comparison is limited to whites. There is a suggestion of a possible east-west trend (higher in the east), but this is minimal and irregular at best. Death rates under 1 year of age by state are shown in Fig. 8.1, with data given in Table A.8.3. By state—and with the constraints imposed by the numbers of deaths —there is no evidence to suggest any appreciable geographic variation

Table 8.2 Average annual death rates per 100,000 population under one year of age for Down's syndrome by color and sex: United States and census regions, 1959-61[a] (ISC code 325.4)

Region	Total			White			Nonwhite		
	Total	M	F	Total	M	F	Total	M	F
United States	4.3	4.3	4.2	4.6	4.6	4.5	2.6	2.7	2.5
New England	4.6	5.4*	3.8*	4.8	5.6*	4.0*	-	-	-
Mid. Atlantic	4.8	4.9	4.8	5.0	4.9	5.2	3.4*	5.1*	1.7*
E. No. Central	4.3	4.1	4.5	4.5	4.2	4.8	2.2*	3.0*	1.5*
W. No. Central	4.3	5.3	3.2*	4.4	5.4	3.4*	1.6*	3.2*	-
So. Atlantic	4.2	4.2	4.1	4.6	5.2	4.1	3.0*	1.9*	4.1*
E. So. Central	4.0	3.0*	5.0	5.1	3.2*	7.1	1.2*	2.4*	-
W. So. Central	4.4	4.0	4.8	4.5	4.0	5.0	3.8*	3.8*	3.8*
Mountain	3.9	4.0*	3.8*	4.0	4.3*	3.7*	2.5*	-	5.1*
Pacific	3.7	4.1	3.3	4.0	4.5	3.4	1.8*	1.2*	2.5*

[a]Number of deaths in Table A.8.2.

Table 8.3 Average annual death rates per 100,000 population under one year of age for Down's syndrome by color, sex and type of county: United States, 1959-61 (ISC code 325.4)

Color & sex	Metropolitan counties			Nonmetropolitan counties
	Total	With central city	Without central city	
Total	4.2	4.1	4.6	4.4
Male	4.4	4.3	4.7	4.3
Female	4.0	3.9	4.5	4.5
White	4.5	4.4	4.8	4.7
Male	4.6	4.6	4.9	4.6
Female	4.3	4.3	4.7	4.8
Nonwhite	2.6	2.6	2.0*	2.7*
Male	2.7*	2.8*	2.1*	2.7*
Female	2.4*	2.4*	2.0*	2.7*

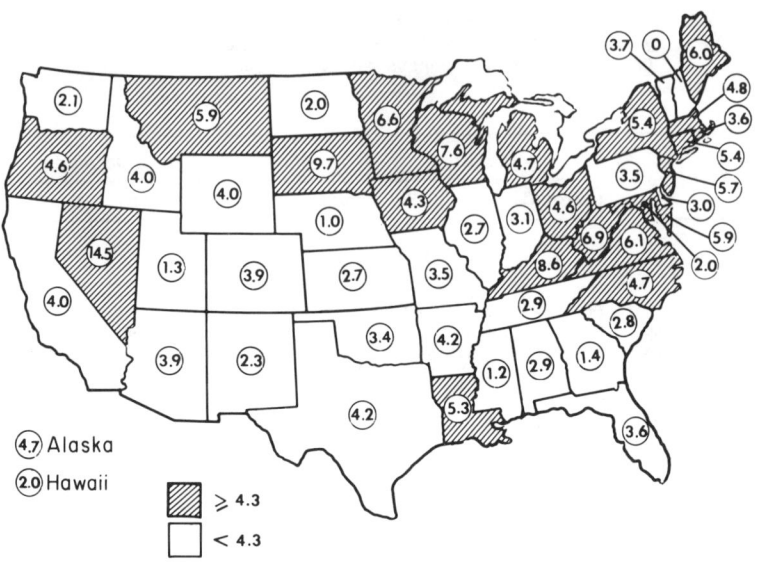

Figure 8.1 Average annual death rates per 100,000 population under 1 year of age for Down's syndrome by state: United States, 1959–61. All but eight rates are based on less than 20 deaths (see Table A.8.3).

in death rates for Down's syndrome in the United States. Most of the rates among the states were concentrated between 3 and 6 deaths per 100,000 population under 1 year of age.

Type of county. Table 8.3 defines the death rates under 1 year of age for Down's syndrome according to color and sex for residents of metropolitan and nonmetropolitan counties, with the former further subdivided according to whether or not the county contained a central city. The overall metropolitan rates are essentially equivalent to the nonmetropolitan rates. Metropolitan counties with central cities had rates somewhat below those without central cities among the whites, and somewhat above among the nonwhites. An apparent male excess in metropolitan counties is counterbalanced by a similar female excess in nonmetropolitan counties.

The differences by type of county within each color-sex group are relatively small and within the bounds of chance fluctuation. Indeed, the rates by type of county are surprisingly close when one considers the possibilities of bias resulting from artifacts of reporting, the small proportion of deaths reported as primary cause, and the small numbers themselves within many of the cells of Table 8.3. As to this

Table 8.4 Cases and incidence rates per 1,000 live births for Down's syndrome: selected surveys, various years, 1935-67

Survey area (source)	Years	Cases	Rate
Rochester, Minnesota (Kurland 1958a)	1945-54	14	1.9
Rochester, Minnesota (Gibson and Kurland, unpublished)	1935-67	36	1.4
Carlisle, England (Brewis et al. 1966)	1955-61	10	1.2
Victoria, Australia (Collmann and Stoller 1962a)	1942-57	1,134	1.5
Seeland, Denmark (Øster 1953)	1938-48	71	1.6
Birmingham, England (Record and Smith 1955)	1942-52	252	1.1[a]
Northamptonshire, England (Pleydell 1957)	1956	86	1.6[a]
WHO, 24 centers (Stevenson et al. 1966b)	1961-64	347	0.9
WHO, 24 centers (Stevenson et al. 1966b)	1961-64	347	0.8[a]

[a] Total births, including stillbirths.

last, there were only 71 deaths under 1 year coded as Down's syndrome among residents of metropolitan counties without central cities in the entire United States during these three years. We should note, however, that the excess of whites over nonwhites in the death rates from Down's syndrome persists in both the urban (metropolitan) and rural (nonmetropolitan) counties. With the exception of the difference by color, the impression remains that the distribution in Down's syndrome deaths is homogeneous.

Morbidity Data

Frequency of Down's Syndrome

Rates per unit number of births provide a useful measure of the frequency of disorders apparent at or shortly after birth. In Table 8.4 are summarized such incidence rates per 1,000 births from several major surveys. Despite the small numbers, the experience at Rochester, Minnesota, and Carlisle, England, are presented not merely in keeping with other chapters of this work, but also because there is no reason to suspect any special bias in these studies that might arise when a specific disease is studied; these were population surveys for a broad range of disorders.

Rochester, Minnesota. Between 1935 and 1967, 36 children with Down's syndrome were born to residents in Rochester, Minnesota (Gibson and Kurland, unpublished data). This provides a rate of about 1.4 per 1,000 births (Table 8.4). With these small numbers, concentrations by year or season were not evident. The 25 males and 11 females provided a male-female sex ratio of 2.3 to 1. However, for a relative frequency of 11 females in 36 cases, the 95-percent confidence interval includes 48 percent females, which in turn is compatible with a male-female ratio as low as 1.1 to 1. The rate of 1.4 for 1935-66 would seem more valid than the 1.9 reported for the decade 1945-53 (Kurland 1958*a*).

Carlisle, England. In Carlisle, England, Brewis and her associates (1966) noted a rate of 1.2 per 1,000 live births, based on 10 affected children born during 1955-61. No breakdown by sex was provided.

Victoria, Australia. An extensive survey was performed by Collmann and Stoller (1962*a* and *b*; 1965) over a sixteen-year period in Victoria, Australia. In this study an urban-rural difference was found, unlike the United States mortality data previously noted. The incidence was higher for urban mothers, although the distributions of the mothers' ages at parturition were similar. The incidence was 1.6 per 1,000 live births for the 770 infants with Down's syndrome born to urban mothers, as opposed to 1.2 per 1,000 for the 364 born to rural mothers (Collmann and Stoller 1962*a*). In another report (Stoller and Collmann 1965), these authors pointed out a cyclic rate in the frequency of this disorder, with peaks approximately eight years apart, the last two of which followed closely the incidence curve for infectious hepatitis. While additional evidence for such a relationship exists (Doxiadis et al. 1970*a* and *b*; Kučera 1970), neither this finding nor Collmann and Stoller's contention of clustering of mongolism has yet received definitive confirmation. This problem is considered in some detail by Lilienfeld and Benesch (1969), with the comment: "From this review of many studies conducted and reported on in the past 10 years, no clear, consistent pattern of temporo-spatial clustering or of seasonal distribution emerges."

Denmark. Øster, in 1953, before the chromosomal basis for this disorder was recognized, reported an extensive survey of Down's syndrome in Denmark and elsewhere. From Seeland, where he considered the rates most accurate, the incidence rate was reported as 1.6 per 1,000 live births for 1938-48.

England. Record and Smith (1955) found that the incidence rate for Down's syndrome was 1.1 per 1,000 total births (live births plus stillborn) in Birmingham, England, for 1942-52. For their 252 cases, a male-to-female ratio of 1.2 to 1 was found. In Northamptonshire, England, Pleydell (1957) found 1.6 per 1,000 total births based on 86 diagnosed cases. In this work rates by sex were not provided.

WHO survey. Although there have been numerous series otherwise emanating from hospitals, an important study under the auspices of the World Health Organization was made by Stevenson and his colleagues (1966*a* and *b*). They have reported the results of a cooperative study of the issue of nearly half a million pregnancies in hospitals from twenty-four centers during 1961-64 (Table 8.5). The centers were located in Australia (2), Brazil, Chile, Colombia (2), Czechoslovakia, Egypt, Hong Kong, India (2), Malaysia (2), Mexico (2), Northern Ireland, Panama, Philippines, Republic of South Africa (3), Spain, and Yugoslavia (2). Because of its importance, births by center are detailed in Table A.8.4.

Among 417,000 single births, there were 347 with Down's syndrome, for a rate of 0.8 per 1,000 total births or 0.9 per 1,000 live births (Table 8.4). Mean age of the mothers was 34.0 years versus 27.3 years for those of all infants not malformed. High frequencies (more than 2 per 1,000 total births) were recorded for Melbourne at the Queen Victoria Hospital (rate 2.1), but the rate was 0.9 for the Royal Women's Hospital in the same city. The only other similarly high rates were from Czechoslovakia (rate 2.0) and Yugoslavia (rates 3.9 and 2.5). The rate in Belfast was 1.1.

Considering the numbers at hand, one would be hard put to define any geographic variation of importance in this study, except for the apparent scarcity of Down's syndrome in Asia. No cases were found in Bombay with almost 40,000 single births, nor in Calcutta with about 19,000 births. There was but one affected birth in the Chinese of Hong Kong for a rate of 0.2. Of the 17 born with the syndrome in Singapore, one was Indian, and the rate for those born of Indian

Table 8.5 Cases and incidence rates standardized for maternal age per 1,000 total (live plus stillborn) single births for Down's syndrome: WHO study, 24 centers, 1961-64

Center	Cases	Rate	Center	Cases	Rate
All centers[a]	347	0.8			
Melbourne, Australia	8[b]	0.9	Singapore, Malaysia	17	0.4
Melbourne, Australia	6[c]	2.1	Mexico City, Mexico	46	2.0
São Paulo, Brazil	11	0.9	Mexico City, Mexico	22	1.7
Santiago, Chile	37	1.3	Belfast, No. Ireland	28	1.1
Bogotá, Colombia	10	0.6	Panama City, Panama	17	1.4
Medellin, Colombia	18	0.8	Manila, the Philippines	17	0.5
Czechoslovakia	27	2.0	Cape Town, Rep. of So. Africa	-[c]	-
Alexandria, UAR (Egypt)	-[b]	-	Johannesburg, Rep. of So. Africa	8	0.8
Hong Kong	1[b]	0.2	Pretoria, Rep. of So. Africa	6	0.6
Bombay, India	-	-	Madrid, Spain	39	1.8
Calcutta, India	-	-	Ljubljana, Yugoslavia	20[b]	3.9
Kuala Lumpur, Malaysia	3	0.2	Zagreb, Yugoslavia	6[b]	2.5

[a]Births by center are listed in Table A.8.4.
[b]Less than 10,000 single births, but more than 5,000.
[c]Less than 5,000 single births, but more than 3,000.

mothers was 0.3 per 1,000, not notably different from the (low) rate of 0.4 among the nearly 40,000 births in that center. In Singapore, over half the mothers were Chinese. Precise ratios for Malaysian and Chinese mothers in Singapore were not available, nor were they in Kuala Lumpur, where the rate too was low (0.2) with about 16,000 births.

In the WHO study, there were 11 cases of Down's syndrome among the 5,000-odd sets of multiple births (10,237 individuals) for a rate of 1.1 per 1,000 total births—which is not appreciably different from the 0.8 per 1,000 for all single births (live plus stillborn).

Summary. The rate for Down's syndrome at birth would seem for the most part to be between 0.9 and 1.6 per 1,000 live births, and perhaps 1.2 would be a reasonable estimate, at least outside Asia. From the available data, there is no convincing evidence of geographic variation in Down's syndrome, although its apparent rarity in Asia—and possibly too in Negroes—suggests the need for further study. On matters such as delayed or missed diagnosis and attention to births out of hospital, for example, the WHO study could give little information.

Other Features of Down's Syndrome

Maternal age. The WHO study provided further evidence for the greatly increased risk of Down's syndrome births with increasing maternal age (Table 8.6). Mothers 20-24 years old at parturition bore 0.3 per 1,000 children with Down's syndrome. The rate increased sharply with each older age group, and attained a rate of almost 17 per 1,000 total births among mothers 45 or older.

Sex. There seemed to be a difference by sex in the frequency of Down's syndrome in the WHO study. There were 155 males in 214,645 births and 192 females in 201,828 with the disorder, or rates of 0.72 per 1,000 for males and 0.95 per 1,000 for females. The male-female sex ratio on the rates was 0.76 to 1, and on the cases 0.82 to 1 (Table 8.7). In New York, Conway and Wagner (1965) noted a similar case ratio of 0.8 to 1, with 616 cases; whereas in Birmingham, England, and in Denmark, case ratios of 1.2 and 1.1 to 1 respectively were recorded. In Rochester, the case ratio was 2.3 to

Table 8.6 Incidence rates per 1,000 total (live plus stillborn) single births for Down's syndrome by maternal age: WHO study of 24 centers, 1961-64

Maternal age	Rate	Maternal age	Rate
Under 15	0.30	30-34	1.63
15-19	0.50	35-39	2.11
20-24	0.32	40-44	6.34
25-29	0.38	45 & over	16.65

Table 8.7 Male-female case ratios in Down's syndrome: selected surveys, various years, 1935-67

Survey area (source)	Years	Total cases	M:F ratio
Rochester, Minnesota (Gibson & Kurland, unpublished)	1935-67	36	2.3[a]
Victoria, Australia (Collmann & Stoller 1962a)	1942-57	1,134	1.0
Denmark (Øster 1953)	1938-48	1,006	1.1
Birmingham, England (Record & Smith 1955)	1948-52	252	1.2
New York City (Conway & Wagner 1965)	1952-62	616	0.8
WHO, 24 centers (Stevenson et al. 1966b)	1961-64	347	0.8[b]

[a] The 95-percent confidence interval includes a sex ratio of 1.1.
[b] Same ratio when based on sex-specific incidence rates.

1, but this is based on a relatively small number of cases. Thus a predilection by sex remains to be proved.

Color. Aside from the WHO survey, the studies thus far do not provide sufficient data to support or refute the excess of white deaths reported for the United States. A study of the 32 persons with Down's syndrome who were born during a ten-year interval in a Washington, D.C., hospital (Parker 1950) revealed a rate of 1.2 per 1,000 births among Negroes (29 cases) versus 1.0 among whites (3 cases), both of which agree with that expected for whites (Table

8.4). Babbott and Ingalls (1962), however, stated that among births in Pennsylvania in 1960 a notable difference was reported between Negroes with Down's syndrome (0.1 per 1,000 births) and whites (0.4). From the numbers and rates cited for all malformations in that study, there would have been approximately 22,000 Negro births and about 185,000 white births in Pennsylvania. The rates for Down's syndrome would then be based on 3 Negroes and about 80 whites. Conway and Wagner (1965) noted that birth reports in New York City over two years indicated rates of 0.4 per 1,000 live births for whites (98 cases) and 0.2 for nonwhites (12 cases). Although both studies support a color difference, in each the rates for whites were about one-third those expected (Table 8.4); such a degree of underreporting for whites makes the color differences recorded tenuous, even if the rather small numbers of nonwhites with Down's syndrome are disregarded.

In the WHO study, South Africa was represented by three centers: Cape Town (where most if not all births were among the Cape Colored), Johannesburg (where the births were for whites), and Pretoria's hospital for Bantu. The rates in the last two were 0.8 for 8 cases in Johannesburg and 0.6 for 6 in Pretoria. No cases were found in Cape Town, but the 95-percent confidence interval based on an observed rate of 0 in 3,051 includes an expectation of 1.2 per 1,000.

The scarcity of Down's syndrome among Asians from the same study has been discussed. The numbers of births recorded were large, but the diagnosis of Down's syndrome in the immediate postnatal period for Asian infants may be difficult unless the physical stigmata are pronounced. Further, the proportion of births in these hospitals to total births in the community needs to be known before the possible bias from this aspect can be estimated.

There is not sufficient evidence to support any predilection for Down's syndrome by color between whites and Negroes from morbidity data, although at least the study of Conway and Wagner (1965) and that of Babbott and Ingalls (1962) provide differences that would agree with the difference found in the United States mortality material. The converse—that is, no difference by color—is suggested by the work of Parker (1950) and the rates for South Africa; further, the incomplete ascertainment suggested for the two studies cited *with* color differences makes less strong the thesis of a differential risk. The deficit among Asians, although striking in the WHO study, needs confirmation from community-wide surveys before it can be accepted. It would appear from the discussions of

Lilienfeld and Benesch (1969) that they came to similar conclusions.

Familial frequency. As part of his study, Øster (1953) provided an extensive review of the literature on Down's syndrome from 1899 to 1952. From published reports he summarized citations of 98 twin-pairs, at least one of whom had Down's syndrome (Table 8.8). Although these data must be considered in the context of potential bias attendant on individual case reports, the collection is of great value. In this survey all 8 sets of monozygous twins were concordant for Down's syndrome and all 34 sets of opposite-sexed twins were discordant. Among the same-sexed dizygous twins, 3 of 21 were concordant. According to Øster, dizygosity was based on the criterion of separate membranes at birth in the case of Russell in 1933, physical appearance of the twins in that of MacKaye of 1936, and both aspects in the report of Jervis in 1943, which account for the three concordant dizygotes. However, none of these features is currently accepted as proof of dizygosity.

If these three instances are accepted as being truly dizygotic, then the possibility of an exogenous precipitant for this disorder, as postulated by Stoller and Collmann (1965), would receive some support. However, susceptibility would have to be limited to the earliest stages of embryogenesis because of the rarity among dizygous twins. The frequency of concordance among monozygous twins would be in accord with this disorder being a chromosomal aberration. A hereditary disorder caused by genetic mutation would seem

Table 8.8 Concordance among twins with Down's syndrome according to zygosity, adapted from Øster's review of literature, 1899-1952

Zygosity	Number of twin pairs				Number of individuals affected		
	Total	Concordant Male	Female	Dis-cordant	Total	Male	Female
Monozygous (MZ)	8	3	5	-	16	6	10
Opposite-sexed dizygous (DZ$_2$)	34	-	-	34	34	18	16
Same-sexed dizygous (DZ$_1$)	21	2	1	18	24	11	13
Same-sexed unknown zygosity	35	4	4	27	43	26	17

Source: Øster 1953.

unlikely, as the antecedents of the propositi seem unaffected and second-generation transmission is exceedingly rare. Øster (1953) reviewed published series, and most of twenty-nine familial instances he accepted were among siblings. In his own Danish experience, Øster found that a sibling with Down's syndrome was subsequently born to six families of the 354 live-born index cases. He considered this to be in keeping with expectations when the age of the mothers and the relation of Down's syndrome to maternal age were considered. From Table 8.8 we see that the frequency in same-sexed twins of unknown zygosity was intermediate between the monozygous and dizygous ratios, with 8 of 35 being concordant for Down's syndrome, suggestive that some of these were indeed monozygous.

Penrose and Smith (1966) extended the study of twins reported by Øster. Of 201 twin-pairs summarized from case reports, 19 were monozygous; and 18 of these were concordant. Concordance was noted in only 1 of 47 same-sexed dizygous twins and in 1 of 80 opposite-sexed dizygous twin-pairs. Of 55 same-sexed twin-pairs of uncertain zygosity, 12 were concordant. Notably, Penrose and Smith accepted only one instance of concordance in definite same-sexed dizygous twins. Although their results provided different ratios of concordance for dizygous twins, the general pattern is similar to that reported earlier by Øster.

Lilienfeld and Benesch (1969) pointed out that multiple cases of mongolism among siblings are usually seen for young mothers, and they agreed with the concept that "familial translocation represented the principal source of multiple cases of mongolism in a family." Elsewhere, they reviewed the frequency of inherited versus sporadic translocation by type. Overall, they believed that the inherited groups represented only 3 percent of those with Down's syndrome but that chromosomal analysis was vital in genetic counseling; "if the patient has a D/G translocation shown to be inherited from a carrier mother, the recurrence risk is probably high, estimated here at 1 in 3."

Comment

Down's syndrome is predominantly the consequence of a sporadic chromosomal aberration which affects males and females equally. There is no evidence of noteworthy geographic variation, at least in the Western Hemisphere, and there is little consistent support for the concept of spatio-temporal clustering—which, however, cannot be ruled out at present.

In the Eastern Hemisphere, there are recorded low rates for births with Down's syndrome from much of Asia, particularly in India. Rates among Chinese in Malaysia and Hong Kong are also low, as is true for the Philippines. Nevertheless, questions of selection bias from these hospital data and incomplete ascertainment for these newborns prevent acceptance of the differences as established. Among Negroes, the deficit noted in United States mortality data is not supported by hospital data for South Africa or Washington, D.C. Studies from Pennsylvania and New York are compatible with such a deficit, but the low rates for whites, at about one-third those otherwise expected, suggest that incomplete ascertainment is at least as good an explanation for the deficit as would be a true difference by color. The question is far from resolved, and further studies are warranted to confirm or deny a color differential in the risk of Down's syndrome.

There is a striking increase in the frequency of this disorder with increasing maternal age, and the rate for Down's syndrome reaches nearly 17 per 1,000 births of mothers 45 or older at parturition.

Death rates in the United States at present are about 0.2 per 100,000 population, all ages, with the rate for those under 1 year of age in excess of 4 per 100,000. Deaths in the first year of life account for about three-fifths of all deaths attributed to Down's syndrome as primary cause of death. However, for the United States in 1955, deaths *with* Down's syndrome (that is, including those listed as contributory cause or associated condition) were more than seventeen times as frequent as those resulting from (that is, underlying cause) the disease. If this ratio still held, deaths among those with Down's syndrome would indeed approximate the reported incidence for this disorder: 1.2 per 1,000 births.

Age-specific death rates decline rapidly after the first year of life and are near 0 per 100,000 at or above age 15. This supports the clinical experience of poor survival in this disease—which, however, in recent years appears to have improved notably. The age-specific death rates may not accurately reflect the course of illness; if as the child gets older he is more likely to succumb from other ills, the already small proportion of deaths for Down's syndrome as underlying cause would tend to become notably less. Thus the dire outlook suggested by these death rates may reflect more properly a declining proportion of deaths coded as underlying cause with increasing age.

9 / CONGENITAL MALFORMATIONS OF THE NERVOUS SYSTEM

John F. Kurtzke
Irving D. Goldberg
Leonard T. Kurland

Although this topic is included within another volume of the APHA monograph series (Shapiro et al. 1968), consideration in that volume is limited largely to the neural malformations as a single entity. We shall present herein a more detailed view of the major malformations of the nervous system, with only a brief introductory statement relative to all congenital anomalies.

Introduction

All Malformations

A survey of the epidemiologic reports on congenital anomalies of all types has been provided by Kennedy (1967). According to the clinical data he reviewed, the rate for major malformations was about 13 per 1,000 live births; estimates from official records of births in the United States and Canada were about 11 per 1,000 live births. The WHO report (Stevenson et al. 1966*a* and *b*) indicated an incidence rate of 13 per 1,000 total births.

In 1963 Hewitt analyzed mortality data from across the United States and found that deaths attributed to congenital defects showed significant east-west variation in two respects: the ratio of males to females for all malformations was higher in the West, and the mortality rate for spina bifida was two or three times higher on the Atlantic coast than on the Pacific coast. To what extent these variations are caused by an artifact in reporting or by an unrecognized genetic or environmental cause is uncertain.

It is of interest that no notable geographic variation in childhood death rates for congenital malformations as a whole was found for whites in the 1959-61 mortality data reported in the Shapiro book. The only differences of note were a somewhat lower rate in nonmetropolitan counties than in metropolitan, and among nonwhites (with much smaller numbers) the death rate for congenital malformations in the South was slightly lower than in other regions. These deviations from uniformity perhaps reflect reporting rather than biologic variations but, for interpretation, need to be considered according to individual entities.

Classification of Congenital Malformations of the Nervous System

The major abnormalities encompassed under congenital defects of the nervous system are those of the neural tube: congenital hydrocephalus, anencephaly, and spina bifida. In the Seventh Revision of the International Statistical Classification, congenital hydrocephalus is coded 752, spina bifida is 751, and anencephaly is included within the category of "monstrosity" as code 750. Aside from these classes and their named inclusions, other congenital malformations of the nervous system and sense organs are to be found within code 753.

Of the 1,109 neural birth defects recorded in the WHO study of twenty-four centers (Stevenson et al. 1966a and b), only a few are not included within the three main categories of anencephaly, spina bifida, and hydrocephalus—although their admixture within these categories is notable (Table 9.1). Monstrosity was not recorded as a named anomaly in that study, but it cannot therefore be assumed that in mortality data most cases coded to 750 are of anencephaly. The death data to be reviewed herein are based on the live-born population at risk and thus exclude fetal deaths and stillbirths. Because most anencephalics are stillborn, only that fraction represented by those who survive birth are retrievable in routine mortality statistics. We have no knowledge as to what proportion of the live-born who die with monstrosity is provided by anencephaly, even though such infants comprise most of the total births (including stillborn) classified as monstrosity.

For ISC code 750, Seventh Revision, the formal inclusions are acephalic monster, anencephalus, hemicephalus, ischiopagus, macrocephalia, megalocephaly, monster, podencephalus, syncephalus, and thoracopagus. Code 751 is designated spina bifida and meningocele and includes encephalocele, meningoencephalocele, meningo(myelo)cele and equivalent terms, and also rachischisis and "malformation of the spinal cord, N.O.S." Congenital hydrocephalus category (code 752) is limited to hydrocephalus and hydroencephalocele, but, as explained below, admixtures of hydrocephalus and spina bifida are variably coded to 751 or 752—or even to other codes. Code 753, as stated, also covers a number of optic defects, but as a primary cause of death it would reflect only the malformations of the nervous system, which include aplasia, dysplasia, hypoplasia, or maldevelop-

Table 9.1 Percentage distribution of congenital malformations of the nervous system by type of malformation: WHO study of 24 centers, 1961-64

Type of malformation	Percent of total
Total	100.0
Anencephaly alone	34.4
Anencephaly and spina bifida	4.9
Hydrocephalus alone	22.9
Hydrocephalus and spina bifida	9.7
Spina bifida alone[a]	20.8
Occipital meningocele	1.4
Other neural tube defects[b]	3.1
Microcephaly	2.4
All other nervous system	0.3
(Number of cases)	(1,109)

[a] With or without spinal meningocele.
[b] Predominantly encephalocele.

ment of brain or spinal cord (not in prior classes), as well as microcephaly and tuberous sclerosis.

Accordingly, the sum of conditions coded to rubrics 750, 751, 752, and 753 can be taken as "congenital malformations of the nervous system" in the death data and is so referred to in this chapter. Code 750 describes a group of defects including anencephaly; code 751 covers spina bifida alone *or* with hydrocephalus; code 752 concerns congenital hydrocephalus alone *or* with spina bifida; and code 753 is a heterogenous collection of other neural anomalies.

Neither the Sixth nor the Seventh Revision of the ISC provided any special criteria or instructions for uniform coding to underlying cause of concurrent spina bifida and congenital hydrocephalus. Thus, depending on the order, location, and wording of these conditions on the death certificate, the underlying cause may have been attributed to either of the two. It was only in 1962 that the United States employed its own four-digit code to indicate under the spina bifida rubric (751) whether this condition was reported with or without mention of hydrocephalus, and to include under congenital hydrocephalus (752) only those deaths occurring without mention of spina bifida. A similar coding procedure was subsequently adopted in the Eighth Revision of the ISC for use in 1968 (World Health Organization 1967).

In any event, it would appear that, prior to these changes, concurrent spina bifida and hydrocephalus were not always uniformly allocated to spina bifida as underlying cause and, since these defects occur frequently in combination, it is difficult to interpret adequately international differences in presently available mortality statistics for these conditions. However, it may be assumed that coding practices in this regard, even prior to 1962, were fairly uniform within the United States under the special instructions and guidelines established by the predecessor agency to the National Center for Health Statistics (National Office of Vital Statistics 1958).

From Table 9.1, one would expect about two-thirds of the deaths coded to spina bifida to reflect spina bifida without hydrocephalus and about one-third spina bifida with hydrocephalus. In the United States for 1962-67, the proportion of code 751 represented by spina bifida alone was almost one-half. Because of the admixtures of even these general classes of neural anomaly, we shall for the most part consider these entities serially within each source of information to be discussed, rather than primarily from the several entities themselves.

Mortality Data

Neural Malformations as Underlying Cause of Death

The frequency with which congenital malformations of the nervous system are coded as the underlying cause of death is high (Table 9.2). For monstrosity, virtually all deaths were so assigned. Four of five deaths from spina bifida were classed as primary in the Netherlands, but only three of five in the United States. Conversely, hydrocephalus was so recorded for half the deaths in the Netherlands, and more than four-fifths in the United States and Norway. For the "other" category, the frequencies were between two-thirds and three-fourths. Thus for this category, most of the deaths among the affected are retrievable from routine mortality statistics.

Table 9.2 Death certificates listing congenital malformations of the nervous system as primary or secondary causes of death, with percent listed as primary cause, by type of malformation: selected countries, various years, 1953-61
(ISC codes 750, 751, 752, 753)

Type of malformation and ISC code	Netherlands 1953-60[a]	Netherlands 1961[b]	United States 1955[c]	Norway 1956-60[d]
Monstrosity (750)				
Total deaths	766	86	1,133	---
Percent primary	99	100	92	---
Spina bifida and meningocele (751)				
Total deaths	1,723	185	2,138	---
Percent primary	83	83	62	---
Congenital hydrocephalus (752)				
Total deaths	1,354	204	2,284	122
Percent primary	58	53	82	88
Other nervous system (753)				
Total deaths	454	90	1,196	---
Percent primary	74	71	67	---

[a] Only one ("most important") secondary cause considered; excludes deaths for 1958 (not available).
[b] Up to 3 secondary causes considered.
[c] Up to 4 secondary causes considered.
[d] All secondary causes considered.

International Comparisons

For the survey of thirty-three countries for various years 1951-58, Goldberg and Kurland (1962) collected data on a number of neurologic disorders. Largely unpublished, though, were the data on congenital malformations of the nervous system. Table 9.3 summarizes the age-adjusted death rates per 100,000 population, all ages, for the twenty-four nations wherein each of the four codes was cited. The sum (codes 750 through 753) then comprises the death rate for malformations of the nervous system for these countries. Details for the rates by sex (where available) and country are in Tables A.9.1 through A.9.4, together with rates from several other lands for spina

Table 9.3 Average annual age-adjusted[a] death rates per 100,000 population for congenital malformations of the nervous system by type of malformation: selected countries, various years, 1951-58

(ISC codes 750, 751, 752, 753)

			ISC codes[b]			
Country	Years	Total 750-753[c]	750	751	752	753
Australia	1954-58	3.0	0.6	1.0	0.8	0.5
Belgium	1954-58	4.2	0.8	1.4	1.4	0.6
Canada[d]	1953-57	5.0	0.7	2.7	1.2	0.4
Chile	1956,58	1.3	0.2	0.4	0.3	0.3
Czechoslovakia	1953-57	2.6	0.5	0.8	0.9	0.5
Denmark	1953-57	2.5	0.3	1.2	0.6	0.3
England and Wales	1953-57	4.6	0.4	3.2	0.6	0.4
Finland	1954-58	3.3	0.8	1.0	1.0	0.4
France	1953-57	1.3	0.1	0.6	0.5	0.2
Iceland	1951-55	2.4	0.4	1.2	0.4	0.3
Ireland	1954-58	6.8	1.2	3.4	1.9	0.3
Israel[e]	1956-58	4.8	0.6	1.7	1.3	1.1
Italy	1953-57	2.8	0.4	1.7	0.6	0.1
Japan	1953-57	0.5	0.03	0.2	0.3	0.04
Mexico	1956	1.1	0.1	0.6	0.4	0.1
Netherlands	1953-57	4.7	1.1	2.1	1.1	0.4
New Zealand[f]	1952-56	3.4	0.3	1.5	1.0	0.5
Norway	1953-57	2.2	0.3	0.9	0.7	0.3
Scotland	1951-55	5.8	0.4	3.4	1.5	0.5
Sweden	1953-57	2.4	0.5	0.9	0.7	0.3
Switzerland	1953-57	3.3	0.4	1.4	1.0	0.4
Union of So. Africa[g]	1953-57	2.7	0.2	0.6	1.1	0.9
United States (total)	1953-57	3.0	0.6	0.9	1.0	0.4
White	1953-57	3.1	0.7	0.9	1.1	0.5
Nonwhite	1953-57	2.0	0.3	0.4	0.9	0.4
Uruguay	1955-57	2.0	0.4	1.0	0.3	0.2

[a] Adjusted to the 1950 census population of the United States.
[b] 750-monstrosity; 751-spina bifida and meningocele; 752-congenital hydrocephalus; 753-other congenital malformations of the nervous system.
[c] Total may not equal sum of individual rubrics due to rounding.
[d] Yukon and Northwest Territories were included in 1956 and 1957 only.
[e] Jewish population only.
[f] Excludes Maori population.
[g] White population only.

bifida. Included there also are the male-female ratios for the age-adjusted death rates.

In Table 9.4 are recorded the numbers of these countries that had the specified sex ratio at that time, according to type of neural malformation. For monstrosity (code 750) and spina bifida (code 751) there is a female preponderance. However, both congenital hydrocephalus (code 752) and other neural malformations (code 753) appear either to predominate in males or—more likely—to be equally distributed by sex.

For all neurologic malformations combined, most countries had death rates between 2 and 4 per 100,000 (Table 9.3). On the low side (less than 2) were France, Chile, Mexico, and Japan. We suspect these low rates reflect primarily reporting inadequacies, as these same

Table 9.4 Number of countries with specified male-female ratio of age-adjusted death rates for congenital malformations of the nervous system by type of malformation: selected countries, various years, 1951-58 (ISC codes 750, 751, 752, 753)

M:F ratio	ISC codes[a]			
	750	751	752	753
1.9	-	-	-	1
1.8	-	-	-	-
1.7	-	-	-	-
1.6	1	1	-	-
1.5	1	-	-	1
1.4	-	-	2	2
1.3	1	1	3	1
1.2	-	1	4	3
1.1	1	-	3	3
1.0	-	3	7	5
0.9	2	4	2	3
0.8	5	7	-	3
0.7	4	12	1	-
0.6	2	1	-	-
0.5	2	-	-	1
0.4	2	-	-	-
0.3	1	-	1	-
0.2	1	-	-	-

Source: See Tables A.9.1-A.9.4.

[a] 750-monstrosity; 751-spina bifida and meningocele; 752-congenital hydrocephalus; 753-other congenital malformations of the nervous system.

countries occupy almost the same ranks for each of the four diagnostic categories. Moderately high rates (between 4 and 5) were recorded for Belgium, England and Wales, the Netherlands, and Israel, in increasing order. Canada had a rate of 5, and Scotland and Ireland, respectively, attained death rates of about 6 and 7 per 100,000.

The range of rates for both monstrosity and for other defects was small. For the former, three-fourths of the countries had rates between 0.3 and 0.8 per 100,000; the highest rates were 1.2 in Ireland and 1.1 in the Netherlands. Monstrosity then would seem to be relatively uniform in geographic distribution. Rates for other defects were mostly between 0.3 and 0.5 per 100,000. Highest were Israel (1.1) and Union of South African whites (0.9). Since the total rates in these countries are close to the median, it would appear that there may be a tendency to code many cases to the nonspecific category.

The rates for hydrocephalus did not show any consistent geographic pattern; the range was small, with most rates between 0.6 and 1.4. The rates were high for Ireland (1.9) and Scotland (1.5).

Far different is the geographic distribution for spina bifida. The range of rates was from 0.2 to 3.4 per 100,000. Rates for most lands were concentrated between 0.8 and 1.7 per 100,000. The lowest rates were for those countries where we have already suggested the likelihood of incomplete reporting (Mexico, France, Chile, U.S. nonwhites, and Japan), or variable coding customs (Union of South Africa). The rates for Canada (2.7) and the Netherlands (2.1) were only a little above those for the majority of the countries.

But note the rates for Ireland (3.4), Scotland (3.4), and England and Wales (3.2). The rate for Northern Ireland was about 3.8 (Table A.9.2). It would appear then that there is an increased risk for spina bifida in the British Isles and Ireland, and especially the latter—both for the Republic and for Northern Ireland. Certainly this warrants further investigation.

United States Mortality, Trend

Death rates for congenital malformations of the nervous system by ISC code were available for 1950-67. Figure 9.1 accumulates for each year the death rates per 100,000 for each of the four entities; the top line represents the rate for all neural malformations combined (codes 750 through 753), and the vertical distance between that line and the one below it for any given year represents the rate for other malformations (code 753), and so forth.

The crude annual death rates for all neural malformations declined by nearly half during this eighteen-year interval. Rates for monstrosity and for other malformations, however, showed virtually no change. The decline up to 1962 was rather evenly divided between spina bifida and hydrocephalus though perhaps at a slightly greater rate for the latter. Between 1962 and 1967, death rates for spina

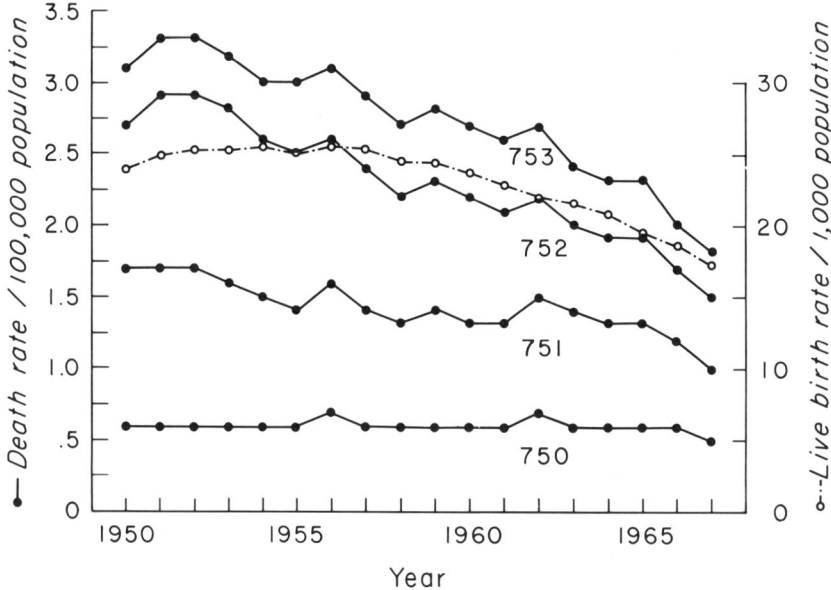

Figure 9.1 Birth rates per 1,000 population and crude death rates per 100,000 population accumulated for monstrosity (code 750), spina bifida (751), congenital hydrocephalus (752), and other congenital neural defects (753) by year: United States, 1950-67. The top line represents annual death rates for all congenital malformations of the nervous system (750 through 753), and the vertical interval between lines represents the death rate for the particular constituent thereof as indicated. The dotted line represents the national live birth rates during this period.

bifida without hydrocephalus declined by 35 percent, while the decrease for hydrocephalus alone was 26 percent.

Further evidence as to the impact of the coding change in 1962 is indicated by the dramatic change between 1961 and 1962 in deaths allocated to these conditions. In this one-year interval, numbers of deaths allocated to spina bifida *increased* by 26 percent, while those attributed to hydrocephalus *declined* by 16 percent. For the subsequent years through 1967, spina bifida deaths regularly exceeded those allocated to hydrocephalus by 7 to 27 percent, as opposed to the excess of hydrocephalus over spina bifida by 2 to 33 percent for 1951-61. We might note further that this coding change also affected the allocation of hydrocephalus undefined. Earlier, only deaths with mention of congenital hydrocephalus or those occurring before 28 days of age were coded to 752, whereas since 1962 all hydrocephalus

Table 9.5 Deaths and death rates per 100,000 population for congenital malformations of the nervous system by type of malformation: United States, 1959-61
(ISC codes 750, 751, 752, 753)

Type of malformation and ISC code	Deaths	Rate Crude	Rate Age adjusted
Total (750-753)	14,448	2.7	1.9
Monstrosity (750)	3,290	0.6	0.4*
Spina bifida and meningocele (751)	3,737	0.7	0.5*
Congenital hydrocephalus (752)	4,790	0.9	0.6
Other nervous system (753)	2,631	0.5	0.4

is assumed to be congenital when in association with other congenital neural malformations, regardless of age.

There is one important aspect still to be mentioned in interpreting the changes in death rates for congenital malformations of the nervous system, for which the only data available were the deaths and crude death rates for all ages. It is obvious that changes in birth rates will affect these crude death rates. Birth rates for the United States did not change appreciably between 1950 (24.1 per 1,000 population) and 1957 (25.3). However, from 1958 on there was a steady decline to a birth rate of 17.8 per 1,000 population in 1967 (National Center for Health Statistics 1969). Thus a decline of 30 percent in birth rates over the last decade in question would explain most of the decline of 40 percent in crude death rates for neural malformations over this same period. However, as seen in Fig. 9.1, it does not seem to account for all the changes.

United States Mortality Data, 1959-61

In 1959-61 in the United States, there were 14,448 deaths coded to malformations of the nervous system as the underlying cause of death (Table 9.5). Crude death rates per 100,000 population, all ages, were 0.6 for monstrosity; 0.7 for deaths allocated to spina bifida, with or without meningocele; 0.9 for those allocated to hydrocephalus; 0.5 for other malformations of the nervous system; and 2.7 per 100,000 for all neural malformations. Age-adjusted rates were slightly lower for each entity.

Rates for deaths, all ages, inadequately reflect the features of these disorders. Because deaths are concentrated in the first year of life, comparisons for death rates under 1 year of age are the most valid. In Table 9.6 are summarized the death rates per 100,000 population under 1 year of age for each type of malformation and for the total, according to color and sex. For deaths under 1 year of age, the rates were similar for the three defined types of malformation, at 27 per 100,000, in contrast to the suggestion of differences provided by death rates, all ages (Table 9.5). The rate for other malformations (code 753) was about half the others, at 13 per 100,000 population under 1 year of age. The sum of these rates is 94 per 100,000.

Age. Age-specific death rates by type of malformation are summarized in Table 9.7, from data in Tables A.9.5 through A.9.8. The greatest number of deaths occurred under 1 year of age. This was most apparent for monstrosity, where all but 26 of the 3,290 deaths took place in the first year of life. The rates for hydrocephalus and

Table 9.6 Average annual death rates per 100,000 population under one year of age for congenital malformations of the nervous system by color, sex and type of malformation: United States, 1959-61
(ISC codes 750, 751, 752, 753)

Color and sex	ISC codes[a]				
	Total 750-753	750	751	752	753
Total	93.5	26.5	27.1	26.9	13.0
Male	84.9	21.2	23.2	26.7	13.8
Female	102.2	31.8	31.1	27.1	12.2
White	99.3	29.0	29.4	27.4	13.5
Male	89.0	23.1	24.7	26.9	14.3
Female	109.9	35.1	34.2	27.8	12.8
Nonwhite	60.2	12.0	14.0	24.3	9.9
Male	61.4	10.2	14.6	25.7	10.9
Female	59.1	13.8	13.4	23.0	8.9

[a]750-monstrosity; 751-spina bifida and meningocele; 752-congenital hydrocephalus; 753-other congenital malformations of the nervous system.

Table 9.7 Age-specific death rates per 100,000 population for congenital malformations of the nervous system by type of malformation: United States, 1959-61
(ISC codes 750, 751, 752, 753)

Age	Total 750-753	ISC codes[a]			
		750	751	752	753
Under 1	93.5	26.5	27.1	26.9	13.0
1-4	3.5	0.0*	0.5	2.0	1.0
5-14	0.8	0.0*	0.1	0.4	0.3
15-24	0.4	0.0*	0.1	0.1	0.2
25-34	0.1	0.0*	0.0*	0.0	0.1
35-44	0.1	0.0*	0.0*	0.0	0.1
45-54	0.1	0.0*	0.0*	0.0*	0.1
55-64	0.0*	0.0*	0.0*	0.0*	0.0*
65 & over	0.0	0.0*	0.0*	0.0*	0.0*

[a]750-monstrosity; 751-spina bifida and meningocele; 752-congenital hydrocephalus; 753-other congenital malformations of the nervous system.

for other defects declined less rapidly with age, but except for the latter, death rates were less than 0.05 per 100,000 for each age group beyond age 24.

Sex. Details as to deaths and death rates by color and sex may also be found in Tables A.9.5 through A.9.8. Our comparisons here will be made for death rates under 1 year of age.

For all neural malformations, the under-1-year death rate was somewhat lower for males (85 per 100,000) than for females (102), but the sex ratio of the rates varied by diagnosis (see Table 9.8). In line with the international comparisons (Table 9.4), there was a definite female excess for monstrosity and for spina bifida, with male-female ratios of 0.7 to 1. Hydrocephalus had a sex ratio of unity—similar to the international ratios—while other malformations indicated a slight male excess at a 1.1 to 1 ratio.

Color. In Table 9.6 were summarized the under-1-year death rates by color, sex, and type of neural malformation. The deaths for nonwhites comprised 10.4 percent of the total at all ages (Tables A.9.5 through A.9.8), and for those under 1 year of age, they were

Table 9.8 Male-female ratios of death rates under one year of age for congenital malformations of the nervous system by color and type of malformation: United States, 1959-61
(ISC codes 750, 751, 752, 753)

Type of malformation and ISC code	M:F ratio		
	Total	White	Nonwhite
Total (750-753)	0.8	0.8	1.0
Monstrosity (750)	0.7	0.7	0.7
Spina bifida and meningocele (751)	0.7	0.7	1.1
Congenital hydrocephalus (752)	1.0	1.0	1.1
Other nervous system (753)	1.1	1.1	1.2

Table 9.9 White-nonwhite ratios of death rates under one year of age for congenital malformations of the nervous system by sex and type of malformation: United States, 1959-61
(ISC codes 750, 751, 752, 753)

Type of malformation and ISC code	W:NW ratio		
	Total	Male	Female
Total (750-753)	1.6	1.4	1.9
Monstrosity (750)	2.4	2.3	2.5
Spina bifida and meningocele (751)	2.1	1.7	2.6
Congenital hydrocephalus (752)	1.1	1.0	1.2
Other nervous system (753)	1.4	1.3	1.4

9.6 percent (1,109 per 11,524). We shall therefore confine the comparisons by color also to death rates under 1 year of age.

As shown in Table 9.9, the ratios of whites to nonwhites for such death rates indicate an overall excess among the whites at 1.6 to 1. The greatest divergence by color is for monstrosity, with a white-nonwhite ratio of 2.4 to 1 and little difference by sex. Spina bifida (2.1 to 1) showed a notable change in this ratio between the sexes at 1.7 to 1 for males and 2.6 to 1 for females, white to nonwhite.

For hydrocephalus, the rates were essentially equal between the colors and between the sexes. The other malformation ratio suggested a slight white excess (1.4 to 1), with ratios equivalent to this for either sex.

Geographic distribution. Deaths and death rates under 1 year of age according to state of residence at death for each type of malformation may be found in Tables A.9.9a and b respectively, and the death rates are drawn in Figs. 9.2 through 9.5. We shall discuss the distribution separately for each type of malformation.

(1) Monstrosity. With a weighted (national) mean death rate of 26.5 per 100,000 under age 1 year, the individual states ranged from rates of 11.6 in Mississippi (20 deaths) to 47.4 in Delaware (16 deaths). About three-fourths of the states had rates of about 18 to 34 per 100,000 under age 1 year. Rates by state (rounded to integers) are drawn in Fig. 9.2, with data for this and the other categories in Tables A.9.9a and b. Most of the states with rates above the mean were concentrated in the northeastern quadrant of the country, and the lowest rates were generally found in the Plains states.

By census region, this geographic variation appears confirmed (Table 9.10). The New England rate of 38 is more than twice that for the Mountain region (17), and the rates for the East North Central (30) and Middle Atlantic (29) regions are also high. Relative proportions are consistent for the two sexes, and for each region and

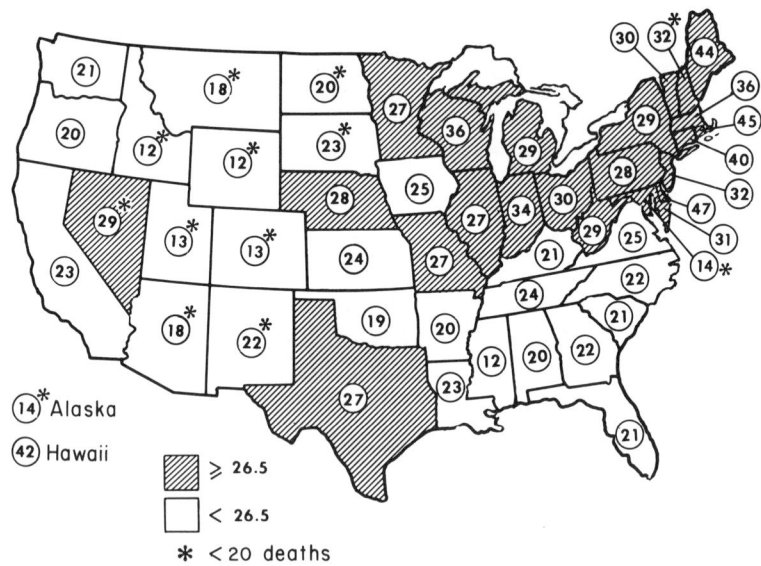

Figure 9.2 Average annual death rates per 100,000 population under 1 year of age for monstrosity by state: United States, 1959–61.

Table 9.10 Average annual death rates per 100,000 population under one year of age for monstrosity by color and sex: United States and census regions, 1959-61[a]
(ISC code 750)

Region	Total			White			Nonwhite		
	Total	M	F	Total	M	F	Total	M	F
United States	26.5	21.2	31.8	29.0	23.1	35.1	12.0	10.2	13.8
New England	38.1	28.3	48.2	39.4	29.4	49.7	3.8*	-	7.8*
Mid. Atlantic	29.4	24.0	35.0	31.3	25.2	37.6	14.4	13.6*	15.1*
E. No. Central	29.9	23.7	36.4	31.8	25.1	38.7	14.4	11.1*	17.6
W. No. Central	26.0	20.0	32.1	26.6	20.9	32.5	16.1*	6.4*	25.9*
So. Atlantic	24.1	19.8	28.5	30.5	24.8	36.5	8.3	7.2*	9.4
E. So. Central	19.5	16.3	22.7	24.2	20.0	28.7	8.0	7.2*	8.7*
W. So. Central	24.6	19.1	30.2	27.6	21.2	34.3	13.3	11.4*	15.2
Mountain	16.5	14.2	18.8	17.0	14.5	19.5	10.1*	10.1*	10.2*
Pacific	23.2	19.6	27.1	23.6	19.6	27.7	20.7	19.3*	22.1*

[a]Number of deaths in Table A.9.10.

either color the female preponderance is evident. Most of the rates for nonwhites are based on less than 20 deaths by sex and region, but even so the sex difference persists, while the geographic variation must be assumed to be unreliable. For every region the rates for nonwhites are much less than those for whites. Deaths by sex and color for each census region are enumerated in Table A.9.10 for this and the other diagnostic categories of malformation.

(2) Spina bifida. The national death rate attributed to spina bifida was 27.1 per 100,000 under 1 year of age, with a range by state of 4.7 (Alaska, with 1 death) to 52.7 (Rhode Island, with 29 deaths). The rate for about three-fourths of the states ranged between 14 and 37 per 100,000. There would seem then to be a somewhat greater variation here than for monstrosity. Figure 9.3 shows the rounded rates by state. The rates for the entire country east of the Mississippi River are, with rare exceptions, much higher than those for the western half. There is a tendency toward a regular gradient that varies inversely with west longitude. This confirms the study of Hewitt (1963), based on earlier mortality data. Thus we have a consistent finding (or a consistent bias), indicating a geographically related variation for spina bifida.

The death rates by census region are supportive (Table 9.11). Highest are rates for the New England (36), East South Central (34),

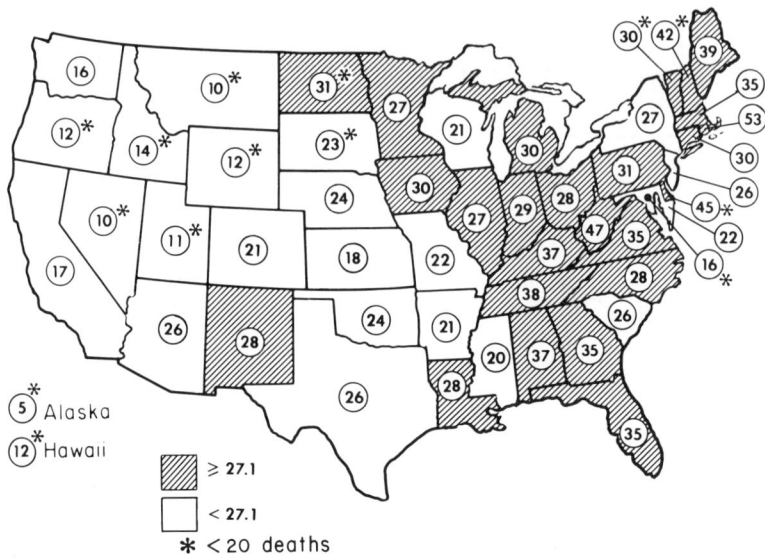

Figure 9.3 Average annual death rates per 100,000 population under 1 year of age for spina bifida by state: United States, 1959-61

and South Atlantic (32 per 100,000) regions. The rates for the Middle Atlantic and East North Central regions, at 28, are next in order. The Pacific rate (16) is less than half the New England rate, and the rate for the Mountain region is also low, at 19 per 100,000. Rates by sex are confirmatory for both colors combined or for whites alone. Again, small numbers preclude reliance on the data for nonwhites. The female predilection is consistent, at least in the rates for whites.

For the entities thus far considered, we have a sex differential (females more often affected), a color difference (rates for whites greater than for nonwhites), and a geographic factor (preponderance in the northeast for monstrosity and in the eastern half of the country for spina bifida). The relation with west longitude is stronger for spina bifida than for monstrosity. It is unfortunate that deaths coded to monstrosity were not subdivided, and that data for these years did not permit the separation of spina bifida with and without hydrocephalus.

(3) Hydrocephalus. The national death rate under 1 year of age for congenital hydrocephalus was 26.9 per 100,000, with a range by states of 8.9 (Delaware, 3 deaths) to 43.0 (District of Columbia, 22

Table 9.11 Average annual death rates per 100,000 population under one year of age for spina bifida and meningocele by color and sex: United States and census regions, 1959-61[a]
(ISC code 751)

Region	Total			White			Nonwhite		
	Total	M	F	Total	M	F	Total	M	F
United States	27.1	23.2	31.1	29.4	24.7	34.2	14.0	14.6	13.4
New England	35.9	26.3	45.8	37.0	27.3	47.0	7.6*	-	15.6*
Mid. Atlantic	28.2	25.5	30.9	30.2	26.5	34.0	12.3	17.8	6.7*
E. No. Central	27.7	22.7	32.7	28.9	23.7	34.2	17.3	14.1*	20.5
W. No. Central	24.9	20.8	29.1	25.9	21.8	30.1	8.1*	3.2*	13.0*
So. Atlantic	31.5	27.6	35.5	38.7	32.3	45.3	13.8	15.6	12.1
E. So. Central	33.7	28.1	39.5	43.4	35.5	51.6	10.4	9.7*	11.1*
W. So. Central	25.8	22.3	29.4	28.0	22.8	33.5	17.5	20.5	14.4*
Mountain	19.1	18.9	19.2	18.0	18.4	17.5	32.9*	25.2*	40.7*
Pacific	16.3	14.9	17.8	17.1	15.6	18.6	10.4*	9.7*	11.1*

[a] Number of deaths in Table A.9.10.

deaths). About three-fourths of the states had rates between 20 and 34 per 100,000. These death rates then appeared more homogeneous than for the prior entities. The highest states were, in order, District of Columbia, Nebraska, Georgia, Virginia, North Carolina, Alabama, and Vermont, accounting for the top one-eighth of the rates. The lowest one-eighth of the rates (listed by increasing death rates) were found for Delaware, Nevada, New Mexico, Hawaii, Idaho, North Dakota, and Colorado. For Colorado only were these low rates based on 20 or more deaths, and it is apparent that the low-rate states are not closely related in space.

The high-rate states comprise the southern "cotton belt," extending somewhat into the northeastern part of the country (Fig. 9.4). The major difference between the rates for hydrocephalus and those for spina bifida by state is that the rates for hydrocephalus in the Northeast are not as consistently high. As we noted previously, monstrosity is concentrated in the Northeast and is rare in the South. One might suspect a real geographic difference among these three entitites—which in turn would suggest differences in cause or precipitants.

By census region (Table 9.12), we see that the highest rates were found for South Atlantic at 32 and East South Central at 31. The western half of the country had the lowest rates at about 22 per

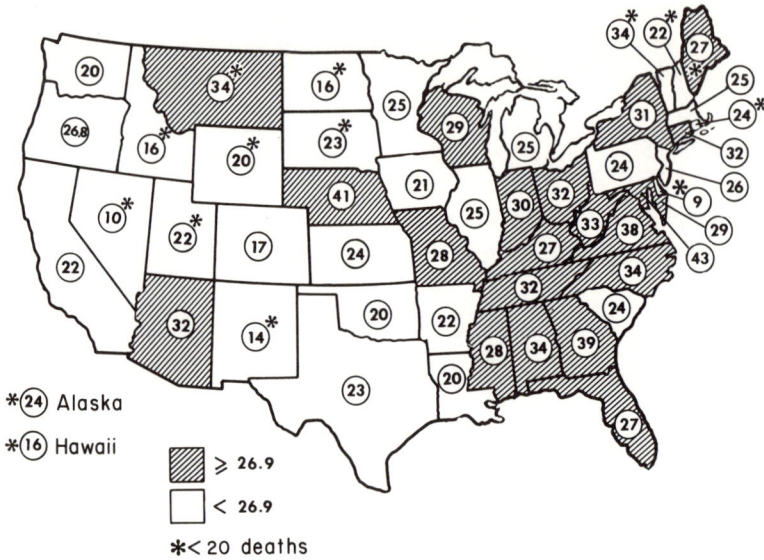

Figure 9.4 Average annual death rates per 100,000 population under 1 year of age for congenital hydrocephalus by state: United States, 1959-61

Table 9.12 Average annual death rates per 100,000 population under one year of age for congenital hydrocephalus by color and sex: United States and census regions, 1959-61[a]
(ISC code 752)

Region	Total			White			Nonwhite		
	Total	M	F	Total	M	F	Total	M	F
United States	26.9	26.7	27.1	27.4	26.9	27.8	24.3	25.7	23.0
New England	27.0	28.8	25.1	26.4	28.5	24.3	42.1*	37.5*	46.8*
Mid. Atlantic	28.0	26.4	29.7	28.2	26.4	30.0	26.6	26.3	26.9
E. No. Central	27.9	27.2	28.5	28.4	27.6	29.2	23.2	23.8	22.7
W. No. Central	25.9	26.2	25.5	26.0	25.9	26.1	24.2*	32.2*	16.2*
So. Atlantic	32.3	31.7	32.8	34.4	32.8	36.0	27.1	29.0	25.3
E. So. Central	30.6	31.5	29.6	33.3	34.2	32.4	23.9	25.0	22.9
W. So. Central	21.8	21.3	22.3	21.9	20.8	23.0	21.6	23.5	19.7
Mountain	21.5	20.8	22.2	21.6	20.4	22.8	20.3*	25.2*	15.3*
Pacific	21.8	23.4	20.0	22.4	24.1	20.6	17.1	18.1*	16.0*

[a]Number of deaths in Table A.9.10.

100,000. This range by region is obviously much smaller than for the prior two entities, as was also indicated by the range for the individual states. Thus while there is reason to suspect a geographic factor related to a high frequency of death reports for hydrocephalus in the Southeast, there is more of a tendency for this entity to be somewhat evenly distributed across the country.

In distribution by sex also, we notice a change from the prior patterns of female preponderance. Hydrocephalus death rates by region were higher for males in four regions and for females in five, with all differences slight. Accordingly, hydrocephalus seems equally distributed by sex and, for each sex, somewhat concentrated in the South, but otherwise tending toward homogeneity.

Another difference from the other disorders is that, by census region, little difference exists between rates for whites and non-whites.

The overall impression for hydrocephalus is one of homogeneity—by sex, by color, and (almost) by geography, although the southeastern states do have a somewhat higher rate.

(4) Other congenital malformations. One would expect the rates in a miscellaneous category to vary only in accord with chance, unless one entity within the group has unique features and itself comprises a large proportion of the group.

For other malformations, the national death rate was 13.0 per 100,000 under 1 year of age, and the range was 4.8 (Nevada, 1 death) to 23.5 (Alaska, 5 deaths). Half the rates were based on less than 20 deaths, so that this wide range may be more explicable on the basis of small numbers than on large geographic variation. More than three-fourths of the states had rates of 8 to 18 per 100,000; the range is small and supports the impression of an even distribution.

The rates by state as drawn in Fig. 9.5 do not appear to represent any consistent pattern, and the data by census region tend to support this. The highest rate was for the Pacific region, at 17 per 100,000 under age 1 year; the lowest was for the East South Central region, at 10. Three regions had rates of 12, and three had rates of 13 (Table 9.13). The Pacific region, while the highest for code 753, was among the lowest for codes 750 through 752, which suggests that part of the geographic variation—at least for code 753—may represent coding artifact. However, for the main types of malformation the geographic differences are too great to attribute much of the variation to their being miscoded under 753 or vice versa. There is then little to suggest noteworthy geographic variation in other neural malformations. By

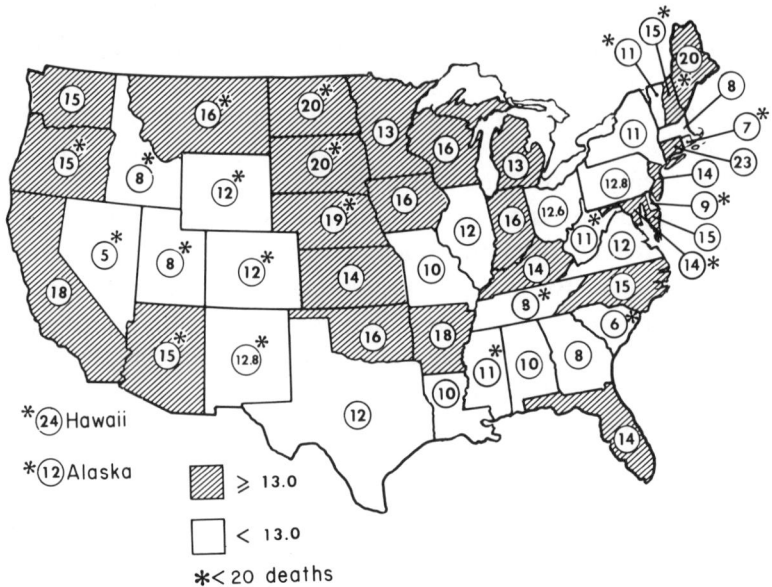

Figure 9.5 Average annual death rates per 100,000 population under 1 year of age for other congenital malformations of the nervous system by state: United States, 1959-61

Table 9.13 Average annual death rates per 100,000 population under one year of age for other malformations of the nervous system by color and sex: United States and census regions, 1959-61[a]
(ISC code 753)

Region	Total			White			Nonwhite		
	Total	M	F	Total	M	F	Total	M	F
United States	13.0	13.8	12.2	13.5	14.3	12.8	9.9	10.9	8.9
New England	13.2	12.9	13.6	13.4	13.1	13.8	7.6*	7.5*	7.8*
Mid. Atlantic	12.0	12.6	11.5	12.3	13.3	11.2	10.1	6.8*	13.5*
E. No. Central	13.3	12.9	13.7	13.7	13.2	14.2	10.3	10.4*	10.3*
W. No. Central	14.0	15.5	12.5	14.3	15.8	12.6	9.7*	9.6*	9.7*
So. Atlantic	11.7	14.0	9.3	12.8	15.2	10.4	8.9	11.1	6.8*
E. So. Central	10.4	9.2	11.6	11.5	9.3	13.8	7.6*	8.9*	6.3*
W. So. Central	12.8	14.5	11.2	13.7	15.1	12.1	9.9	12.1*	7.6*
Mountain	11.7	11.7	11.7	11.0	11.4	10.6	20.3*	15.1*	25.4*
Pacific	16.8	19.0	14.5	17.2	19.1	15.2	13.4	18.1*	8.6*

[a]Number of deaths in Table A.9.10.

sex, there is neither consistent nor notable variation; by color, there is at best a modest underrepresentation of nonwhites (regardless of region).

(5) Interrelationships among types of malformation. The distributions of congenital malformations of the nervous system, when viewed in Figs. 9.2 through 9.5, show some apparent similarities and differences. The distribution by state for other malformations (code 753) differs notably from the rest. The main groups, however, tend to show a concentration in the eastern half of the country: predominantly Northeast for monstrosity (code 750), Southeast for hydrocephalus (code 752), and both Northeast and Southeast for spina bifida (code 751). Superficially, hydrocephalus and spina bifida appear more similar in distribution than any other pair.

Visual impressions, however, can be misleading. Accordingly, the distributions of the death rates by state for each type of malformation were tested formally for correlations between each pair. The Pearson product-moment coefficient of correlation was calculated, with the results given in Table 9.14. The only relationship with statistical significance was that between monstrosity (code 750) and spina bifida (code 751) ($P < 0.001$). The correlation of 0.53 was

Table 9.14 Correlations of death rates under one year of age for specified types of congenital malformations of the nervous system occurring in the states: United States, 1959-61
(ISC codes 750, 751, 752, 753)

Malformation groups compared (ISC codes)[a]	Correlation coefficient[b] (r)	Coefficient of determination[c] (r^2)	Significance level[d]
750 and 751	0.531	0.282	$P<0.001$
750 and 752	-0.067	0.004	NS
750 and 753	0.008	0.000	NS
751 and 752	0.172	0.030	NS
751 and 753	-0.177	0.031	NS
752 and 753	0.126	0.016	NS

[a] 750-Monstrosity; 751-spina bifida and meningocele; 752-congenital hydrocephalus; 753-other congenital malformations of the nervous system.

[b] Pearson (product-moment) correlation coefficient.

[c] Proportion of variance in one malformation group that is associated with variance in the other.

[d] Probability that correlation coefficient is different from zero (NS - not significant, $0.20 < P < 0.975$).

sufficient to explain one-fourth of the variance in either variable as associated with the variance of the other ($r^2 = 0.28$).

The next highest positive coefficient of correlation was between spina bifida and hydrocephalus ($r = 0.17$), and the only noteworthy negative coefficient correlation was that between spina bifida and other malformations ($r = -0.18$). However, these coefficients are not significantly different from zero ($P > 0.20$). Even if they were significant, the associations would explain only 3 percent of the variance. The earlier suggestion that code 753 tended to be recorded reciprocally with the major types thus receives only minimal support. Of special interest was the lack of significant association between spina bifida and hydrocephalus, despite the apparent similarities in Figs. 9.3 and 9.4.

With the similarities by inspection, testing for these same relationships with the Spearman rank-order correlation method was also done, because as a nonparametric measure it avoids the concern as to whether the assumptions underlying the Pearson coefficient of correlation have all been met. However, the results were similar, with only the monstrosity and the spina bifida distributions showing a significant association ($r_s = 0.47$), while that for spina bifida and hydrocephalus was still not significant ($r_s = 0.25, P \sim 0.07$).

It is unfortunate that the data for monstrosity could not be subdivided according to individual clinical entities, or at least for anencephaly. As will be further discussed, anencephaly and spina bifida seem to share a number of epidemiologic characteristics. We have already noted that anencephaly should comprise the greatest bulk of the *births* attributed to monstrosity, but that most anencephalics are stillborn. However, we suspect that insofar as code 750 seems to behave as a single entity rather than as a group of pathologically unrelated disorders (as is code 753), it is likely a reflection of anencephaly.

(6) Sum of malformations. Despite the lack of any suggestion of negative correlation between pairs of malformations, some of the geographic variation discussed might result from coding variations in different states. If this is the case, then the distribution of all malformations combined would appear more homogeneous than the constituents thereof. In Fig. 9.6 are the rates by state for deaths under 1 year of age, again rounded to integers, for the sum of the four categories we are considering. The concentration from Maine to Florida east of the Mississippi River is noteworthy. The death rates ranged from 50.0 for Idaho to 129.7 for Maine. All of New England

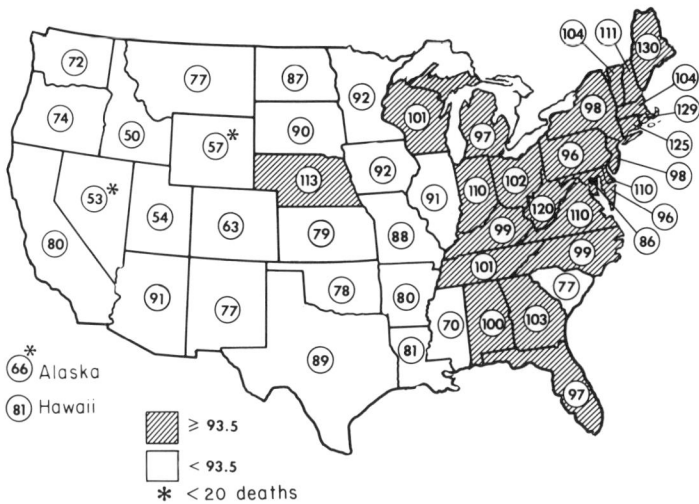

Figure 9.6 Average annual death rates per 100,000 population under 1 year of age for all congenital malformations of the nervous system by state: United States, 1959–61

had rates in excess of 100. In the eastern third of the country, only South Carolina, at 77.0, and the District of Columbia, at 86.1, were below the national mean rate of 93.5.

Accordingly then, the geographic variations appear worthy of further investigation as to possible reasons for their preponderance in the eastern states.

Type of county. Whether residence at death was in a metropolitan or a nonmetropolitan county is of relevance in seeking urban-rural differences in these disorders, as has occasionally been posited.

(1) Monstrosity. In Table 9.15 are the death rates under 1 year of age for monstrosity. For the United States as a whole, there is a slight preponderance of monstrosity deaths reported for residents of metropolitan counties as opposed to nonmetropolitan, at 28 versus 24 per 100,000. The difference is present for each color and for each sex.

Within the metropolitan counties, there is little difference in the overall rates between those with and those without central cities (28 vs 29 per 100,000), and the differences by sex or color are discrepant. Thus the *degree* of urbanization within the metropolitan counties does not seem to be a factor.

Table 9.15 Average annual death rates per 100,000 population under one year of age for monstrosity by color, sex and type of county: United States, 1959-61 (ISC code 750)

Color & sex	Metropolitan counties			Nonmetropolitan counties
	Total	With central city	Without central city	
Total	28.1	27.9	29.0	23.6
Male	22.7	22.1	25.1	18.6
Female	33.7	33.8	33.0	28.7
White	30.6	30.8	30.2	26.1
Male	24.7	24.2	26.3	20.4
Female	36.9	37.6	34.2	32.0
Nonwhite	13.6	13.8	11.3*	9.2
Male	11.4	11.9	6.2*	8.1
Female	15.8	15.8	16.2*	10.2

It is this lack of a regular gradient from the most urban to the most rural counties that leads us to question the meaning of the metropolitan-nonmetropolitan difference, which is statistically significant beyond the 0.1-percent level for the United States as a whole. We suspect that incomplete ascertainment in the more rural regions may be responsible for much of the difference.

(2) Spina bifida. Here the impression is opposite to that for monstrosity, with the nonmetropolitan death rates at 28 exceeding the metropolitan at 26 per 100,000, a difference significant at the 5-percent level (Table 9.16). This difference persists regardless of sex or color. Again, however, the differences *within* the metropolitan counties for those with and without central cities are not at all consistent, and for females and white males, the lowest rates were recorded for metropolitan counties without central cities.

(3) Hydrocephalus. The pattern by type of county for congenital hydrocephalus death rates is similar to that for spina bifida. The metropolitan rate at 26 per 100,000 is significantly less ($P < 0.05$) than the nonmetropolitan rate at 28. The only divergence from this finding was for nonwhite females, whose metropolitan rate was 25 versus 20 for the nonmetropolitan (Table 9.17). Once again the subtypes of the metropolitan counties did not provide rates that

Table 9.16 Average annual death rates per 100,000 population under one year of age for spina bifida and meningocele by color, sex and type of county: United States, 1959-61
(ISC code 751)

Color & sex	Metropolitan counties			Nonmetropolitan counties
	Total	With central city	Without central city	
Total	26.3	26.3	26.3	28.3
Male	22.3	22.2	22.6	24.8
Female	30.5	30.6	30.2	32.0
White	28.7	29.0	27.3	30.6
Male	23.8	24.1	22.9	26.2
Female	33.7	34.2	31.9	35.2
Nonwhite	13.2	13.3	12.3*	15.5
Male	13.3	12.8	18.6*	16.9
Female	13.1	13.7	6.1*	14.0

Table 9.17 Average annual death rates per 100,000 population under one year of age for congenital hydrocephalus by color, sex and type of county: United States, 1959-61
(ISC code 752)

Color & sex	Metropolitan counties			Nonmetropolitan counties
	Total	With central city	Without central city	
Total	26.1	26.2	25.6	28.3
Male	25.6	26.0	24.0	28.6
Female	26.6	26.5	27.3	27.9
White	26.5	26.8	25.5	28.9
Male	26.0	26.7	23.7	28.4
Female	27.0	26.8	27.3	29.4
Nonwhite	24.0	23.7	27.6	24.9
Male	23.2	22.7	28.9*	30.2
Female	24.8	24.7	26.4*	19.7

Table 9.18 Average annual death rates per 100,000 population under one year of age for other congenital malformations of the nervous system by color, sex and type of county: United States, 1959-61
(ISC code 753)

Color & sex	Metropolitan counties			Nonmetropolitan counties
	Total	With central city	Without central city	
Total	12.0	11.9	12.3	14.8
Male	12.5	12.3	13.0	16.1
Female	11.5	11.5	11.6	13.3
White	12.5	12.5	12.6	15.3
Male	12.8	12.8	13.1	16.8
Female	12.2	12.2	12.1	13.8
Nonwhite	9.0	9.1	8.2*	11.4
Male	10.2	10.0	12.4*	12.1
Female	7.8	8.2	4.1*	10.8

suggest urban-rural gradients, since for the most part it was the metropolitan county without central city for which the lowest rates were reported.

(4) Other congenital malformations. In accord with the last two prior groupings, other congenital malformations of the nervous system were recorded more often from nonmetropolitan counties: 15 per 100,000 versus 12, significant beyond the 0.1-percent level (Table 9.18). There was little difference, however, according to the type of metropolitan county.

Thus only for deaths allocated to monstrosity was the death rate significantly higher in metropolitan counties, while for each of the other categories of neurologic malformation the rate was higher in nonmetropolitan counties. There was no regular gradient of risk from most urban to most rural types of county, because the only demonstrable differences were between the dichotomy of metropolitan versus nonmetropolitan. Even though the differences noted for the death rates were significant statistically, they were not of great magnitude, being less than 5 per 100,000 under 1 year of age for monstrosity and only 2 or 3 per 100,000 for the other categories of malformation. Accordingly, these data do not afford much evidence for ruralization or urbanization as major risk factors in neural malformations.

Morbidity Data

We can now consider malformations of the nervous system under the much more appropriate categories of anencephaly, spina bifida, and hydrocephalus. Relative frequencies for these and the other neural abnormalities from a large series were listed at the beginning of this chapter in Table 9.1. The admixture of even the three main classes is appreciable, but very few of the significant neural defects are *not* included therein—perhaps 7 percent in all. Our attention then will be limited to the three main groupings.

Incidence Rates among Births

The largest series collected at one time under reasonably standardized methods, and from many different areas of the world, is the WHO study of twenty-four centers (Stevenson et al. 1966a and b). The composition of this study has been detailed in Chapter 8 (Down's syndrome), and the number of births by center is recorded in Table A.8.4.

Table 9.19 shows the incidence rates per 1,000 total (live plus stillborn) births. These data exclude about 5,000 sets of multiple births and refer only to the approximately 417,000 single births which took place in hospitals for 1961-64 in these centers.

In this study, there were twenty-five individuals with defects of the nervous system among twenty-four sets of affected twins. This included one pair of females, one of whom had spina bifida alone and the other spina bifida with hydrocephalus. If we count each individual among the 5,022 pairs of twins, the rate for hydrocephalus was 0.7 per 1,000 births, from four with hydrocephalus alone and three with hydrocephalus and spina bifida. The latter, together with two with spina bifida and anencephaly, added to the seven with spina bifida alone, provided a rate of 1.2 per 1,000 births for spina bifida. Nine anencephalics with the two who also had spina bifida gave a rate of 1.1 per 1,000.

Comparison with rates for the single births in the same study suggests that twinning results in neither an excess nor a deficit of neural tube anomalies (Table 9.20).

Detail as to the rates by center and neural tube abnormality for the

Table 9.19   Cases and incidence rates[a] per 1,000 total (live plus stillborn) single births for congenital malformations of the nervous system by type of malformation: WHO study of 24 centers, 1961-64

Type of malformation	Cases	Rate[a]
Total	1,109	2.66
Anencephaly alone	382	0.92
Anencephaly and spina bifida	54	0.13
Hydrocephalus alone	254	0.61
Hydrocephalus and spina bifida	108	0.26
Spina bifida (with or without spinal meningocele)	231	0.55
Occipital meningocele	16	0.04
Other neural tube defects[b]	34	0.08
Microcephaly	27	0.06
All other nervous system	3	0.01

[a]Rates standardized for maternal age.
[b]Predominantly encephalocele.

Table 9.20   Incidence rates[a] per 1,000 total (live plus stillborn) births for major congenital malformations of the nervous system among single-born and twin-born infants by type of malformation: WHO study of 24 centers, 1961-64

Type of malformation[b]	Single born	Twin born
Hydrocephalus	0.9	0.7
Spina bifida	0.9	1.2
Anencephaly	1.1	1.1
(Number of cases)	(1,029)	(25)

[a]Rates standardized for maternal age.
[b]Rate for each type of malformation includes those persons who also have one or both of the other defects.

CONGENITAL MALFORMATIONS / 197

WHO study is provided in Table A.9.11. Differences between that table and others presented are caused by the rounding of rates.

There are many other studies on the frequency at birth of malformations of the nervous system. The major ones are summarized in Table 9.21 according to whether the rates refer to total births (live plus stillborn), live births, or stillbirths (numerator) among total births (denominator). The following discussion is based on Tables A.9.11 and 9.21.

Major malformations of the nervous system. Incidence rates per 1,000 single total births in the WHO study ranged from 0.6 for Calcutta to 10.2 for Belfast (Table A.9.11). The second highest rate

Table 9.21 Total number of cases and incidence rates per 1,000 births for congenital defects of the neural tube by type of defect: selected community surveys, various years, 1935-67

Survey area (source)	Years	Total cases (neural tube)	Rate			
			Total neural tube	Hydro-cephalus	Spina bifida	Anen-cephaly
			Rate per 1,000 total (live plus stillborn) births			
WHO, 24 centers[a] (Stevenson et al. 1966b)	1961-64	1,079	2.6	0.9[b]	0.9[b]	1.1[b]
South Wales (Laurence 1966)	1956-62	835	8.1	0.5	4.1[b]	3.4
Southampton Borough, England (Williamson 1965)	1958-62	90	6.0	0.9	3.2	2.0
Birmingham, England (Leck & Millar 1963)	1957-61	536	5.3	---	3.2[b]	2.6[b]
Birmingham, England (Leck 1963, 1966)	1940-65	1,966	4.7[c]	---	2.6[c]	2.2
Victoria, Australia (Collmann & Stoller 1962a,b)	1942-57	292	1.8	0.6	0.6	0.7
Liverpool, England (Smithells 1962; et al. 1964, 1965)	1960-63	438	6.8[d]	---	3.5	3.3[d]
Northamptonshire, England (Pleydell 1957)	1944-55	168	3.2	0.5	1.9	0.9
Rochester, Minnesota (Gibson & Kurland, unpubl.)	1935-67	85	3.2	1.8[b]	2.0[b]	0.9[b]
			Rate per 1,000 live births			
Rochester, Minnesota (Kurland 1958a)	1945-54	25	3.4	2.2[b]	←1.2[b]→	
Carlisle, England (Brewis et al. 1966)	1955-61	36	4.2	1.8[b]	3.3[b]	0.2
			Rate among stillbirths per 1,000 total births			
Scotland (McKeown & Record 1951)	1939-46	3,325	4.4	1.4	0.5	2.5
Scotland (Leck 1963)	1951-60	4,304	4.4	1.3	0.3	2.9
Birmingham, England (McKeown & Record 1951)	1940-47	579	3.7	0.7	0.8	2.2

[a]Single births only; rates standardized for maternal age.
[b]Rate includes those who also have one or both of the other types of neural tube defects.
[c]Spina bifida for 1950-65 only.
[d]Anencephaly for 1960-62 only.

was that for Alexandria, at 7.9. All other rates were less than 4 per 1,000 and most were between 1 and 3. The overall rate was 2.6 per 1,000 for neural tube defects and 2.7 per 1,000 when other neurologic anomalies were included.

The ranges for total births from other sources were 1.8 to 8.1 per 1,000. The highest was for South Wales, followed by Liverpool (6.8) and Southampton Borough (6.0), both of England. Rates in Birmingham, England, were 4.7 and 5.3 for two periods, but in Northamptonshire, England, the rate was only 3.2. This was about the same as the rate for Rochester, Minnesota. The low rate of 1.8 per 1,000 was recorded for Victoria, Australia. (References are provided in Table 9.21.)

Based on live births from two community surveys, rates were 3.4 for Rochester, Minnesota, and 4.2 for Carlisle, England. Rates for stillbirths per 1,000 total births are also about 4 per 1,000 from Scotland and from Birmingham, England.

For neural malformations as a whole, there is evidence of considerable geographic variation. Rates in the British Isles are generally high but rather scattered (South Wales, Southampton Borough, Liverpool), and maximal in Belfast. In the other lands, only the rate for Alexandria seems notably high (WHO study). Especially low rates were recorded for Calcutta; Medellín, Colombia; and Manila, but the numbers of cases reported are small.

From Table 9.21, one might expect rates of 2 to 8 per 1,000 births, centering at about 4 per 1,000, which may serve as a reasonable base-line value from which to judge noteworthy variations. Our information thus far suggests, however, that the various neural malformations have differing characteristics. Therefore we need attend to the individual entities, insofar as individual features can be defined for disorders that are so often concomitant.

(1) Hydrocephalus. Rates for hydrocephalus alone were mostly 0.5 to 0.9 per 1,000 (Table 9.21) and averaged 0.6 in the WHO study, with a range of 0.1 for Calcutta to 2.0 for Alexandria (Table A.9.11). In Melbourne, the rate was 1.6 at one hospital, but 0.8 at the other. The next highest rate was for Belfast at 1.2. The three South African hospitals representing respectively Colored, white, and Bantu patients, had rates of 0.8, 0.5, and 1.1 each. The lowest rates besides Calcutta were for Singapore; one Mexico City center; Santiago, Chile; Medellín, Colombia; Hong Kong; Manila; and Madrid (all at 0.2 and 0.3). Thus low rates were scattered geographically. In Asia, the rates for Bombay (0.7) and Kuala Lumpur (1.0) and in

South America, those for São Paulo (1.0) and Bogotá (0.9) were above the average.

For hydrocephalus with spina bifida, the rates for each of the centers were at or below 0.6 per 1,000 total births, except for Belfast with 1.6 and one Melbourne center with 1.1 (Table A.9.11). The rates for hydrocephalus with or without spina bifida from Table 9.21 were 0.9 as the average for the twenty-four WHO centers and 1.8 for Rochester, Minnesota, both based on total births—that is, live plus stillborn. The rate when based on live births alone was little different, being 2.2 in Rochester and 1.8 in Carlisle, England.

Thus hydrocephalus alone probably accounts for a rate just under 1 per 1,000 births, and with spina bifida a little more than 1. Hydrocephalus alone, from the available data, would seem uniform in geographic distribution throughout the world. This is in keeping with our tentative interpretation of relative homogeneity among deaths from hydrocephalus in the United States. The addition of coincident spina bifida to this category did not appreciably alter this interpretation (except for Belfast).

(2) *Spina bifida.* The range of the rates for spina bifida with or without other malformations was appreciable, ranging from 0.6 to 4.1 per 1,000 total births (Table 9.21). Highest rates were for South Wales and Liverpool. In the WHO study (Table A.9.11), spina bifida alone had a high rate of 2.6 in Belfast and low rates of 0.0 in Manila, and 0.1 in Bogotá, Calcutta, and Singapore. For spina bifida with hydrocephalus, only Belfast at 1.6 and Melbourne at 1.1 had rates of more than 0.6. For spina bifida with anencephaly, no center had a rate that exceeded 0.6. For all centers combined, the rates (and proportions) for spina bifida were 0.6 alone, 0.3 with hydrocephalus, and 0.1 with anencephaly. Rates for all spina bifida were highest in Belfast (4.6 per 1,000 births)—more than twice as high as the next ranking centers: Melbourne at 2.2 (the other Melbourne rate being 1.2) and Alexandria at 2.0. All others had rates less than 2 per 1,000, with the lowest from several (but not all) South American centers and several (but not all) Asian centers. The rates in South Africa were 0.8 for Colored, 0.9 for white, and 1.2 for Bantu.

We see, therefore, that the rates for spina bifida seemed to vary notably with geography, with maximal values in parts of the United Kingdom, especially in Belfast.

(3) *Anencephaly.* Per 1,000 total births, anencephaly alone or combined with other neural defects accounted for rates of 0.7 (Victoria) to 3.4 (South Wales) (Table 9.21). The rate for anen-

cephaly alone in the WHO study averaged 0.9 per 1,000 (Table A.9.11), but only two centers had high rates: Alexandria (3.2) and Belfast (4.1). Rates for all anencephaly, alone or with other defects, were high only in Belfast (4.5) and Alexandria (3.8). No other center attained a rate of 2 per 1,000 for anencephaly with or without spina bifida. Penrose (1957) has reported that the incidence rates at birth in Europe for anencephaly and spina bifida (but not Down's syndrome) were highest in Ireland and western Great Britain, and that the rates decreased as one proceeded eastward on the continent of Europe.

When based on live births alone, anencephaly rates would be expected to be low, as was the case in Carlisle, England, where the rate of 0.2 contrasts with the much higher rates for total births from six centers of England and Wales (Table 9.21). Anencephalic *stillbirth* rates in Scotland (2.5 and 2.9 per 1,000 total births) were somewhat higher than the Birmingham rate of 2.2, though all were much more in keeping with rates for the United Kingdom based on total births than those based on live births alone. This is what prevents assurance as to the proportion contributed to monstrosity deaths (code 750) by anencephaly.

(4) Interrelationships among types of malformation. Previously, we discussed such interrelationships insofar as their distribution by state from death data would permit. We found a highly significant correlation between monstrosity and spina bifida distributions, but no other pairs showed evidence of association.

The WHO series permits a similar assessment from morbidity data, from the distributions of each entity by center among the twenty-four centers. This assessment is limited by the small number of cases (see Table A.9.11). Comparisons were made for the rates based on the 254 cases of hydrocephalus alone, the 231 of spina bifida alone, and the 382 of anencephaly alone. The Pearson product-moment coefficient of correlation of the rates among the centers was calculated for each pair of malformations: spina bifida and anencephaly, spina bifida and hydrocephalus, and anencephaly and hydrocephalus. The results are set forth in Table 9.22.

A highly significant association was found between spina bifida and anencephaly ($r = 0.75$). More than half the variance in the distribution of one of these can then be explained by the variance of the other ($r^2 = 0.57$). We may recall that the only significant association found for the distributions by state in the mortality data was between spina bifida and monstrosity.

Table 9.22 Correlations of incidence rates among total (live plus stillborn) single births for specified congenital malformations of the nervous system occurring alone in 24 areas: WHO study of 24 centers, 1961-64

Malformation groups compared[a]	Correlation coefficient[b] (r)	Coefficient of determination[c] (r^2)	Significance level[d]
H and SB	0.445	0.198	$P < 0.05$
H and A	0.526	0.277	$P < 0.01$
SB and A	0.752	0.566	$P < 0.001$

[a] Hydrocephalus alone (H), spina bifida alone (SB), anencephaly alone (A), as shown in Table A.9.11.
[b] Pearson (product-moment) correlation coefficient.
[c] Proportion of variance in one malformation group that is associated with variance in the other.
[d] Probability that correlation coefficient is different from zero.

Unlike the death data, distributions for hydrocephalus and anencephaly were significantly associated in the WHO series ($r = 0.53, P < 0.01$), and even hydrocephalus and spina bifida revealed a positive relationship ($r = 0.45, P < 0.05$). Practically speaking, hydrocephalus and anencephaly are mutually exclusive entities, so that their correlation here may be more a reflection of coding or diagnostic variation by center.

From these associations, then, we note a relation between distributions of spina bifida and anencephaly and between spina bifida and monstrosity. The results from the morbidity and the mortality data were discrepant in terms of associations between the pairs of the other entities: positive from the morbidity data, and unrelated from the mortality distributions. We have considered other evidence, such as the sex ratios, which indicates that hydrocephalus behaves differently from spina bifida and anencephaly. Accordingly, the evidence of association for hydrocephalic births with the others should be viewed cautiously.

Sex Ratios in Neural Malformations

From the international comparisons of death data recorded previously, we noted a definite excess of females for monstrosity and for spina bifida, whereas hydrocephalus and other neural malformations showed little difference by sex, or at most a possible excess of males. For the United States deaths, 1959-61, there was also a female preponderance for monstrosity and for spina bifida; rates were essentially equal by sex for hydrocephalus and minimally higher in males for other malformations. Death data for 1962-67 in the United States indicated a male-female ratio of 1.2 to 1 on the rates (all ages) for hydrocephalus alone, but a ratio of 0.8 to 1 for spina bifida, either alone or with hydrocephalus.

Table 9.23 shows sex ratios for each individual type and combination of neural tube malformation from the two series that permitted such detail, the WHO series (Stevenson et al. 1966a and b) and that from Rochester, Minnesota (Gibson and Kurland, unpublished data). They are compared with the sex ratios recorded for the three main categories of malformation (alone or combined) from Scotland (McKeown and Record 1951). The data from Rochester, however, must be considered in the light of the small numbers of cases. The rank order of the sex ratios in both the WHO and the Rochester

Table 9.23 Male-female ratios among total (live plus stillborn) births with neural tube defects by type of defect: selected surveys, various years, 1935-67

Type of defect	WHO study[a] (1961-64)		Scotland[b] (1939-46)		Rochester[c] (1935-67)	
	M:F ratio	No. of cases[d]	M:F ratio	No. of cases	M:F ratio	No. of cases
Hydrocephalus						
alone	1.33	252	---	---	0.73	19
with spina bifida	0.96	108	---	---	0.56	28
total	1.21	360	1.04	---	0.62	47
Spina bifida						
alone	0.82	229	---	---	0.43	10
with anencephaly	0.42	54	---	---	0.11	10
total	0.79	391	0.76	---	0.37	52[e]
Anencephaly						
alone	0.54	381	---	---	0.08	14
total	0.52	435	0.36	---	0.09	24

[a] 24 centers, single births only (Stevenson et al. 1966a,b).
[b] Registrar-General (McKeown and Record 1951).
[c] Rochester, Minnesota (Gibson and Kurland, unpublished data).
[d] Excludes cases with sex undertermined.
[e] Includes 4 with microcephaly.

series is virtually equivalent, even though females predominated for each type of defect in Rochester.

From the WHO study, there is a clear male predominance for hydrocephalus alone. The male-female ratio falls to just under unity when hydrocephalus is combined with spina bifida. Spina bifida alone in that series shows a male-female ratio of about 0.8 to 1. When found with hydrocephalus, this ratio is almost unity, but when seen with anencephaly, there is a great female excess, the male-female ratio being 0.4 to 1.

Anencephaly alone in the WHO data was twice as common in females, with a male-female ratio of 0.5 to 1. That anencephaly with spina bifida is even lower (0.4) may be explained by a happenstance of small numbers—or perhaps by the presence of two additive risk factors to which females are especially susceptible. In Rochester no such discrepancy was found, and the former explanation might seem the more likely. The data for Scotland do not permit separation of the defects occurring alone versus those in combination. Nevertheless, they support the female predominance for spina bifida and anencephaly and a male excess for hydrocephalus.

In general, then, it seems likely that anencephaly is much more common in females, spina bifida has a modest female excess, and hydrocephalus a modest male excess. This would suggest that hydrocephalus at least is epidemiologically an entity distinct from the others. This was also our impression from the mortality data. Separation of anencephaly from spina bifida is not so clear; these entities seem to share a number of common features, in addition to coexistence in many of the affected.

Secular Trends in Anencephaly

There has been considerable interest, especially in the past decade or so, in the changing frequencies of these malformations with time. Most attention has been focused on spina bifida and anencephaly. Because large inconsistencies remain among the various studies, we shall consider only the data for anencephaly. Our assertion that the rates for spina bifida tend to parallel those for anencephaly can be tested from the cited references. Incidentally, we have the general impression, from the sparse data available, that rates for hydrocephalus may not be as variable with time as those for anencephaly.

The studies to be considered are summarized in Table 9.24 and drawn in Fig. 9.7. Cases for the first three studies in Table 9.24 were

Table 9.24 Peak years in secular trends of incidence rates among total (live plus stillborn) births for anencephaly: selected surveys, various years, 1920-65

	Survey area and symbol (Figure 9.7)	Years	Number of cases	Trend: peak years
A	Berlin, Germany	1930-54	918[a]	1945-49
B	Hamburg, Germany	1930-63	196[a]	1930-34[b]
C	Göttingen, Germany	1930-54	45[a]	1941-45
D	Birmingham, England	1940-65	1,130	1940-41[b] 1956-57
E	Melbourne, Australia	1942-57	106	no trend[c]
F	Halifax, Canada	1946-55	74	1949-52[c]
G	Charleston, S.C., USA	1946-55	34	(?)1951-55[b,c]
H	Boston, Mass., USA	1920-65[d]	202	1930-34
I	Providence, R.I., USA	1920-65[e]	323	1930-34 (?)1940-44
J	Boston, Mass., USA	1930-65[f]	305	1930-34[b] (?) 1946-49

Source: Lenz 1965 (Surveys A,B,C); Leck 1966 (Survey D); Collmann and Stoller 1962a(Survey E); Alter 1963a (Surveys F,G); MacMahon and Yen 1971(Surveys H,I); Naggan 1969 (Survey J).

[a]Estimated from incidence rates and total births.
[b]Peak in first or last period covered in the study.
[c]Based on centered moving average of biennial rates.
[d]Study period extended from 1875, with 268 cases.
[e]Study period extended from 1885, with 349 cases.
[f]Part of this series included in study (H) of MacMahon and Yen.

approximated from the rates and births in each period. Because of the small numbers of cases in the studies labeled E, F, and G, biennial rates were first calculated from the cases and births, and from these a centered moving average of each two consecutive biennial periods was recorded. The data for the studies labeled H and I extended back to 1875 and 1885, respectively. The former recorded the experience at the Boston Lying-in Hospital, which was also one of the two resources for the last study, J. In Table 9.24, we have attempted to identify the type of trend for each study, with notation of the time for the peak rate or rates. Where the peak rate

CONGENITAL MALFORMATIONS / 205

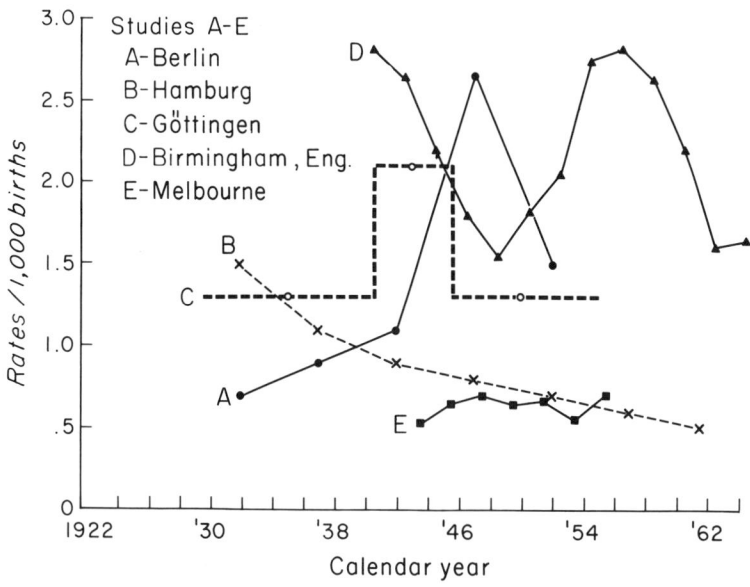

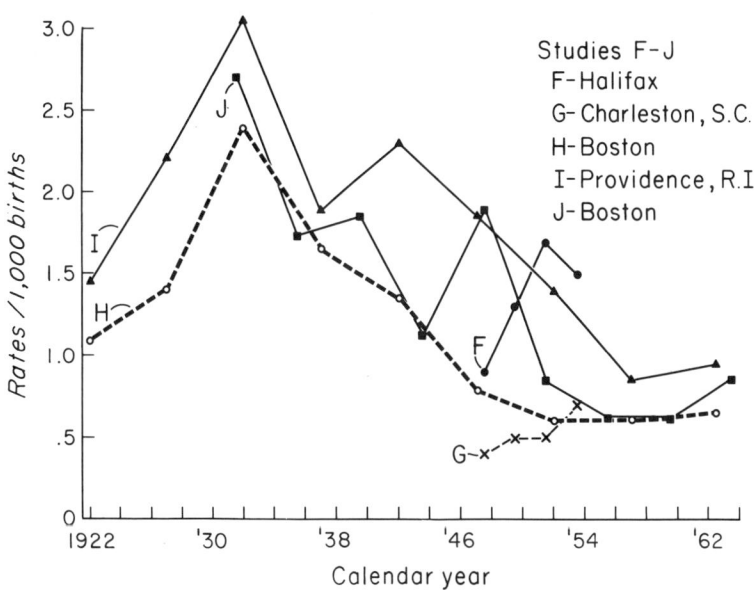

Figure 9.7 Rates per 1,000 total births for anencephaly by year: selected surveys, various years, 1920–65. Rates are taken from surveys in Table 9.24.

occurred in the first or the last period for the study in question, this too has been identified.

In the United States there is a well-defined peak value in 1930-34 for rates for anencephaly (studies H, I, and J). That this was the first period for one study (J) may well be the reason its author (Naggan 1969) thought the rates thereafter were declining with time. It is of some interest that the rates for Hamburg (study B) follow the same pattern as seen in study J. We may recall the declining death rates for spina bifida and hydrocephalus noted earlier for the United States during the period 1950-67 (Fig. 9.1). This might be considered evidence for the same trend, as most of the studies previously cited also included analyses for spina bifida, which had essentially the same patterning with time.

A peak in the first period was also found for Birmingham, England, for 1940-41 (study D). This *could* be part of the same decline from the early 1930s seen for those works just considered. A somewhat later peak (1941-45) was found for Göttingen (study C), which may match a slight secondary peak in Providence, Rhode Island (study I). Later, we found a peak for Berlin (study A) in 1945-49, which coincides with a secondary peak from one study in Boston (study J) but not present in the other Boston survey (study H). The Halifax rate seems to peak at 1949-52 (study F); the very slight change in Charleston, South Carolina (study G), is similar in time to this last study. No notable changes over admittedly short periods were found in Melbourne, Australia (study E), and perhaps the Charleston rates (study G) too should be considered to have not changed with time.

There is only one study that clearly indicates a bimodal curve with striking peaks: that for Birmingham, England (study D), which starts at a maximum for 1940-41, then declines almost by half by 1948-49, and increases again to the same high level by 1956-57, only to decrease once more to the same nadir in 1962-63. Peak-peak and valley-valley intervals are each about sixteen years in duration.

Various explanations for the phenomena have been offered. Mac-Mahon and Yen (1971) considered this an unrecognized epidemic temporally related to the Great Depression in the United States. Lenz (1965) thought the war might be a factor for the peak in Berlin and Göttingen, but left unexplained the lack of any similar peak in Hamburg at that time. Naggan (1969) thought the Boston data indicated a declining rate with time for anencephaly, as we have previously noted. However, the peak in the early 1930s was not observed in Göttingen, and the Birmingham sixteen-year periodicity has not been observed elsewhere.

Thus the evidence at present indicates that there are indeed striking secular changes in rates for anencephaly (and spina bifida). There is no evident temporal, geographic, or sequential explanation that is satisfactory for all these studies. Certainly it would seem premature to consider that anencephaly is a disappearing disorder, and neither the depression, the war, nor any other obvious factor explains all the varied configurations found. This would seem a most fruitful area for further epidemiologic inquiry.

Comment

Congenital malformations of the nervous system represent an important source of morbidity and mortality, particularly in the perinatal period. The ISC coding in use for the period in question divided this group into monstrosity, spina bifida, congenital hydrocephalus, and other malformations. There were no special instructions for coding concurrent spina bifida and hydrocephalus in the United States until 1962, when their allocation was defined in a fashion later adopted in the Eighth Revision of the ISC (World Health Organization 1967). In the Eighth Revision also, anencephaly has been differentiated out from the monstrosity group, a rubric no longer used. We suggest that spina bifida be subdivided into that with hydrocephalus, that with anencephaly, and that occurring alone; perhaps one further subgrouping of spina bifida with other congenital neural malformations may also be in order. An additional category that occurs often enough to be separate is microcephaly. In the Eighth Revision both it and encephalocele are four-digit subcodes of other malformations.

Should these changes be accomplished, mortality data routinely available would in a short while be sufficient to clarify many of the questions this chapter has covered (such as the interrelationships among these entities, their sex ratios, and color differences) and some which have not been discussed (relation to maternal age, and correlates of variations in geographic distribution).

International mortality data on malformations of the nervous system indicate a notable female preponderance for monstrosity and spina bifida. For hydrocephalus and other malformations, the difference if any is slightly toward more males involved. In the United

States, 1959-61, monstrosity and spina bifida also predominated in females, hydrocephalus had a sex ratio of unity, and other malformations showed a slight male excess. Later mortality data in the United States did support a modest male preponderance for hydrocephalus without spina bifida. Morbidity data indicated a female excess for anencephaly and spina bifida, and hydrocephalus was generally somewhat more common in males.

Differences by color were found in the United States mortality statistics of 1959-61, with a white preponderance for monstrosity and spina bifida, and much less of a white excess for other malformations. However, the rates for hydrocephalus were essentially equal by color or sex. Limited morbidity data from South Africa suggest there is no difference in risk for any neurologic malformation according to color.

Geographic variation was noteworthy in the United States. Other malformations had a rather small range, and high-rate states were scattered, both suggesting no more than chance variation. Although hydrocephalus death rates were higher in the southeastern United States, the range in rates was modest. However, monstrosity death rates were notably high in the northeastern states, and the rates for spina bifida deaths similarly were high in virtually all eastern states. When tested formally, distributions for monstrosity and spina bifida showed a highly significant correlation, but no pair of the other combinations of the four categories showed any significant association. We believe that the largest single entity in the category of monstrosity is anencephaly, but most anencephalics would *not* be included in standard mortality data because most are stillborn.

A similar assessment of geographic distribution in the WHO study of births in twenty-four centers (with, however, many fewer cases) indicated that the strongest correlation was between anencephaly and spina bifida. All three correlations (including hydrocephalus and anencephaly) were statistically significant (at least at the 0.05 level), and each was higher than the corresponding correlations from the mortality data. Whether the two relationships for hydrocephalus reflect artifacts of coding practice or of small samples must be considered. This seems likely for hydrocephalus with anencephaly at least, as these disorders, practically speaking, are mutually exclusive.

Noteworthy changes with time in the frequency of neural malformations have been recorded. The United States mortality rates (all ages) decreased by nearly half between 1950 and 1967, owing almost entirely to parallel declines in the frequencies of hydrocephalus and spina bifida. The declining number of births accounts for at least part of this change. Generally, though, it has been variations in the frequency of anencephaly (and spina bifida) that have received the most attention.

In the United States and in parts of Europe, the peak incidence for anencephaly seems to have occurred in the early 1930s. In other parts of Europe, peaks have been described for several separate periods between 1940 and 1960, without much consistency. And there is one area—Birmingham, England—where a sixteen-year cycle (peak-peak or valley-valley) has been described. In essence, then, explanation for these variations, which are large, remains a worthy topic for future epidemiologic inquiry.

As to geographic variations on a cross-sectional basis, we wonder whether one man's trough was another's apex. Still, there appear to be striking variations. Coffey and Jessop (1957) noted that 6 per 1,000 hospital births in Dublin were of anencephalics. In the WHO study, Belfast far outranked the other centers in the incidence rates of anencephaly and spina bifida, but was not nearly so much above the mean for hydrocephalus (Stevenson et al. 1966b). Bostonians of Irish descent had much higher rates for anencephaly or spina bifida than those of Jewish descent (3.1 per 1,000 total births vs 0.8), according to Naggan and MacMahon (1967). There is some evidence from the international mortality comparisons, and from the individual morbidity studies, that other parts of the British Isles also may share in this predilection—particularly Scotland, South Wales, and some (but not all) parts of England. However, the excess in the non-Irish sections is not so great. And hydrocephalus seems less variable than anencephaly and spina bifida. The rather high rates (including hydrocephalus) noted in Alexandria would also seem worth probing further. We have not been able to define any geographic area where the data consistently indicate an excessively *low* rate for any or all of the malformations of the nervous system. But this whole topic remains a fertile field for the epidemiologic plow.

10 / OTHER SPECIFIC NEUROLOGIC DISORDERS

John F. Kurtzke
Leonard T. Kurland

In this chapter we shall discuss neurologic disorders for which no special mortality tables based on 1959-61 deaths in the United States were available, with one exception (herpes zoster, code 088). The mortality statistics for a number of neurologic diseases are of limited value, either because they seldom lead to death (as in the case of herpes zoster), or because they are not separately coded in the Sixth and Seventh Revisions of the International Statistical Classification (ISC).

In the Eighth Revision of the ISC (World Health Organization 1967) and in the International Classification of Diseases, Adapted (ICDA) (National Center for Health Statistics 1968a), which went into effect in 1969, more diseases have been assigned specific code numbers. Some of these are four-digit codes, and it is still uncertain whether they will be retrievable from routine mortality data on an international scale. As mentioned previously, disorders such as stroke and brain tumor are discussed in other volumes of this APHA monograph series.

The entities to be considered here will be grouped under the headings of spinal cord affections, selected neuropathies, and familial diseases. Discussion of a given disorder generally is limited by the availability of appropriate population-based information as to its frequency and not necessarily by the intrinsic medical or social importance of the disease.

Spinal Cord Affections

This section will be limited to those diseases of the spinal cord in which heredity is believed to play a minor role; a later section is concerned with the "heredofamilial" disorders.

Syringomyelia

Syringomyelia and syringobulbia (Eighth Revision ICDA, code 349.0) are disorders in which the typical findings are segmental involvement of the spinal cord or the lower brain stem, with sensory dissociation (loss of pain and temperature, and preservation of touch) and variable involvement of the long tracts (pyramidal, sensory). Trophic disturbances are common. Poser (1956) recommended that syringomyelia be limited "to an abnormal cavity within the brain stem, the pons, the medulla, or the spinal cord [but not] to cystic lesions resulting from trauma, myelomalacia, hematomyelia, or other external agents."

In his review of concomitant syringomyelia and spinal cord tumor, Poser (1956) indicated that at autopsy one of every six cases of syringomyelia was associated with an intramedullary tumor. The precise pathophysiology in the development and enlargement of the syringomyelic cavity (syrinx) remains unknown. Syrinx is often found in association with congenital defects of the bone or nervous system, but the question remains as to whether this is a developmental anomaly, the result of hydrodynamic forces through a patent central canal of the spinal cord, or an unusual neoplasm. The relative roles of heredity and environment are also unclear.

The disorder may first become manifest in childhood or in the senium, but in most instances, symptoms begin in early adult life—at an average age of 25 to 35 years (Poser 1956; McIlroy and Richardson 1965). Males and females appear to be equally affected. The course is generally protracted, and long periods of no change may be intermixed with those of rather rapid deterioration. Death is often the result of intercurrent illness. The efficacy of surgical treatment has not been fully demonstrated, and radiotherapy has not altered the course.

The population survey of Rochester, Minnesota, based on records from the Mayo Clinic and affiliated hospitals, revealed one case of syringomyelia in the resident population in 1955 (Kurland 1958a). This provides a prevalence rate of 3 per 100,000 population. In the study by Brewis and her associates (1966) of Carlisle, England, there were 6 patients alive on prevalence day in 1961, for a prevalence rate of 8 per 100,000. There were 16 cases in Iceland in 1963, according to Gudmundsson (1968b), thus reflecting a prevalence rate of 9 per 100,000 population. These rates, based on very few cases, do not differ significantly, and no other estimates of prevalence have been found.

Based on the ten years 1954-63, the average annual incidence rate for the diagnosis of syringomyelia in Iceland has been estimated at 0.3 per 100,000 population (Gudmundsson 1968b).

Dorsolateral Sclerosis

Subacute combined degeneration of the cord is a disorder characterized by involvement of the lateral columns (pyramidal tracts) and posterior columns, and the patient presents with spastic paraparesis and proprioceptive sensory deficit predominantly of the lower limbs. Most instances are found in association with pernicious anemia, although the anemia often occurs without neurologic dysfunction and at times the neurologic signs may even antedate the anemia. Furthermore, pernicious anemia may cause peripheral neuropathy, optic atrophy, or dementia, with or without spinal cord involvement. In the Eighth Revision of the ICDA, dorsolateral sclerosis is listed under pernicious anemia (code 281.0). Pernicious anemia itself is said to show a "30 percent familial occurrence," with at least one parent, sibling, child, or parent's sibling of probands affected, according to Mosbech (1953).

Not all dorsolateral sclerosis can be attributed to pernicious anemia. Some cases are found in association with folate deficiency; diabetes mellitus has been suspected in others; Jamaican neuropathy shows similarities in the involvement of the spinal cord; and in some, no cause can be identified.

The average annual incidence rate for dorsolateral sclerosis (all definite cases) in Rochester, Minnesota, was 3.3 per 100,000 population (Kurland 1958a). In Carlisle, England, the annual incidence rate for this entity was 2.1 per 100,000 (Brewis et al. 1966). Most of the cases in both series were associated with pernicious anemia (Table 10.1).

The prevalence rates for dorsolateral sclerosis were 26 per 100,000 in Rochester and 25 per 100,000 in Carlisle. In both series males and females were represented in approximately equal numbers. In Rochester, the average age at prevalence day was 71 and the average age at onset was 60. In Carlisle, the maximal age-specific prevalence was found for those "over 70 years of age" (Brewis et al. 1966).

Jamaican Neuropathy

The progressive illness described by Cruickshank (1961) and by Montgomery and his colleagues (1964) as Jamaican neuropathy is primarily an affection of the spinal cord, with pyramidal tract and posterior column signs. In some patients, optic nerve involvement or deafness is present. Pathologically, meningomyelitic changes were

Table 10.1 Cases and average annual incidence and point prevalence rates per 100,000 population for dorsolateral sclerosis with or without pernicious anemia: Rochester, Minnesota, and Carlisle, England, various years, 1945-61

Survey area (source)	Years	Incidence		Prevalence[a]	
		Cases	Rate	Cases	Rate
		Total series			
Rochester, Minnesota (Kurland 1958a)	1945-54	10	3.3	8	26.4
Carlisle, England (Brewis et al. 1966)	1955-61	10	2.1	18	25.3
		With pernicious anemia			
Rochester, Minnesota (Kurland 1958a)	1945-54	8	2.7	8	26.4
Carlisle, England (Brewis et al. 1966)	1955-61	8	1.6	12	16.9
		Without pernicious anemia			
Rochester, Minnesota (Kurland 1958a)	1945-54	2	0.7	-	-
Carlisle, England (Brewis et al. 1966)	1955-61	2	0.4	6	8.4

[a]Prevalence day was at the end of the period cited.

noted in some patients. The disorder is common in Jamaica and neighboring islands, with more than two hundred cases described (Montgomery et al. 1964). Still, no epidemiologic inquiry has been reported. The illness (or illnesses) is presumably nutritional in origin. Although it may be limited geographically, as its title suggests, there may be similar disorders elsewhere that have not yet been detected. The possibility exists that this disorder could be a form of folate deficiency, which according to Grant and his colleagues (1965) may cause similar dysfunction.

Subacute Myelo-Optico-Neuropathy (SMON)

In many parts of Japan, since about 1956, a peculiar neuromyelopathy (noted particularly in patients with acute or chronic gastrointestinal disorders) has occurred; some of its clinical features are similar to those of Jamaican neuropathy. This entity has been referred to as subacute myelo-optico-neuropathy (SMON). The signs

Table 10.2 Percentage distribution of cases according to age at onset for Japanese myeloneuropathy by sex, with male-to-female ratio of the cases: Nagoya, Japan, 1956-69

Age at onset	Total	Male	Female	M:F ratio
All ages	100.0	100.0	100.0	0.6
0 - 9	-	-	-	-
10 - 19	2.8	4.1	2.0	1.3
20 - 29	11.6	11.7	11.5	0.6
30 - 39	20.3	22.9	18.9	0.8
40 - 49	20.1	20.9	19.6	0.7
50 - 59	25.4	24.3	26.1	0.6
60 - 69	14.7	12.3	16.1	0.5
70 & over	5.1	3.8	5.9	0.4
(No. of cases)	(752)	(292)	(460)	

Source: Adapted from Sobue et al. 1971.

and symptoms are referable to the posterior and lateral columns of the spinal cord. Rather characteristic features include sensory changes, particularly paresthesias in the distal lower extremities, at times motor disturbances (usually flaccid muscle weakness of the legs), and occasionally optic nerve involvement. Pathologically, there is involvement of the posterior and lateral columns, peripheral nerves, and optic nerves. During 1956-69 Sobue and his associates (1969; 1971) observed 752 cases in Nagoya, and Toyokura and his colleagues (1969) studied "a large number" in Tokyo. To 1970, 44 patients were ascertained in one hospital in Niigata (Tsubaki et al. 1971). The disease occurs mostly in urban centers, with occasional cases noted in the surrounding countryside.

An analysis of a clinical series at Nagoya University Hospital indicated that the cases occurred throughout adulthood with the largest number in the age group 50-59 years; there were no cases in the group under age 10 (Table 10.2). There was a preponderance of females (male-female sex ratio about 0.6 to 1).

Various causes have been suggested, including a virus (Inoue et al. 1971), but Tsubaki and his associates (1971) have recently presented evidence implicating the widespread use of clioquinol (iodochlorhydroxyquinoline, hydroxyquinoline, chinoform) as an intestinal antiseptic. The removal of this drug from the market in Japan has apparently been associated with a decrease in incidence of the disease. Abnormalities of cyanide detoxification and other pharmaceuticals used in the treatment of intestinal parasites and dyspepsia are also agents which may deserve study (Marsden and Knight 1971).

Further clinical and pathologic correlations of SMON, Nigerian funicular myelopathy, Jamaican neuropathy, and other tropical neuropathic syndromes, in conjunction with meaningful population studies, are clearly in order.

Some Muscular Atrophies

In addition to the hereditary polyneuropathies and motor neuron disease, Dyck and Lambert (1968) described four instances of a "Charcot-Marie-Tooth type" of progressive spinal muscular atrophy. There were no familial cases. The disease was characterized by symmetric distal atrophy and weakness of all four limbs, with no clinical or electrodiagnostic evidence of peripheral nerve involvement, nor presumably of polymyositis. The course was exceedingly protracted.

Selected Acute Neuropathies

Bell's Palsy

Bell's palsy is included under the Eighth Revision, ICDA, as code 350. It is an acute paralysis of the facial muscles due to involvement of the facial nerve without apparent cause, although viral, postinfectious, and autoimmune mechanisms have been suggested. In clinical series (Taverner 1955, 1965; Jepsen 1965), this entity tends to comprise only half the cases of peripheral facial nerve paralysis. Other causes of facial palsy are poliomyelitis, Guillain-Barré syndrome, sarcoidosis, diabetic neuropathy, multiple sclerosis, and local trauma and infections.

In hospital experience Bell's palsy is found in patients of every age, but mostly those in midadult life. Males and females are about equally affected, the right and left sides are similarly involved, and only rarely is the condition bilateral (Taverner 1955).

Several population studies of Bell's palsy have been made, but the reported incidence rates fluctuate widely, possibly because of differ-

Table 10.3 Cases and average annual incidence rates per 100,000 population for Bell's palsy by sex: selected surveys, various years, 1955-67

Survey area (source)	Years	Cases	Rate Total	Male	Female	M:F ratio
Rochester, Minnesota (Hauser et al. 1971)	1955-67	121	22.8	20.1	25.0	0.8
Reykjavik, Iceland (Gudmundsson 1970)	1960-67	90	12.1	8.4	15.9	0.5
10 general practices, England (Melotte 1961)	1957-59	23	24.2	25.2[a]	23.1[a]	1.1
Carlisle, England (Brewis et al. 1966)	1955-61	63	13.0	---	---	---

[a] Estimated.

ences in case ascertainment and in criteria for inclusion (Table 10.3).

In the survey of Carlisle, England, 1955-61, Brewis and her colleagues (1966) found 63 cases and reported an incidence rate of 13 per 100,000 for "definite" idiopathic facial paralysis. No categorization by sex was presented.

A study of Bell's palsy was carried out in Rochester, Minnesota, for 1955-67 (Hauser et al. 1971). The average annual incidence rate, based on 121 cases, is about 23 per 100,000 population, with little difference by sex (males 20.1, females 25.0). Age-specific rates were lowest for those less than 10 years old, increased until the fourth decade, and did not vary by age groups thereafter. There was no seasonal variation by age or sex or for the total group.

Similar findings as to incidence (24 per 100,000), sex, and season were noted over a 2½-year period in the late 1950s by Melotte (1961), who collected 23 cases from ten general practices in England.

In contrast to these rates, Gudmundsson (1968a) originally stated that he had encountered only 55 cases of Bell's palsy in Iceland during 1960-67, for an incidence rate of 4 per 100,000. Although he at first believed that he had seen all or most cases of Bell's palsy in that interval, he discovered many more through checking his colleagues' records, the total being 108 (Gudmundsson 1970). By limiting consideration to the cases from the Reykjavik area, he then calculated an annual incidence rate of 12 per 100,000 from the 90 cases seen during 1960-67, with the male-female ratio approximately 0.5 to 1 (8.4 males vs 15.9 per 100,000 females). The recalculated rate brings the incidence rate for Bell's palsy in Iceland up to that recorded for Carlisle, England. But these rates are half those of the two other surveys. Since one of the studies with the two higher rates is also from England, the differences noted may be a reflection of difference in methodology or in completeness of case ascertainment rather than of true geographic variation.

In none of the clinical or population series previously mentioned nor in most of the neurologic literature is there evidence for familial Bell's palsy. Alter (1963b) reported that in one-fourth of patients hospitalized in Israel for Bell's palsy, other members of the same generation, or of previous generations, had been affected. In some instances examinations or medical records revealed that a relative had had facial palsy, but in many, the evidence was limited to the patient's history. Alter believed that the pattern was consistent with transmission as a single autosomal dominant trait with low penetrance. He cited a small number of reports of familial Bell's palsy from the United States, Germany, Spain, and France, dating from 1919 to 1959.

Two additional reports in the 1960s were referred to by DeSanto and Schubert (1969) in their own description of 10 cases of Bell's palsy within three generations of a large family (63 members). One of those was the report of Kakar and his associates (1966), who concluded that the trait, as described in several families with Bell's palsy, was recessive. In the family reported by DeSanto and Schubert, Bell's palsy appeared as a dominant trait with incomplete penetrance, if each case was acceptable as "idiopathic" disease. Three were members affected during their teens, and four were affected when they were between 20 and 25 years of age. A preponderance of so many young persons (none of whom was known to have been then examined neurologically) might raise some question as to diagnosis. The presumption of a genetic influence perhaps affecting the facial canal or the nerve itself may be premature; however, further investigation into familial aggregation of Bell's palsy appears warranted. As to differences by sex, the population studies, in contrast to the hospital series, suggest a female predilection; but numbers are as yet too few for this difference to be considered definitive.

Trigeminal Neuralgia

Tic douloureux comprises attacks of very brief but severe and recurrent pain in the distribution of one or more branches of the trigeminal nerve. There is no sensory defect on examination, and the remainder of the nervous system seems unaffected. Although tic douloureux is coded separately (Eighth Revision ICDA, code 351), the code also includes terms that have clinically different connotations.

The study of Rochester, Minnesota, for 1945-54 revealed an average annual incidence rate of 4 per 100,000 population (Kurland 1958a). Age at onset ranged from 28 to 93, with a mean of 58 years; most persons were in the sixth and seventh decades of life. No sex predilection was seen. In Carlisle, England, during 1955-61, there were 10 cases, for an incidence rate of 2 per 100,000. Brewis and her colleagues (1966), in contrasting this rate with that of Rochester, conceded that underreporting was a likely explanation for the difference. Most of the patients in Carlisle were 60 to 75 years old.

Familial cases were not encountered in either series. Pratt (1967) referred to clinical series of tic douloureux with a "familial incidence varying from nil to 6 percent."

Herpes Zoster

The classic case of "shingles," as it is known to the layman, is characterized by pain and vesicular rash in a dermatomal distribution. There seems little doubt that the varicella-zoster virus is the agent responsible for the disease (Seiler 1949), but the mechanism of its production is unknown.

One current hypothesis is that the virus is acquired during clinical or subclinical varicella, and that it lies dormant in cells of the posterior root ganglion until or unless some change in the environment (reduction of varicella antibody, death of the cell, concomitant disease) permits replication and release of the pox virus. Because the disorder is so readily recognized, medical attention is usually limited to the general practitioner, and the specialist sees mostly the refractory or complicated cases.

Average annual incidence rates available for herpes zoster are summarized in Table 10.4. Hope-Simpson (1965) recorded an annual rate of 3.4 per 1,000 population from his practice in Cirencester, England, between 1947 and 1962. McGregor (1957) with a similar survey found an annual rate of 4.6 per 1,000 in Hawick, Scotland,

Table 10.4 Cases and average annual incidence rates per 1,000 population for herpes zoster by sex: selected surveys, various years, 1945-62

Survey area (source)	Years	Cases	Rate			M:F ratio
			Total	Male	Female	
Cirencester, England (Hope-Simpson 1965)	1947-62	192	3.4	3.6	3.2	1.1
Hawick, Scotland (McGregor 1957)	1948-55	81	4.6	4.9	4.4	1.1
Rochester, Minnesota (Kurland 1958a)	1945-54	248	0.8	0.7	0.9	0.8
Edinburgh, Scotland (Seiler 1949)	1947-48	246	2.0^a	2.0^b	2.0^b	1.0

[a] Estimated by Seiler.

[b] Calculated from percentages of cases and population by sex.

from 1948 to 1955. In Rochester, Minnesota, 1945-54, Kurland (1958a) noted a rate of 0.8 per 1,000 population. Taking the 246 cases seen in 1947-48 by a proportion of the local physicians in Edinburgh, Seiler (1949) *estimated* an annual incidence of 2 per 1,000. As may be seen in Table 10.4, there is no appreciable difference by sex in the incidence rates for herpes zoster in these communities. That this holds too for individual ages is indicated by the data of McGregor (1957) and Kurland (1958a) (see Table 10.5).

Age-specific attack rates for zoster increase notably with increasing age and peak in the oldest age group, as shown in Fig. 10.1. Incidence rates are low in early childhood, range near 2 per 1,000 from adolescence to about age 35 or so, then increase steadily thereafter. This interpretation is from the studies of Hope-Simpson (1965) and McGregor (1957). That of Kurland (1958a) seems to follow this pattern but at a much lower level.

Attack rates that have varied from 1 to 5 per 1,000 population would seem difficult to explain. Actually, the rates for Cirencester and Hawick (Fig. 10.1 and Table 10.4) are reasonably close, near 4 per 1,000; and the rate of 2 reported by Seiler (1949) was admittedly an estimate. The discrepant value is that for Rochester. It is apparent from Fig. 10.1 that an explanation for this discrepancy does *not* lie in different-aged populations, because the Rochester rate is much below the others at every age. Although these studies may provide evidence of a true geographic difference in the incidence of

Table 10.5 Cases and average annual incidence rates per 1,000 population for herpes zoster by age and sex: Hawick, Scotland, 1948-55, and Rochester, Minnesota, 1945-54

Survey area and age	Cases	Rate		
		Total	Male	Female
Hawick, Scotland				
All ages	81	4.6	4.9	4.4
0 - 4	-	-	-	-
5 - 14	4	2.4	2.7	2.1
15 - 44	16	2.2	2.7	1.7
45 - 64	37	8.1	10.1	6.5
65 & over	24	10.4	8.9	11.6
Rochester, Minnesota				
All ages	248	0.8	0.7	0.9
0 - 14	9	0.1	0.1	0.1
15 - 34	58	0.6	0.5	0.7
35 - 54	61	0.8	0.7	0.9
55 - 69	76	1.9	1.5	2.2
70 & over	44	2.4	2.2	2.5

Source: McGregor 1957 (Hawick); Kurland 1958a (Rochester).

herpes zoster between the United Kingdom and the United States, there is another factor to be considered before this can be accepted.

Although a disease frequency equal to or exceeding that of any other community survey thus far has generally been found for Rochester, Minnesota (not only because of diagnostic skill but also because of complete enumeration), we may have an exception with herpes zoster since all patients may not have been seen at the various facilities of the Mayo Clinic. Both Hope-Simpson and McGregor had general practices in their communities, and such cases are more than likely to be seen initially by the family physician. The proposed extension of the Rochester study to cover 1945-69 may clarify this question and also the question of possible cyclic or periodic variations in the incidence of this disease. There were no obvious secular trends with time in the studies of McGregor or Hope-Simpson. There was a suggestive seasonal variation in spring and fall in the Rochester study, and this was similar to that found in Seiler's study. However, no seasonal variation was noted in the other studies.

Clinically, the thoracic dermatomes, as a unit, were the most commonly involved in both population surveys (Seiler 1949; Kurland

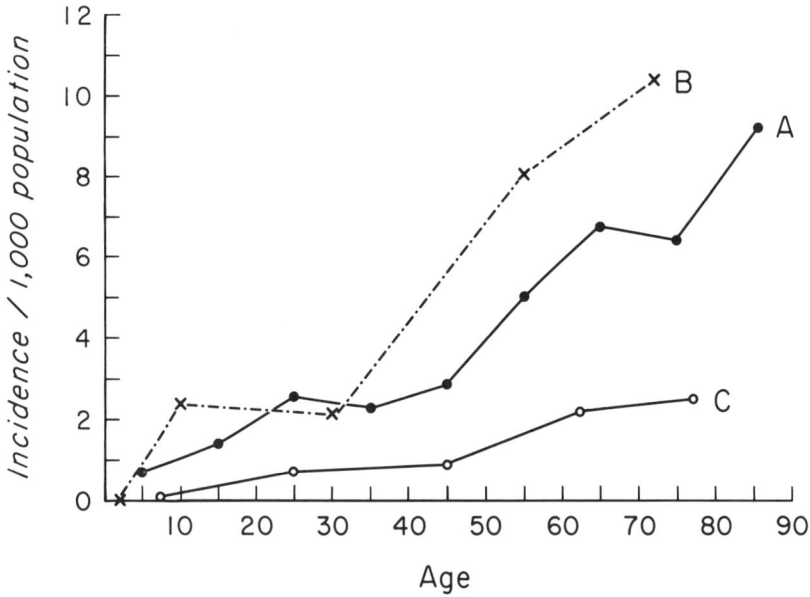

Figure 10.1 Average annual age-specific incidence rates per 1,000 population for herpes zoster: Cirencester, England, 1947–62 (*A*); Hawick, Scotland, 1948–55 (*B*); and Rochester, Minnesota, 1945–54 (*C*). (Source: Hope-Simpson 1965, McGregor 1957, and Kurland 1958*a*.)

1958*a*; McGregor 1957; Hope-Simpson 1965) and in hospital case series (Boughton 1966; Bamford and Boundy 1968).

Postherpetic neuralgia refers to persistent pain after the acute attack. Pain persisting more than four weeks after onset was recorded in 7 percent of the Rochester cases. Recurrent attacks of herpes zoster were noted in 3 percent of cases in two series (Seiler 1949; Kurland 1958*a*) and in 4 percent in another (Hope-Simpson 1965).

Association between herpes zoster and underlying malignancy, particularly of the lymphoid system (Merselis et al. 1964), has been known for some time. In Rochester, 13 of the patients were found to have a concurrent malignancy, whereas only 3 would be expected to have such a malignancy on the basis of the age-specific cancer prevalence rates.

Guillain-Barré Syndrome

Infectious neuronitis, or the Landry-Guillain-Barré-Strohl syndrome (Eighth Revision ICDA, code 354), is a disorder characterized by the acute or subacute onset of a predominantly motor disturbance in the limbs, and occasionally in the cranial and truncal musculature. Less severe sensory deficits are seen in the limbs and are most often distal, whereas the weakness may be greater proximally. When death ensues, it is generally from respiratory (ventilatory) insufficiency. The most typical laboratory abnormality is an elevated level of cerebrospinal fluid protein—which, however, may not appear until convalescence, may be evanescent, and bears little relation to the severity of illness. The cause is unknown, but hypotheses of viral and immune mechanisms have been offered (Melnick and Flewett 1964; Wiederholt et al. 1964; Leneman 1966; McFarland and Heller 1966; Ravn 1967).

In Olmsted County, Minnesota (Lesser et al., unpublished data), 29 cases with onset during 1935-67 were diagnosed, for an average annual incidence rate of 1.6 per 100,000. The average annual rate per 100,000 was 1.3 for 1935-55 and 2.0 for 1956-67. Although the higher rate in recent years may mirror a true increase in incidence, it is believed to be a reflection of better case ascertainment resulting from increased awareness of the clinical features and the effects of vaccine in the elimination of poliomyelitis, which at times resembles the Guillain-Barré syndrome (Table 10.6).

The 1955-61 survey of Carlisle, England (Brewis et al. 1966), revealed 3 cases, for a rate of 0.6 per 100,000. In Iceland (Gudmundsson 1969) from 1954 to 1963, there were 13 cases, for an average annual incidence rate of 0.7 per 100,000; 8 of the patients

Table 10.6 Cases and average annual incidence rates per 100,000 population for Guillain-Barré syndrome: selected surveys, various years, 1935-67

Survey area (source)	Years	Cases	Rate
Rochester, Minnesota (Kurland 1958a)	1945-54	3	1.1
Olmsted County, Minnesota (Lesser et al. unpubl.)	1935-67	29	1.6
Carlisle, England (Brewis et al. 1966)	1955-61	3	0.6
Iceland (Gudmundsson 1969)	1954-63	13	0.7
Guam (Chen et al. 1968)	1960-66	5	1.8

were males. On Guam during 1960-66, 5 cases (3 males, 2 females) were diagnosed, for an average annual incidence rate of 1.8 per 100,000 (Chen et al. 1968).

From clinical series, a male preponderance seems likely. The male-female case ratio was 2.2 to 1 at the Mayo Clinic (Weiderholt et al. 1964) and 1.3 to 1 in Copenhagen (Ravn 1967). However, cases are too few in the available population surveys to define a sex difference in incidence rates; and, as usual, the bias in hospital series is unknown. There is no apparent age predilection; infants as well as those 80 or older are affected. The case-fatality ratio in Iceland was 15 percent (Gudmundsson 1969). There was a suggestion of seasonal variation in this disorder (Melnick and Flewett 1964), but it has not been uniformly noted in degree, season, or even existence (Weiderholt et al. 1964; McFarland and Heller 1966; Ravn 1967).

Other Familial and Presumably Hereditary Disorders

The incidence and distribution of hereditary disorders are largely the result of their natural mutation rate, fertility, mode of transmission, population size at the time of introduction of the affected into the gene pool, and factors of chance in migration and "genetic drift." There remains, however, the possibility that environmental factors may exist which affect the mutation rate, the age at onset, or the rate of progress in these disorders. An epidemiologic inquiry into possible environmental factors may help not only to answer these questions but also to provide data on the socioeconomic impact of the illnesses.

Huntington's Chorea

This disorder is manifested by progressive mental deterioration and adventitious movements of choreiform nature. Pathologic changes are maximal in the basal ganglia (especially the caudate nucleus) and in the cerebral cortex. Treatment of parkinsonism with levodopa may produce choreo-athetotic movements (Cotzias et al. 1969; Mena et al. 1970). Clinical evidence has revealed that the choreiform movements of Huntington's disease can be diminished by high doses of reserpine, and administration of this agent in schizophrenics has produced a parkinsonistic state. Detailed investigation of brain catecholamine metabolism is in order for this disease.

Huntington's chorea is used as the classic example of an autosomal dominant trait with high penetrance (Myrianthopoulos and Rowley 1960). Accordingly, equal involvement by sex is expected and indeed found in all studies reviewed. Age at onset varies but is believed by some to be reasonably constant within a given family, whereas others contend that in succeeding generations a younger age of onset can be anticipated (Merritt 1967). If this is true, average age at onset should be lower in the most recent studies. From community surveys at present, an age at onset somewhat under 40 is likely (Table 10.7), which does not differ from earlier (hospital) series. It is likely that "anticipation" has resulted from the more accurate delineation of early symptoms in families under medical observation; thus the illness in such instances only seems to have begun at younger ages in the later generation.

The largest series in a defined population is that of Brothers (1964). In Fig. 10.2 is the cumulative percentage frequency curve for age at onset and age at death in that series. Mean age at onset was 37.2 years (Table 10.7) and median age 36 years (Fig. 10.2). In 90 percent of the cases, the illness began at or over the age of 20; and in about half of the cases, it began between age 28 and age 44. In only

Table 10.7 Average age at onset and average duration of illness for Huntington's chorea: selected surveys, various years to 1965

Survey area (source)	Years	Mean age at onset[a]	Duration in years[a]
Victoria, Australia (Brothers 1964)	to 1963[b]	37.2 (206)	12.3[c] (97)
Victoria, Australia (Brothers 1964)	to 1963[b]	36[d] (206)	13[c,d] (123)
Cornwall, England (Bickford & Ellison 1953)	to 1951[b]	42.8 (21)	--- (---)
Suburban London, England (Heathfield 1967)	1965	45.1 (80)	7.6[e] (80)

[a] Number of cases in parentheses.

[b] Study refers to historical data for those who died before prevalence day.

[c] Duration (years), onset to death.

[d] Median value, calculated from Figure 10.2.

[e] Duration (years), onset to prevalence day for survivors.

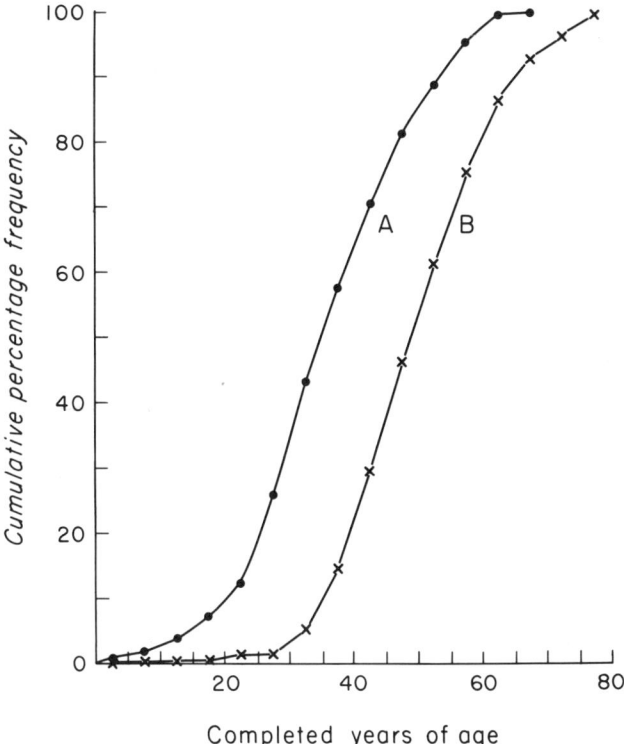

Figure 10.2 Cumulative percentage frequency for Huntington's chorea by age at onset (A), and by age at death (B): Victoria, Australia, various years to 1963 (Source: Brothers 1964.)

one-sixth of the cases did the illness begin at 50 years or older. The curves were equivalent for each sex. Mean duration of illness from onset to death is about twelve years. In Victoria the duration in two-thirds of the cases was between seven and eighteen years (Brothers 1964). Taken from median ages at onset and death, duration would be thirteen years (Fig. 10.2).

Because the disease is invariably fatal, and when reported on the death certificate likely to be correct, it would be worthwhile to have mortality statistics for this entity. Although irretrievable in the past, with the new code for Huntington's chorea (Eighth Revision ICDA, code 331.0) perhaps the future will provide such information. From a special survey, this disease was reported as cause of death at a rate of 0.2 per 100,000 population for Canada in 1951 (Kurland 1958a).

The prevalence rate for Huntington's chorea in different communities may be expected to vary greatly because of the effect of a few

Table 10.8 Cases and prevalence rates per 100,000 population for Huntington's chorea: selected surveys, various years, about 1951-65

Survey area (source)	Year	Cases	Rate
Rochester, Minnesota (Kurland 1958a)	1955	2	6.7
Carlisle, England (Brewis et al. 1966)	1961	2	2.8
Iceland (Gudmundsson 1969)	1963	5	2.7
Victoria, Australia (Brothers 1964)	c.1963	138	4.6
Cornwall, England (Bickford & Ellison 1953)	c.1951	19	5.3
Northamtonshire, England (Pleydell 1954)	1954	13	4.9
Minnesota (Pearson et al. 1955)	c.1954	---	5.4
Suburban London, England (Heathfield 1967)	1965	81	2.5
Poland (Cendrowski 1964)	c.1964	---	4.1

large family constellations which may have been present and influenced the decision to conduct an investigation in a particular area. Available studies are summarized in Table 10.8.

During 1960-66, when the indigenous population of Guam was being observed for all neurologic diseases, no cases of Huntington's disease were diagnosed (Chen et al. 1968). In Rochester, Minnesota (Kurland 1958a), there were two siblings with the disease in 1955, for a prevalence rate of nearly 7 per 100,000. Rates for the surveys of Carlisle, England (Brewis et al. 1966), and of Iceland (Gudmundsson 1969) were both about 3 per 100,000 population. Brothers and Meadows (1955), in a preliminary study, found 57 living patients in Victoria, Australia, for a prevalence rate of 3 per 100,000. The more complete work by Brothers (1964) resulted in a prevalence rate of almost 5 per 100,000, based on 138 cases in Victoria. Brothers cited this as an "incidence of current cases" but clearly meant a prevalence rate. In Tasmania, all 86 known cases originated from a woman who had emigrated from Somerset, England, in about 1848 (Brothers 1964).

Bickford and Ellison (1953) found 19 cases of Huntington's chorea in Cornwall, England, for a prevalence rate of 5 per 100,000. Pleydell (1954) calculated a rate of 5 per 100,000 for Northamptonshire from 13 patients. A rate of more than 5 per 100,000 was estimated for the State of Minnesota by Pearson and his associates (1955). In a large suburban area outside London, Heathfield (1967) found 81 patients, for a prevalence rate of nearly 3 per 100,000. Cendrowski (1964), in a brief report, noted a prevalence of 4 per 100,000 in Poland.

On these bases the prevalence rate of Huntington's chorea was between 3 and 7 per 100,000 population. The lower rates were recorded for small series (Brewis et al. 1966; Gudmundsson 1969) and for one (Heathfield 1967) in which ascertainment may well have been incomplete. Perhaps 5 or 6 per 100,000 would be a likely estimate. If a prevalence rate of 6 per 100,000 is accepted and the average duration after onset is about twelve years, as indicated by these studies (Bickford and Ellison 1953; Pleydell 1954; Brothers and Meadows 1955; Pearson et al. 1955; Brothers 1964; Heathfield 1967), one would expect an average annual incidence rate of 0.5 per 100,000 population. For the ten years 1955-64, it was found that the incidence rate in Rochester was 0.5 per 100,000 based on two new cases (Kurland and Choi, unpublished data). The incidence rate should equal the mortality rate, if all deaths are ascertained; the death rate in Canada was 0.2 versus the estimated incidence rate for Rochester of 0.5.

Wilson's Disease

Hepatolenticular degeneration, described by Wilson, is a disorder characterized by liver involvement (cirrhosis), neurologic symptoms of variable types of extrapyramidal dysfunction, together with dementia and a pigment deposition in the cornea called the Kayser-Fleischer ring. Any of these features may be absent in a given patient. The disease is essentially progressive, and fatal if untreated. Onset of symptoms is usually in adolescence or early adult life, but it has been recorded to begin "at the age of four and as late as the fifth decade" (Merritt 1967). There may be a slight male preponderance. The clinical changes may be considered a manifestation of chronic copper toxicity, and most (but not all) patients have a deficit of ceruloplasmin, a copper-binding serum protein (Kurtzke 1962; Merritt 1967). Generally, the disorder has been considered a familial one, and Pratt (1967) indicated that it is likely to be transmitted as an autosomal recessive trait.

No routine data are available from mortality statistics, although Wilson's disease is now coded separately (code 273.3). In the special survey of death certificates for Canada in 1951, the annual mortality rate was calculated at 0.3 per 1,000,000 population (Kurland 1958a).

In a disorder as scarce as Wilson's disease, it is not surprising that thus far no cases have been recorded in Rochester, Minnesota (Kurland 1958a; Kurland and Choi, unpublished data), or Carlisle, England (Brewis et al. 1966). There were 3 patients with Wilson's disease in Iceland in 1963, according to Gudmundsson (1969), for a prevalence rate of 1.6 per 100,000 population (95-percent confidence limits on this rate were 0.3 and 4.7 per 100,000). In the ten years (1954-63) of Gudmundsson's survey, 3 new cases were discovered, for an average annual incidence rate of 0.2 per 100,000. This is almost ten times higher than the 1951 Canadian mortality rate for this disease. All the Iceland cases were siblings, and the parents were second cousins. One of the patients was a twin, and the heterozygote twin was unaffected. The consanguinity might lead to caution in extrapolating the Icelandic rates to other communities, but even these would indicate that the disease is rare. In Iceland, the age at onset ranged from 16 to 26.

Hereditary Ataxias

This is a heterogeneous group of disorders in which classification is complicated by the existence of formes frustes and the occurrence in some families of several types of ataxia. In the new Eighth Revision coding, the hereditary ataxias are allocated in code 332, with Friedreich's ataxia (code 332.0) and Marie's ataxia (code 332.1) as subdivisions. The major types of hereditary ataxias, as adapted from Greenfield's classification (1954), are Friedreich's spinocerebellar degeneration, Marie-Sanger cerebellar ataxia with spasticity, olivopontocerebellar atrophy, and ataxia with atrophy of Lévy and Roussy. A separate category of parenchymatous cerebellar degeneration might be added to this list. Inheritance for these entities varies by type and may follow any of several patterns (Pratt 1967).

In Gudmundsson's study (1969) in Iceland, two patients, siblings whose parents were first cousins, were observed to have hereditary ataxia, resulting in a prevalence rate of 1.1 per 100,000. In Carlisle (Brewis et al. 1966), 5 cases of "cerebellar ataxia" provided a prevalence rate of 7 per 100,000, but it is not known whether any were familial. During 1960-66, no cases of Friedreich's ataxia were diagnosed on Guam. Two patients from one family had spinocerebellar ataxia. Seven patients with spinal pyramidal system involvement (spastic paraplegia) were seen; three were siblings, the others apparently were unrelated. Familial spastic paraplegia is considered by some a variant of the hereditary ataxias. On that basis, and including the paraplegics, the rate for hereditary "ataxia" on Guam (all types) would be about 24 per 100,000; while for the true spinocerebellar cases, the rate would be 5 per 100,000 (Chen et al. 1968). There was no obvious association of these hereditary ataxias with the amyotrophic lateral sclerosis that is highly prevalent on Guam. A likely estimate for the prevalence of the cerebellar ataxias then may be about 5 per 100,000. None of the cited rates differs significantly because of the small numbers.

Hereditary Neuropathies

Various inherited disorders of peripheral nerves have been described (including amyloid neuropathy, sensory neuropathy, and others), but the only one that seems relatively common is Charcot-Marie-Tooth disease or peroneal muscular atrophy (Eighth Revision ICDA, code 330.1). Various families show transmission as "autosomal dominant, autosomal recessive, x-linked dominant and x-linked recessive modes of inheritance" (Pratt 1967).

On Guam, 1960-66, 12 patients with peroneal muscular atrophy were observed. Eight of these were from two families. Two patients experienced onset of the disease during the study period. Nine were alive on Guam when prevalence was measured in 1967, for a prevalence rate of 23.7 per 100,000 (Chen et al. 1968). There was no indication of an association of hereditary neuropathies with amyotrophic lateral sclerosis on the island. In the Rochester study, no cases were observed (Kurland 1958a). Herndon (1954), in North Carolina, estimated that the prevalence rate based on his survey was at least 5.4 per 100,000. In Iceland, 3 patients were alive on prevalence day, for a rate of 1.6 per 100,000 (Gudmundsson 1969).

Dystonia Musculorum Deformans (DMD)

This is a basal-ganglion disease (Eighth Revision ICDA, code 331.1) characterized by adventitious movements of a slow, writhing, twisting nature, maximal in the trunk. It is a progressive disorder, and mental deterioration is common in the late stages. An alternative label is torsion dystonia (TD).

A detailed monograph concerning 121 cases in a rural region of northern Sweden has been published by Larsson and Sjögren (1966). All cases were traced to three ancestral couples, and inheritance was as an "autosomal monohybrid dominant trait." Clinical types of involvement were the hyperkinetic, the myostatic or rigid, and the abortive form. This isolate, while providing information on clinical and genetic features, gives little indication of the overall prevalence rate. Although generally considered a disease of childhood, in this Swedish series the *mean* age at onset was 37, with almost 80 percent of the patients experiencing onset between the ages of 28 and 52.

A more customary age at onset was provided by Zeman and Dyken (1967) who collected 162 cases from greater Indianapolis, Indiana. The median age at onset was at 9, and 90 percent had become symptomatic by 18 years of age.

Recently, Eldridge and his associates (1967) have contested the idea that inheritance is uniformly dominant in this disorder and hold that "there is also an autosomal recessive form which has its onset usually between 5 and 15 years of age, runs a rapid and severe course and is relatively frequent in families with European Jewish ancestry." The basis of this conclusion was their evaluation of 63 families with DMD collected from several neurologic clinics in the United States. Twelve of these families (three Jewish or part Jewish) showed DMD compatible with dominant inheritance. There were 51 families with a recessive pattern and 27 were Jewish. The average age at onset of 15 years among the non-Jewish families with the dominant form of DMD was higher than the average age of 9 to 10 found for the other three groups (dominant form in those of Jewish ancestry and recessive form in both Jewish and non-Jewish families) (see Table 10.9). The differences that they cited according to clinical site or severity do not appear to be adequate to segregate the four groups.

The evidence is strong that there is indeed a recessive form of DMD; whether this is peculiar to the Ashkenazim Jews may be questioned. One major source for the above data was a neurosurgical clinic in New York where fourteen of the sixteen families were

Table 10.9   Age at onset for dystonia musculorum
deformans by mode of transmission and
ethnic origin, with number of cases by sex:
selected areas and years, United States

Mode of transmission[a] and ethnic origin	Age at onset		Number of cases		
	Mean	Range	Total	Male	Female
"Dominant" non-Jewish	15.1	5-40	44	26	18
"Dominant" Jewish	8.5	6-11	5	3	2
"Recessive" non-Jewish	9.7	2-35	26	14	12
"Recessive" Jewish	9.8	4-16	34	18	16

Source: Modified from Eldridge et al. 1967.

[a]Differentiation is between families with DMD in multiple generations (= "dominant") and in single generations (= "recessive"); latter is "probably heterogeneous" (Eldridge et al. 1967, p. 783).

Jewish, and where, apparently, most of the cases of the recessive type were obtained. Another source was a Maryland center with an interest in certain genetic isolates in the Pennsylvania-Ohio region, from which many of the cases of the dominant type may have arisen; none of these cases would have involved Jewish families. An exhaustively detailed study of this disorder has even more recently been provided by Eldridge (1970).

No cases of DMD have been found in the major population surveys (Kurland 1958a; Brewis et al. 1966; Gudmundsson 1968b, 1969; Kurland and Choi, unpublished data). One might surmise then that DMD is as rare as Wilson's disease. Eldridge (1970) has estimated a prevalence of 3 per 1,000,000 for the United States, including 25 per 1,000,000 for Jewish, and 0.3 per 1,000,000 for Negro citizens of this country.

11 / CEREBRAL PALSY

Irving D. Goldberg
Nung Won Choi
Leonard T. Kurland
John F. Kurtzke

In this and the following chapters consideration is given to classes of dysfunction defined by the end result of various pathogenetic mechanisms rather than to individual diseases or syndromes. Cerebral palsy (CP) is one of these heterogeneous classes of neurologic dysfunction that has been defined, inter alia, as "those disorders of uncertain or unknown etiology arising during the perinatal period—that is, from conception to the end of the neonatal . . . period [under 28 days] —affecting the motor function of the brain and in which the dysfunction is recognized prior to the end of infancy (two years)" (Kurland 1957a). Recognition by age 2 is not always practical, because the less severe varieties require sufficient mental and motor development for adequate testing.

Although the symptoms and signs of CP vary, the cases can be divided roughly into three groups according to whether the major damage is to the primary motor system, the basal ganglia, or the cerebellar pathways. On this basis they can be classified as spastic, athetoid, or ataxic. There is no clear dividing line among the three types and admixtures are the rule rather than the exception. In addition, there may be signs of damage to other parts of the central nervous system, with resultant sensory defects, dysphagia, apraxia, or hemianopsia. Intellectual defects are not uncommon.

Mortality Data

The categorization of deaths from CP is essentially twofold, depending on the age at death. In the Sixth and Seventh Revisions of the ISC (World Health Organization 1957), one would use code 351 for death at 28 days of age or over, and code 760 for death before 28 days.

Code 351 includes such diagnoses as cerebral infantile palsy, cerebral spastic infantile paralysis, cerebral spastic infantile paraplegia, Little's disease, paralysis due to birth injury (intracranial and spinal), porencephaly, spastic diplegia and paralysis, and infantile or congenital diplegia, hemiplegia, monoplegia, paraplegia, and tetraplegia. This code includes all residuals of intracranial and spinal injury at birth, present or causing death at ages 28 days and over, but excludes the current (neonatal) intracranial and spinal birth injuries (code 760). It also excludes spastic types of paralysis not infantile or congenital (code 352). In this chapter we shall refer to code 351 as ICP (infantile cerebral palsy).

Code 760 includes birth injury of the brain and spinal cord, congenital paralysis (cerebral), traumatic brain hematoma, intracranial and intraspinal hemorrhages, brain edema, rupture of brain or compression during birth, and tentorial tear due to injury at birth (with or without immaturity). This code excludes residuals of intracranial and spinal injury at birth, present or causing death at age 28 days and over (code 351). In this chapter we shall refer to code 760 as NCP (neonatal cerebral palsy).

International Comparisons

Goldberg and Kurland (1962) presented an international comparison of age-adjusted mortality rates for a number of neurologic disorders from thirty-three countries in the 1950s. As part of that endeavor, data on the CP deaths were collected but not published. Data from twenty-three countries for cerebral spastic infantile paralysis (ISC code 351) are noted in Table A.11.1, and from twenty-one countries for intracranial and spinal injury at birth (code 760) in Tables A.11.2 and A.11.3 (Goldberg and Kurland, unpublished data).

Death rates for ICP per 100,000, age adjusted to the 1950 United States census population, for males ranged from 0.04 in Mexico to 1.0 in Japan. The range for females was from 0.08 in Mexico to 0.9 in Japan. Among the countries listed the median rate was 0.4 for males and 0.3 for females. There was a slight preponderance of males in the adjusted rates for almost all countries.

Since all deaths from NCP occur in the first 28 days of life, it would have been desirable to base the rates for NCP on live births or the population under 1 year of age. However, from available information (Goldberg and Kurland, unpublished data), the youngest group on which these rates could be based was the population under 5 years of age. These data are shown in Table A.11.2 and serve to illustrate the variation in death rates among these countries. The under-5-year death rates for NCP were notably higher than the age-specific or total death rates for ICP. Among males, the under-5-year death rate for NCP ranged from 9.8 per 100,000 in Japan to 62.2 in the Netherlands; among females, it varied from 5.9 in Japan to 38.9 in Sweden. Among these countries the median rate was 49.7 for males and 28.7 for females. In each country there was a notably higher mortality for males, at a level of about 1.6 to 1 in the male-female ratio of the under-5-year rates. Rates for all ages reflect the same sex pattern but serve to illustrate the tenfold greater magnitude of deaths from NCP as opposed to deaths from ICP (Table A.11.3).

Multiple-cause data on the frequency of CP as a secondary as well as a primary cause of death from the United States, Norway, and the Netherlands are shown in Table A.11.4 for various years between 1953 and 1961. In Norway all secondary causes were included, in the United States up to four secondary causes, and in the Netherlands (1961) up to three secondary causes were considered, so that these multiple-cause statistics are roughly comparable. Among the death certificates listing ICP as a cause of death, this condition was listed as a secondary cause in 42 percent of the certificates in Norway, 51 percent in the United States, and only 19 percent in the Netherlands. It is interesting to note in Table A.11.1 that despite the much greater relative frequency with which ICP was recorded as a primary cause in the Netherlands than in Norway, the age-adjusted rate in Norway (0.7) was somewhat higher than that in the Netherlands (0.5). For the NCP category, multiple-cause data were not available for Norway, but for the other two countries NCP was recorded as a primary cause of death in more than 90 percent of the death certificates in which this condition was listed.

United States Mortality Data, Trend for ICP and NCP

Mortality data for the United States show a marked difference in the trends for infantile as opposed to neonatal cerebral palsy. Between 1949 and 1967, the crude death rate (all ages) for ICP remained constant at a level of 0.4 per 100,000 population each year except for 1949 (0.5) and 1966-67 (0.3). The average annual age-adjusted death rate (all ages) was also 0.4 for 1949-51 and 1959-61.

In contrast to the stable death rate for ICP, the under-1-year death rate for neonatal cerebral palsy showed a steady and marked decline during 1949-61. This rate dropped from 175.8 per 100,000 children

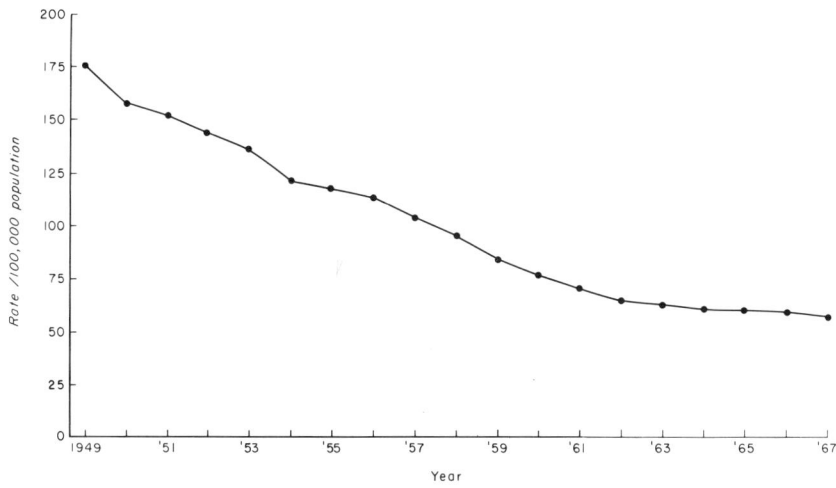

Figure 11.1 Death rates per 100,000 population under 1 year of age for neonatal cerebral palsy (intracranial and spinal injury at birth) by year: United States, 1949-67

under 1 year of age in 1949 to 70.9 in 1961 and to 59.4 in 1967, as depicted in Fig. 11.1. This decrease may be a result of improved obstetric care or of improved prognosis and survival beyond the neonatal period.

United States Mortality Data, 1959-61: ICP

The deaths and death rates for ICP in the United States in 1959-61 are presented in Table 11.1. Rates for all ages were 0.4 per 100,000 for both sexes combined, with 0.5 for males and 0.3 for females. The crude rates were slightly higher for nonwhites, whereas there was no difference by color when the rates were age adjusted.

Age. The highest rates were noted for white and nonwhite children who were less than 1 year of age. The rates dropped sharply in the age group 1-4 years, gradually declined until the age group 35-44 years, and then leveled off (Fig. 11.2). Almost one-fifth of the total deaths occurred before the first birthday, and three-fourths occurred before 15 years of age, as seen from Table 11.1.

Sex. In general, slightly higher rates were noted for males of both color groups in the United States (Table 11.1), and this sex

Table 11.1 Deaths and average annual death rates per 100,000 population for infantile cerebral palsy (cerebral spastic infantile paralysis) by age, color and sex: United States, 1959-61
(ISC code 351)

Age	Total			White			Nonwhite		
	Total	Male	Female	Total	Male	Female	Total	Male	Female
	Number of deaths								
All ages	2,184	1,231	953	1,874	1,049	825	310	182	128
Under 1	378	206	172	307	166	141	71	40	31
1-4	454	267	187	379	228	151	75	39	36
5-14	664	361	303	579	308	271	85	53	32
Under 15	1,496	834	662	1,265	702	563	231	132	99
15-24	319	193	126	273	165	108	46	28	18
25-34	145	81	64	136	74	62	9	7	2
35-44	88	48	40	80	43	37	8	5	3
45-54	47	29	18	40	25	15	7	4	3
55-64	42	20	22	38	17	21	4	3	1
65 & over	46	26	20	42	23	19	4	3	1
Unknown	1	-	1	-	-	-	1	-	1
	Crude death rate								
All ages	0.4	0.5	0.3	0.4	0.4	0.3	0.5	0.6	0.4
Under 1	3.1	3.3	2.8	2.9	3.1	2.7	3.9	4.4	3.4
1-4	0.9	1.1	0.8	0.9	1.1	0.7	1.1	1.1	1.0
5-14	0.6	0.7	0.6	0.6	0.7	0.6	0.6	0.7	0.5
Under 15	0.9	1.0	0.8	0.9	1.0	0.8	1.0	1.1	0.9
15-24	0.4	0.5	0.3	0.4	0.5	0.3	0.5	0.7	0.4*
25-34	0.2	0.2	0.2	0.2	0.2	0.2	0.1*	0.2*	0.0*
35-44	0.1	0.1	0.1	0.1	0.1	0.1	0.1*	0.1*	0.1*
45-54	0.1	0.1	0.1	0.1	0.1	0.1*	0.1*	0.1*	0.1*
55-64	0.1	0.1	0.1	0.1	0.1*	0.1	0.1*	0.1*	0.0*
65 & over	0.1	0.1	0.1	0.1	0.1	0.1*	0.1*	0.2*	0.1*
	Age-adjusted death rate								
All ages	0.4	0.4	0.3	0.4	0.4	0.3	0.4*	0.5*	0.3*
Under 15	0.8	0.9	0.8	0.8	0.9	0.7	0.9	1.0	0.8

difference corresponds to the mortality data from various parts of the world, as shown in Table A.11.1.

Geographic distribution. Although average annual age-adjusted death rates varied but slightly among the nine census regions, they were slightly higher in the southern regions for children less than 15 years of age (Table 11.2). The higher rates noted in the South Atlantic and East South Central regions were generally a reflection of those for both colors and sexes.

Death rates by state for children under 15 are delineated in Fig. 11.3 and Table A.11.5. About half the states were represented by less than 20 deaths each, and these were mostly concentrated at both ends of the range of the rates. The suggestion of a southern cluster

CEREBRAL PALSY / 237

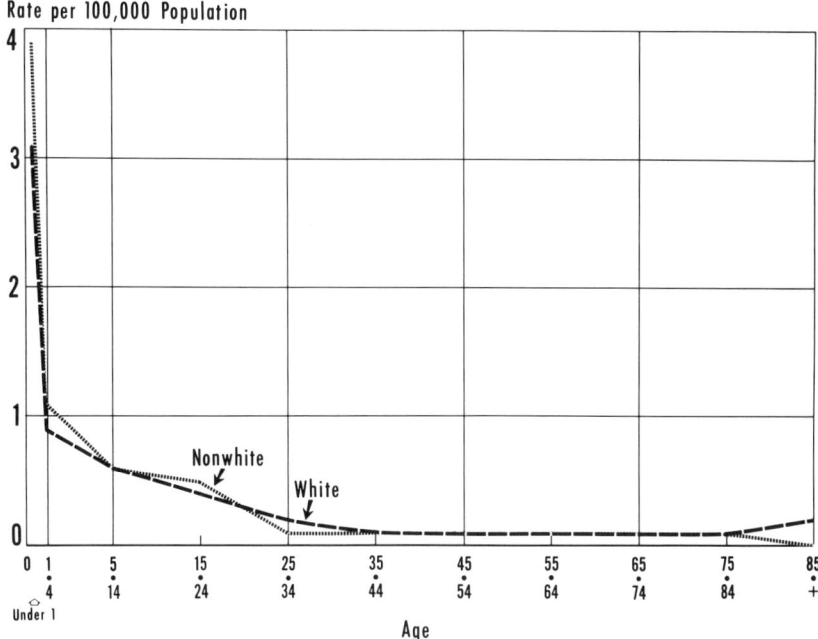

Figure 11.2 Average annual age-specific death rates per 100,000 population for infantile cerebral palsy (cerebral spastic infantile paralysis) by color: United States, 1959-61

Table 11.2   Average annual age-adjusted death rates per 100,000 population under 15 years of age for infantile cerebral palsy (cerebral spastic infantile paralysis) by color and sex: United States and census regions, 1959-61
(ISC code 351)

Region	Total			White			Nonwhite		
	Total	M	F	Total	M	F	Total	M	F
United States	0.8	0.9	0.8	0.8	0.9	0.7	0.9	1.0	0.8
New England	0.7*	0.8*	0.6*	0.6*	0.8*	0.6*	0.5*	0.9*	-
Mid. Atlantic	0.7	0.7	0.7	0.7	0.7	0.7	0.7*	1.0*	0.5*
E. No. Central	0.9	1.0	0.8	0.9	1.0	0.8	1.0*	1.0*	1.0*
W. No. Central	0.9	1.0	0.8*	0.9	1.0	0.8*	1.1*	1.1*	1.2*
So. Atlantic	1.0	1.2	0.8	1.0	1.2	0.8*	1.0	1.3*	0.8*
E. So. Central	1.1	1.0	1.1*	1.1	1.1*	1.1*	1.0*	0.9*	1.1*
W. So. Central	0.9	1.0	0.7	0.9	1.0	0.7	0.7*	0.8*	0.7*
Mountain	0.8	0.9	0.8	0.8*	0.8*	0.8*	0.9*	1.4*	0.5*
Pacific	0.5	0.6*	0.5*	0.5	0.5*	0.5*	0.5*	0.8*	0.3*

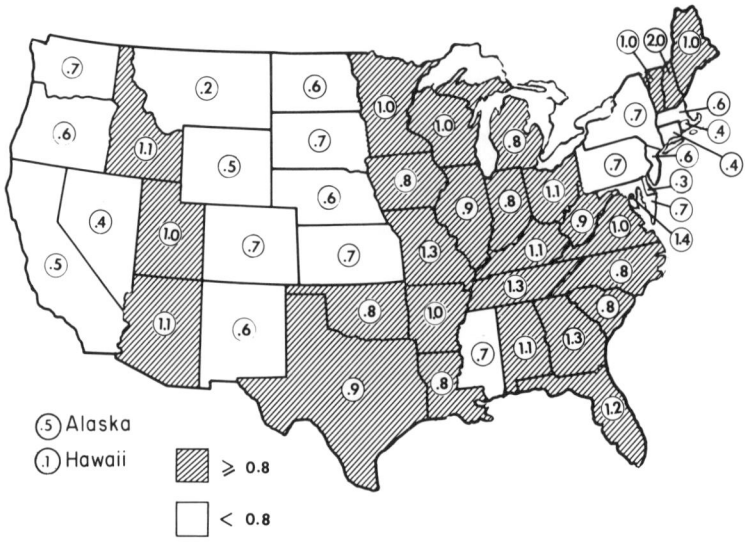

Figure 11.3 Average annual age-adjusted death rates per 100,000 population under 15 years of age for infantile cerebral palsy (cerebral spastic infantile paralysis) by state: United States, 1959–61. Rates that do not meet the standard of reliability or precision as defined in Notes on Tables and Figures are indicated by an asterisk (*) in Table A.11.5.

by census region does not seem to be borne out by the rates under 15 for the individual states; although there was no consistent pattern in the distribution of rates by states, the states with the lower rates (0.7 or less) seem to cluster in the western portion of the country as well as in the Middle Atlantic (New Jersey, New York, and Pennsylvania) and southern New England states.

Color. Slightly higher death rates were found for nonwhites of both sexes in the under-1-year age group, otherwise there was no apparent difference by color. Evaluation of color differences by geographic region was limited by the small number of nonwhites (Table 11.2).

Type of county. There was a slight excess in nonmetropolitan counties over metropolitan counties for both sexes in the under-15 age-adjusted death rate for ICP (Table A.11.6). This pattern held for most of the individual geographic regions.

CEREBRAL PALSY / 239

United States Mortality Data, 1959-61: NCP

Neonatal cerebral palsy is by definition limited to death within the first 28 days of life. In 1959-61 in the United States, there were 9,629 deaths so ascribed, 59 percent coded to 760.0 (neonatal injury) and the remainder to 760.5 (premature birth). Death rates for injury at birth based on populations under 1 year old and for all ages for 1959-61 are shown in Table 11.3. These represent a considerable decrease from earlier rates, as noted previously.

Sex. Regardless of color and geographic area, considerably higher rates were noted for males than for females (Table 11.4). For the total United States, the male-female ratio in the under-1-year rates was slightly greater for whites than for nonwhites (1.8 to 1 vs 1.5 to 1). Male-female ratios for code 760 were slightly greater than those previously noted for ICP code 351.

Color. The under-1-year death rate for nonwhites was almost twice

Table 11.3 Deaths and average annual death rates per 100,000 population under one year of age and all ages for neonatal cerebral palsy (intracranial and spinal injury at birth) by color and sex: United States, 1959-61

(ISC code 760)

Color and sex	Deaths under 1 year[a]	Rate	
		All ages (crude)	Under 1 year
Total	9,629	1.8	78.1
Male	6,120	2.3	97.6
Female	3,509	1.3	57.8
White	7,405	1.6	70.6
Male	4,784	2.0	89.4
Female	2,621	1.1	51.0
Nonwhite	2,224	3.6	120.8
Male	1,336	4.5	145.6
Female	888	2.8	96.1

[a] All deaths occurred in children under 28 days of age.

Table 11.4 Average annual death rates per 100,000 population under one year of age for neonatal cerebral palsy (intracranial and spinal injury at birth) by color and sex: United States and census regions, 1959-61

(ISC code 760)

Region	Total			White			Nonwhite		
	Total	Male	Female	Total	Male	Female	Total	Male	Female
United States	78.1	97.6	57.8	70.6	89.4	51.0	120.8	145.6	96.1
New England	70.7	94.8	45.8	67.6	91.8	42.7	149.1	172.4	124.9*
Middle Atlantic	83.9	103.5	63.7	75.7	93.9	56.8	149.5	182.4	116.9
East North Central	68.8	87.4	49.6	63.6	81.2	45.4	112.5	141.2	84.3
West North Central	61.5	78.2	44.2	57.2	73.6	40.2	132.3	154.4	110.2
South Atlantic	83.4	105.9	60.4	77.8	98.6	56.2	97.3	124.3	70.5
East South Central	77.2	94.6	59.3	70.4	89.0	51.0	93.7	108.7	78.9
West South Central	96.8	116.3	76.7	79.9	99.2	59.8	159.4	180.7	138.2
Mountain	71.8	92.1	50.9	70.9	91.1	50.0	83.6	106.0	61.1*
Pacific	81.7	100.5	62.1	73.1	91.7	53.6	148.1	169.1	126.7

that for whites of corresponding sex, and the all-ages crude rate for nonwhites was more than twice that for whites in each sex (Table 11.3). This white-nonwhite difference is somewhat greater than that observed in the death rates for ICP (code 351) noted earlier.

Geographic distribution. There was no obvious geographic pattern in the United States on the basis of the death rates for children under 1 year of age in the nine geographic regions, as shown in Table 11.4.

Type of county. The death rates for children under 1 year of age were slightly higher in metropolitan counties than in nonmetropolitan counties for both color groups combined, and this pattern held for all but the New England and East South Central regions (Table A.11.7). With respect to color, the excess in the rates for nonwhites as compared with whites was greater in metropolitan counties than in nonmetropolitan counties.

Morbidity Data

The results of various studies on the incidence and prevalence of cerebral palsy are shown in Tables 11.5 and 11.6, respectively. In Rochester, Minnesota, Kurland (1958a) reviewed all cases of central nervous system disorders diagnosed and coded in the Mayo Clinic records for 30,000 residents of the community of Rochester for 1945-54. For CP, more than thirty diagnostic categories were retrieved, including the following: Little's disease, cortical paralysis, cerebral infantile or birth or childhood paralysis, diplegia or hemiplegia, mental retardation, tremor, chorea, athetosis, and extrapyramidal disease or syndrome. From this list, cases that fit the definition of CP (Kurland 1957a) were ascertained.

There were 74 cases in which an abnormality of cerebral motor function presumably developed within the neonatal period and was first noted during infancy. About one-third (27 cases) of these cases were classified as CP as follows: 12 hemiplegic, 4 monoplegic, 8 "spastic," 1 basal ganglion syndrome, and 2 ataxic.

During the period of the study, 3 of the 12 hemiplegic and 6 of the 8 spastic patients had been born in Rochester; the annual incidence rate represented by these two groups combined was 1.2 per 1,000 births (Table 11.5). This was considered a minimal estimate. (Note that the correct denominator of 7,300 births is used for this rate instead of the 14,200 as published.)

Table 11.5 Cases and average annual incidence rates per 1,000 live births for cerebral palsy: selected surveys, various years, 1925-63

Survey area (source)	Years	Cases	Rate
Rochester, Minnesota (Kurland 1957a; 1958a)	1945-54	9	1.2
Carlisle, England (Brewis et al. 1966)	1955-61	13	1.5
Denmark (Hansen 1960)	1925-53	2,820	1.3
Iceland (Gudmundsson 1967a)	1954-63	235	2.2
Østfold, Norway (Andersen 1954)	c 1953	33	1.9
Edinburgh, Scotland (Ingram 1955)	1935-52	208	2.0
Denmark (Hansen 1960)	1925-29	321	0.9
	1930-34	357	1.1
	1935-39	433	1.3
	1940-44	528	1.3
	1945-49	599	1.4
	1950-53	582	1.9

Twenty-one of the 27 Rochester patients were alive at the end of the study period. The prevalence rate thus was about 0.7 per 1,000 total population, or 1.6 per 1,000 population less than 20 years of age (Table 11.6). The age distribution of the patients living in Rochester on prevalence day (December 31, 1954) was as follows: 0-9 years, 7; 10-19 years, 7; 20-29 years, 3; and 30 or older, 4.

Brewis and her associates (1966) in Carlisle, England, reported an incidence rate for CP of 1.5 per 1,000 live births. This was based on 8,528 live births from 1955 through 1961, among whom 13 were subsequently diagnosed as suffering from CP. On prevalence day the 24 living patients represented a rate of 1.4 per 1,000 population less than 14 years of age, or 0.3 per 1,000 for all ages.

The reader is referred especially to the work of Hansen (1960), which includes detailed discussion of the problems of definition and field research of CP, comparisons of clinical types of motor dysfunction, and data from about 4,000 patients in Denmark. Hansen's study covered approximately thirty years. There was an increase in incidence from 0.9 per 1,000 births (1925-29) to 1.9 per 1,000 (1950-53), which could be interpreted as a better salvage rate rather

Table 11.6 Cases and prevalence rates per 1,000 population, all ages and childhood ages, for cerebral palsy: selected surveys, various years, 1953-62

Survey area (source)	Year	Cases	Rate All ages	Rate Childhood
Rochester, Minnesota (Kurland 1957a, 1958a)	1954	21	0.7	1.6[a]
Carlisle, England (Brewis et al. 1966)	1961	24	0.3	1.4[b]
Denmark (Hansen 1960)	1955	2,621	0.6	1.6[a]
Iceland (Gudmundsson 1967a)	1962	224	1.2	2.1[a]
Østfold, Norway (Andersen 1954)	1953	77	0.4-0.8[c]	1.5[a]
Östergöttland, Sweden (Herlitz and Redin 1955)	1954	96	0.4	2.1[d]

[a] Under 20 years of age.

[b] Under 14 years of age.

[c] Confirmed (0.4) versus diagnosed (0.8).

[d] Ages 2-11 years inclusive.

than any true change in frequency. As of 1955 the prevalence rate was 0.6 per 1,000 general population. The case ratio was 56 males to 44 females. Age-specific prevalence rates were maximal at 1.8 per 1,000 at ages 2-4, declined somewhat thereafter to age 30, and were much lower at older ages. Hansen's findings indicated an increased risk for CP with: (*a*) mothers 35 years old or older; (*b*) firstborn, twins, and prematures; (*c*) prior abortions and stillbirths; (*d*) difficult deliveries; (*e*) "cerebral symptoms in the neonatal period"; and (*f*) birth in the last quarter of the year.

Gudmundsson (1967*a*) in Iceland found a prevalence of 1.2 per 1,000 general population, with 224 patients. The male-female ratio was 1.5 to 1. He did not consider maternal age or the season to be factors, but concurred essentially in previously mentioned findings (*b*) through (*e*) of Hansen. The annual incidence rate was essentially stable during the ten years, at 2.2 per 1,000 live births.

Andersen (1954) surveyed the county of Østfold, Norway, and from the 33 cases of children aged 5-9 years estimated an incidence rate of 1.9 per 1,000 live births; this group was chosen as having the maximal age-specific prevalence rate. For the total alive at the time, he calculated a prevalence rate of 1.5 per 1,000 population under 20 years old. The prevalence rate for all ages would be 0.4 per 1,000 for the 77 cases he confirmed by examination, or 0.8 for the 134 total cases diagnosed. In Edinburgh, Scotland, Ingram (1955) noted a rate of 2.0 per 1,000 births for 1935-52, with 208 cases of CP. Herlitz and Redin (1955) in Östergöttlands Län, Sweden, calculated a childhood prevalence rate of 2.1 per 1,000 population of 2-11 year olds, or a total population prevalence rate of 0.4 per 1,000.

These studies showed considerable uniformity in the frequency of CP. Between 1 and 2 cases per 1,000 live births can be expected, maximal prevalence is in early childhood at about 2 per 1,000 on an age-specific basis, and the general prevalence rate is about 0.6 per 1,000 total population. There appeared to be a slight excess of CP in males over females. Survival much beyond age 30 for those with CP is greatly diminished when compared with expectation for the general population. These conclusions are drawn from studies of white populations in advanced centers of Norway, Sweden, Denmark, Iceland, England, Scotland, and the United States, and should not be extrapolated to regions far different in socioeconomic, medical, or racial composition. The common feature to the predisposition for CP seems to be the survival of the infant after birth trauma or anoxia, or both; yet there may well be other conditions that predispose to the brain damage whose signal is cerebral palsy.

Comment

An attempt was made to evaluate population selectivity for mortality from cerebral spastic infantile paralysis, and from intracranial and spinal birth injuries as indexes of distribution of cerebral palsy in the United States. In 1959-61 in the United States, the death rate for the former (ISC code 351), both crude and age adjusted, was 0.4 per 100,000. With respect to ISC code 760, the crude death rate was 1.8 per 100,000 total population, all ages, and 78.1 per 100,000 children under 1 year of age. Rates were higher for males and for the nonwhite population. There was no evidence of meaningful variation in geographic distribution. These statements hold for both infantile CP (code 351) and neonatal CP (code 760).

Morbidity data from among socioeconomically advanced regions of the Western Hemisphere, and limited to whites, indicated a rather uniform incidence and prevalence—and hence distribution—for CP.

Between 1 and 2 cases per 1,000 births, a childhood prevalence rate of about 2 per 1,000 population, and a prevalence rate for all ages of about 0.6 per 1,000 population seemed to be likely estimates as to frequency. Survival was much diminished, and age-specific prevalence rates beyond age 30 were low. For detailed data based on a large series of CP cases, those of Hansen (1960) in Denmark are unparalleled.

12 / BLINDNESS
Hyman Goldstein

Few data have been compiled that can be used for comparisons among countries on the demographic characteristics of blind persons or the causes of blindness. Estimates of the number of bilaterally blind throughout the world at the present time have ranged from 10,000,000 to more than 14,000,000, or prevalence rates of 320 to 450 per 100,000 population (Wilson 1965).

Definition

The lack of comparability among various studies results in part from the variability in the definition of blindness. The following definition of economic blindness (actually, that of "severe visual impairment") was used as a standard in the Model Reporting Area for Blindness Statistics (MRA): distant visual acuity of 20/200 or less in the better eye, with best correction; or visual field no greater than 20 degrees in diameter regardless of acuity (in the better eye) (National Institute of Neurological Diseases and Blindness 1963). The causes of blindness in the MRA studies—to which extensive attention will be paid in this chapter—were categorized from the "Standard Classification" developed by the Subcommittee on Classification of the Committee on Operational Research of the National Society for the Prevention of Blindness. The "major affection" groups in this classification are glaucoma (primary and noncongenital), myopia, keratitis, other affections of the cornea or sclera, cataract, uveitis, retrolental fibroplasia (RLF), retinal degeneration, other retinal affections, optic nerve atrophy, multiple affections (of those listed), other, and unknown. There is also a separate "major cause" grouping that consists of infection, injury or poisoning (or both), neoplasm, diabetes, senile degeneration, vascular diseases, other general diseases, prenatal influence, multiple causes, "unknown to science," and not reported or determined.

Glaucoma, a state characterized by an increase in intraocular pressure, may be either secondary to other disease or injury of the orbital contents or "primary." The latter is divided into the narrow-angle "congestive" glaucoma, which may be acute or chronic, and the wide-angle "simple" glaucoma of the elderly. Only the primary form is included as a "major affection."

Keratitis refers to inflammation of the cornea. Among the major specific infections in this group is trachoma, which is "a chronic follicular keratoconjunctivitis... caused by a Rickettsia-like organism, *Chlamydia trachomatis*" (Allen 1963).

Cataract, an opacification of the lens, also is varied in type and cause. Two subdivisions are developmental and degenerative. The latter includes senile (capsular) cataract; traumatic (direct force, radiation, heat, electricity); complicated (from other eye infections); and systemic (diabetes, myotonic dystrophy, parathyroid disease, toxins, and so forth). Diabetes itself is responsible for a characteristic juvenile cataract, as well as for increased risk of senile cataract (Adler 1957; Allen 1963).

Retrolental fibroplasia (RLF) is in essence high-oxygen poisoning in premature infants. It appeared de novo in the early 1940s and was "the chief cause of blindness in infants" (Adler 1957) by the middle of the 1950s. The Yearbook of Ophthalmology reviewed a number of papers on RLF in the 1957-58 edition; one paper on RLF was published in the 1958-59 issue, but none was reported thereafter. At the present time the disorder should be infrequently encountered because of the specialized facilities for the care of premature infants and the increased knowledge of the role of oxygen in causation of the affliction.

The *retinal degenerations* vary in type and in age of patient affected, and *optic atrophy* results from many neurologic and ophthalmologic disorders. Thus all the classes except RLF refer to groups of conditions and, at best, may be taken as the starting point in future investigations into the epidemiology of blindness. Even so, this is by far the most extensive and systematic classification that has been used in seeking the population characteristics of disorders of vision.

Survivorship of the Blind

Rogot and his fellow-workers (1966), with about 20,000 blind registrants in Massachusetts during 1940-59, indicated that longevity among the blind was somewhat below that of the general population. Among males, survival was close to that of the general population for persons age 5-24, but was less favorable for those over 24 years of age. Survival among females was close to expectation only for those less than 15 years old and was notably less for those age 25-74.

A study of mortality rates of insurance policyholders who were totally blind revealed different data:

The 1951 Impairment Study of the Society of Actuaries, covering the period 1935-50, found that totally blind persons accepted for life insurance experienced [mortality] rates of only 76 percent of those among standard life insurance risks. This reflects both the careful selection of blind applicants and their increasingly effective training in self-care. The markedly low rate of accidental death among the insured blind has been attributed to the greater restriction of their activities, their more sheltered lives, and the consequent reduction of exposure to accidental hazards (Metropolitan Life Insurance Company 1966).

Belloc and her associates (1957) collected follow-up data on 530 white blind persons with primary glaucoma who were recipients of aid to the blind in California during a five-year period. At age 40, the survivorship for both males and females was significantly less than expected; but at age 65, the decrease was significant only for males. Comparison with nonblind recipients of Old Age Assistance revealed that the elderly males and females of this group had the same survival rates as did the blind. Thus the decrease in survivorship from normal expectation for the elderly blind may be related to socioeconomic status rather than to visual deficit per se.

Incidence and Prevalence of Blindness in the United States

Early attempts to estimate the frequency of blindness in this country were in essence fruitless. Incorporation of this question in the census questionnaires was given up after 1930. Attempts at ascertaining the number of blind in the United States by the National Health Survey were made in 1935-36 and during the period July 1957 through June 1958. For the latter period a nationwide household survey of a representative sample of the population was conducted, using as a definition of blindness the "inability to read ordinary newsprint even with the aid of glasses."* The full definition included, as blind, persons who were (a) 6 years old or older and by or for whom a negative response was given to the question: "Can

---

*A near vision of 14/35 is adequate for a person to read newsprint, usually 8-point type, provided there are no other problems. This is equivalent to a distant visual acuity of 20/50. A definition of blindness embodying visual acuities ranging from 20/50 downward would include persons who are not legally blind as well as some who are not even "partially seeing" as defined (National Society for the Prevention of Blindness 1966).

you read ordinary newspaper print with glasses?" or (b) less than 6 years of age (or 6 or older but who had never learned to read) and who were reported as being blind or in terms indicating no useful vision in either eye (Health Statistics, National Health Survey 1959).

The 1957-58 National Health Survey arrived at an estimated number of 960,000 blind persons in the United States, or a prevalence rate of 5.7 per 1,000 population (Health Statistics, National Health Survey 1959). No attempt was made to validate the "blindness" diagnosis. The rate greatly exceeded rates previously produced by any census or by the 1935-36 National Health Survey. The rate was almost three times that otherwise estimated for economic blindness at that time. Such overestimation might be the result largely of reliance on respondents' replies to a question that embodied a rather general definition of blindness. In view of the definition employed, National Health Survey officials now refer to the above estimates as pertaining to "severe vision impairment," not to blindness. However, because the acuity could have been as good as 20/50 within this study, the data should perhaps be accepted as an estimate of persons who claimed some visual impairment, but not necessarily a severe one (National Society for the Prevention of Blindness 1966).

Another National Health Survey—July 1959 through June 1961—produced an estimated prevalence of 5.6 per 1,000 population with severe visual impairment in the United States (Health Statistics, National Health Survey 1962). A still later National Health Survey—July 1963 through June 1965—indicated a rate of 6.6 per 1,000 population (National Center for Health Statistics 1968b). The methods of study were essentially the same as those used in the 1957-58 study.

Another survey of binocular visual acuity among adults had been conducted under the National Health Survey in 1960-62 (National Center for Health Statistics 1964). The data were derived from direct examination of 6,672 persons aged 18 to 79, representing about 86 percent of the sample referred for examination. A standardized single-visit examination was given each examinee by medical and other staff members in the specially designed mobile units used for the survey. The data on visual acuity were the first to be collected for a national probability sample of the adult population in the United States.

The study showed that 0.8 percent of those tested with correction were unable to read at the 20/100 level—that is, they had a maximal central visual acuity of 20/200. If visual acuity of 20/200 were used as the definition of blindness, this sample would indicate a "blindness" prevalence rate of 8 per 1,000 of the adult population age 18-79. For males, the rate was 5 per 1,000; for females, 10 per 1,000. Among males, the rate increased steadily with age from 0 per 1,000 in the age group 18-24 until it reached a peak of 17 per 1,000 in the 65-74 age group, and then decreased slightly in the age group 75-79. Among females, the rate decreased from 5 per 1,000 in the age group 18-24 to a low of 1 per 1,000 in the age group 35-44, and then increased steadily, reaching a peak of 50 per 1,000 in the oldest age group, 75-79 years.

The report stated that the proportion of persons with such severe visual impairment was too small to give reliable statistics for this segment of the population. Furthermore, it added that neither the testing nor the examination procedures were sufficient to provide the basis for making a more precise estimate of the prevalence of blindness. There were additional factors that make the findings difficult to evaluate: (a) the oldest age groups were not included, that is, those 80 or older, for whom the highest blindness rates have been found in other studies; (b) response among the ill and infirm was unknown, and these are the groups that might have had more visual impairment; and (c) "usual" correction rather than "best" correction was used.

Schools for the Blind

For students in schools for the blind, there are usually reliable medical and family histories. However, since studies of such students are usually limited to certain residential schools, the results cannot be generalized to all such residential schools or more particularly to the ever-growing number of students now being educated in special classes of the regular public school system. Further, no generalization concerning the distribution of causes of blindness in students may be made to the blind population of all ages.

Kerby (1950; 1952; 1958), Berens and his associates (1955), and Hatfield (1963) carried out a series of surveys during 1945-59 of blind students in residential schools and day classes for the blind. They showed that the blindness rate caused by infectious diseases had decreased markedly with time, mostly because of decreases in incidences of ophthalmia neonatorum and syphilis. The rate from injuries also had decreased, but to a lesser extent. However, there was an increased incidence of retrolental fibroplasia, and by 1950 this accounted for approximately half the cases of blindness in children of preschool age. The incidence of blindness resulting from prenatal influence* increased slowly in this period and accounted for about 48 percent of the cases by 1959.

Hatfield (1963) compared estimated blindness prevalence rates for school-age children in her study with those found in previous studies of schoolchildren and indicated that the rate had increased almost 61 percent between 1933-34 and 1958-59 (Table 12.1), primarily because of the great increase in the prevalence of retrolental fibroplasia among schoolchildren. More recent data would be expected to show a reversion to the earlier rates, with the decline of RLF.

Other Estimates

A number of studies have attempted to estimate the prevalence of blindness, incorporating data arising from governmental aid to the blind and various state registers of the blind. Using all available information, Hurlin (1953; 1962) estimated the prevalence of blindness by state. His rates per 1,000 population for the United States as a whole were 1.98 as of July 1, 1952 and 2.14 for 1960. These rates represented the following estimates of the number of blind people in the country: 308,000 in 1952 and 385,000 in 1960.

Model Reporting Area for Blindness Statistics

The need for uniform data on reported cases of blindness and on causes of blindness led to the formation of the Model Reporting Area for Blindness Statistics (MRA) in 1962. The basis for the MRA concept was that states with blindness registers would voluntarily agree to collect, on a uniform basis, certain specified data on each reported blind person and make those data available annually to the National Institute of Neurological Diseases and Blindness (NINDB)

---

*Conditions in the prenatal influence category are those which are hereditary and those which are "congenital" (present at birth), but whose exact cause has not been determined or is unspecified. The group includes the congenital malformations (such as coloboma and absence of a part or all of the eye), congenital cataracts and glaucoma, albinism, and hereditary retinal degeneration (such as retinitis pigmentosa). Excluded from the category of prenatal influence are conditions caused by prenatal infections (such as syphilis and toxoplasmosis), rubella in the mother during pregnancy, and hereditary neoplasms (such as retinoblastoma) (National Society for the Prevention of Blindness 1966).

Table 12.1 Estimated rates per 100,000 enrolled pupils for blindness among school-age children by cause: United States, selected residential schools for the blind, city school systems and state departments of education, specified years, 1933-59

Cause	1933-34	1943-44	1954-55	1958-59
All causes	21.2	21.9	19.9	34.1
Infectious diseases	6.1	5.0	1.5	1.3
Toxoplasmosis	---[a]	---[a]	0.1	0.3
Rubella	---[a]	---[a]	0.1	0.2
Ophthalmia neonatorum	2.3	2.3	0.3	0.1
Syphilis	1.1	1.1	0.3	0.1
Tuberculosis	0.1	0.0	0.1	0.1
Measles	0.2	0.2	0.0	0.0
Other	2.4	1.4	0.6	0.5
Injuries	1.6	1.5	1.0	0.8
Poisonings	0.0	0.0	3.8	11.3
Excessive oxygen (RLF)	---[a]	---[a]	3.8	11.3
Other	0.0	0.0	0.0	0.0
Tumors	0.5	0.8	1.0	1.2
General diseases[b]	0.3	0.3	0.1	0.6
Prenatal influence[c]	10.8	12.1	11.2	16.3
Not reported	1.9	2.2	1.3	2.6
(Number in study)	(2,702)	(3,749)	(4,426)	(7,757)

[a] Cause not separately classified.

[b] Diseases affecting the body as a whole or a particular system such as diabetes mellitus, diseases of the central nervous system, metabolic diseases, senile degeneration, etc.

[c] Diseases or conditions which have their effect on the development of the eyes or causing defects during embryonic life prior to birth. These include developmental abnormalities and defects of the eye of genetic origin and those due to certain infections, diseases, and toxins.

for analysis and publication in the annual statistical reports of MRA. It was believed that this would help the states in fulfilling administrative and service needs and possibly furnish uniformly collected data for research purposes.

Each of the thirty-five states maintaining blindness registers in 1961 was evaluated by the Biometrics Branch, NINDB, as to its capacity and willingness to satisfy MRA standards. The Biometrics Branch also undertook to act in a coordinating and technical capacity and agreed to furnish consultation and other assistance to the states accepted into MRA.

MRA Standards

The following are the standards (National Institute of Neurological Diseases and Blindness 1963) of MRA to which each member state agreed: first, to follow a standard definition of blindness—that is, visual acuity of 20/200 or less in the better eye with best correction, or visual acuity of more than 20/200 if the widest diameter of the field of vision subtends an angle no greater than 20 degrees; second, to include on their registers all residents whose visual acuity is within this definition, irrespective of need or desire for service and without any exclusion on the basis of age, race, or any other factor; third, to collect at least the following minimal information: (*a*) date and type of addition (whether new addition or re-addition) to the MRA register; (*b*) county of residence or equivalent; (*c*) date of birth; (*d*) sex; (*e*) race; (*f*) age at onset of blindness; (*g*) date of eye examination leading to certification of blindness; (*h*) discipline of examiner; (*i*) degree of vision; (*j*) site or type (or both) of affection and cause of blindness; and (*k*) date of and reason for removal from MRA register; fourth, to use the Standard Classification of Causes of Severe Vision Impairment and Blindness and its accompanying Index of Diagnostic Terms developed by the Subcommittee on Classification of the Committee on Operational Research of the National Society for the Prevention of Blindness (see previous definition of blindness); fifth, to remove from the register any person who had died, moved out of state, or recovered vision beyond the MRA definition of blindness by means of an annual clearance to determine the residence and blindness status of every person on the register; and sixth, to forward annually to NINDB decks of verified punch cards of persons newly reported during the year as well as those remaining on the register at the end of the year. Names are not requested in order to preserve anonymity.

Cause-of-blindness data for newly reported blind persons (first additions to the register) first became available from MRA states in 1963 following training workshops for the registry personnel and a quality-control program instituted by NINDB.

Cause-of-blindness data were accepted from MRA states for tabulation and analysis only if the examinations were by ophthalmologists or eye-ear-nose-and-throat (EENT) specialists. However, the certification of a person's meeting the definition of blindness on the basis of visual acuity or field of vision could be made by any person qualified to take the measurements. Cause data were submitted by ophthalmologists and EENT specialists on about 92 percent of all first additions in 1965 and 1966 (National Institute of Neurological Diseases and Blindness 1966; 1969). The Model Reporting Area for Blindness Statistics represents the largest segment of the United States population on which blindness data under a uniform definition and with uniform classification of causes of blindness have been collected.

Data on first additions to the MRA were available from thirteen states in 1965 and from fourteen in 1966 (National Institute of Neurological Diseases and Blindness 1966; 1969). In addition, data for those remaining on the register at the end of the year were made available. The findings for 1966 only will be presented, the prior year being essentially the same. The MRA states are not necessarily representative of the country as a whole with respect to demographic, racial, or other characteristics. However, they do represent the best data currently available on causes of blindness and characteristics of the blind in one-fifth of the United States population.

MRA Rates and Percentages, 1966

Table 12.2 shows the incidence and prevalence rates per 100,000 population of MRA states in 1966 for all additions to the register and for the total on the register at the end of the year. All additions include first additions and re-additions. The latter are newly reported persons who had formerly been on the register, but who had been removed because of recovered vision, migration from the state, and so forth. In this study their number is negligible. The first additions therefore comprise the reported incidence. Because of interstate variation in age and race composition of the respective populations, age standardization of the rates by race is desirable and is expected to be calculated for 1969-71 data.

MRA Incidence

Rates for additions generally remained low for the group under 45 years old and increased sharply thereafter, with the highest rates observed for the group 85 or older (Table 12.3). ("Age" here refers to age of registrant in year of registration, not age at onset of blindness.) There was little difference by sex until age 65 or older, when the rate was higher for females. There was a slight preponderance for females in the overall rates. The age-sex-color-specific rates shown, however, should be regarded with caution because of the

Table 12.2 Rates per 100,000 population for all additions to blindness register (reported incidence) and for total on register at end of year (reported prevalence): MRA[a] by state, 1966

State	Reported incidence rate	Reported prevalence rate
MRA total	15.3	146.7
Connecticut	14.0	118.2
Georgia	---	113.7
Kansas	16.7	145.0
Louisiana	10.5	168.9
Massachusetts	18.7	180.3
New Hampshire	21.2	155.0
New Jersey	9.2	105.7
New Mexico	6.7	252.7
North Carolina	23.3	208.7
Oregon	23.0	126.2
Rhode Island	8.8	120.9
South Dakota	17.1	135.6
Utah	14.8	124.1
Vermont	19.2	169.1
Virginia	14.2	128.4

[a]Model Reporting Area for Blindness Statistics, United States.

unknown reliability of the estimated population base for a noncensus year. In each age group the rates for nonwhites were considerably greater than those for whites, and the overall rates for nonwhites were about twice those for whites.

The category of "unknown" extent of vision includes persons presumably blind by definition, but who could not be examined adequately because of age or other reasons, or for whom there was no report of actual visual acuity. About 30 percent of whites and 35 percent of nonwhites either were totally blind or had visual acuity no greater than 5/200. A higher percentage of nonwhites than whites had restricted fields and on this basis were classified as being blind (Table 12.4).

About 20 percent of all those less than 5 years old were reported as having no vision. Another 42 percent in this age group had an "unknown" extent of vision, probably because of the difficulty of examining the very young (Table 12.5). In the remaining age groups

Table 12.3 Rates per 100,000 population for all additions[a] to blindness register (reported incidence) by age, color and sex: MRA[b], 1966

Age[c]	Total			White			Nonwhite		
	Total	Male	Female	Total	Male	Female	Total	Male	Female
All ages	15.3	14.3	16.3	13.4	12.4	14.3	22.4	20.8	23.9
Under 5	3.5	4.9	3.1	d	d	d	d	d	d
5-19	5.0	5.5	4.4	4.2	4.7	3.7	6.2	6.4	6.0
20-44	5.1	5.8	4.4	4.3	5.0	3.6	9.8	10.1	9.4
45-64	18.6	19.4	17.9	14.7	15.7	13.8	51.0	48.1	53.7
65-74	41.8	39.4	43.9	34.8	33.4	36.0	96.8	85.4	107.0
75-84	137.6	128.2	144.6	127.1	118.8	132.9	205.6	178.8	228.9
85 & over	342.4	318.1	354.2	329.7	296.9	349.1	d	d	d

[a] See Table 12.4 for number of additions by color and Table 12.5 for number by age.

[b] Model Reporting Area for Blindness Statistics, United States. Includes data on all additions for 14 states in 1966. (See Table 12.2)

[c] Age at registration in MRA state.

[d] Rate not computed when estimated population was less than 25,000 or when percentage with unknown information, such as race, was 10 percent or more.

Table 12.4 Percentage distribution of all additions to blindness register by degree of vision in better eye by color: MRA[a] total, 1966

Degree of vision	Total	White	Nonwhite
Total	100.0	100.0	100.0
Absolute blindness	5.2	4.9	6.9
Light perception	9.1	8.7	9.4
Light projection	1.2	1.2	1.8
Less than 5/200	15.7	15.5	17.6
5/200 to less than 10/200	9.9	10.6	6.4
10/200 to less than 20/200	18.2	18.8	14.8
20/200	27.7	28.2	26.4
Restricted field	5.7	5.5	7.7
Unknown	7.3	6.7	9.0
(Number of additions)	(5,684)[b]	(4,373)	(1,000)

[a] Model Reporting Area for Blindness Statistics, United States. Includes data on all additions for 14 states in 1966. (See Table 12.2)

[b] Includes 5,471 first additions, 213 re-additions, and 311 persons of unknown color.

Table 12.5 Percentage distribution of all additions to blindness register by degree of vision in better eye by age[a]: MRA[b] total, 1966

Degree of vision	All ages	Under 5	5-19	20-44	45-64	65-74	75-84	85 & over
Total	100.0	100.0	100.0	100.0	100.0	100.0	100.0	100.0
Absolute blindness	5.2	20.7	5.3	7.0	5.3	5.2	2.9	3.4
Light perception	9.1	21.3	7.3	8.3	8.6	10.7	8.2	9.2
Light projection	1.2	2.0	0.4	1.0	1.2	1.7	1.4	1.2
Less than 5/200	15.7	4.7	6.1	14.0	16.9	20.6	16.1	17.7
5/200 to less than 10/200	9.9	2.0	8.1	7.2	10.5	9.3	11.4	11.9
10/200 to less than 20/200	18.2	3.3	18.8	17.8	19.3	17.4	18.6	18.5
20/200	27.7	4.0	40.5	28.4	24.9	25.5	30.5	27.1
Restricted field	5.7	-	2.4	10.0	9.3	5.2	4.2	2.4
Unknown	7.3	42.0	11.1	6.4	4.1	4.2	6.8	8.6
(Number of additions)	(5,684)[c]	(150)	(506)	(613)	(1,368)	(921)	(1,276)	(654)

[a] Age at registration in MRA state.
[b] Model Reporting Area for Blindness Statistics, United States. Includes data on all additions for 14 states in 1966. (See Table 12.2)
[c] Includes 5,471 first additions, 213 re-additions, and 196 persons of unknown age.

the largest percentage was found in the 20/200 category. The fairly high percentage of persons reported with vision of exactly 20/200 probably indicates a lack of either precise measurement or careful reporting, particularly because this level of acuity is the criterion for distinguishing the "legally" blind.

The data on causes have certain limitations. Despite efforts to achieve uniformity, there are differences in interpretation of principles of classification and errors in coding. Also the variation in diagnostic skills among states or localities may account for some of the differences (Goldstein 1966).

There were no appreciable differences between the sexes according to major affection groups, except for a preponderance of males in the group with optic nerve atrophy and a slight preponderance of females in the group with cataract (Table A.12.1). A comparison by color, however, showed marked differences for three major affections. The percentage of nonwhites with glaucoma was more than twice that of whites (21 percent vs 9 percent), whereas the percentage of nonwhites with retinal degeneration was one-third that of whites (7 percent vs 21 percent). The group of "other retinal affections" also showed a somewhat higher percentage for whites (15 percent) than for nonwhites (13 percent). It is not known to what extent variations in age distributions by color account for these differences. Blindness resulting from glaucoma is often a sign of lack of medical care and these differences by color may represent medical utilization rather than disease frequencies.

In general, higher percentages of glaucoma, cataract, and retinal degeneration were found among new registrants in the older age groups than in the younger ones (Table A.12.2). Cataract, however, was frequent in persons of all ages. The percentage of persons with optic nerve atrophy was relatively high in the young, in whom most neurologic disorders might be expected. The instances of retrolental fibroplasia reported among persons 5 years old or older probably represented delayed reporting of blindness, since this affection is known to appear shortly after birth.

The category of 20/200 visual acuity accounted for the largest percentage of each of the major affection groups, except for retrolental fibroplasia and glaucoma (Table A.12.3). Of persons with retrolental fibroplasia, one-third to one-half either were totally blind or had only light perception. About one-fourth of all first additions with glaucoma had a field of vision restriction of 20 degrees or less, and one-tenth of those with optic nerve atrophy were similarly affected. Field loss was uncommon in the other categories.

The percentage of males in whom the cause was "injuries and poisonings" was higher than the corresponding percentage among females, regardless of color (Table A.12.4). A similar pattern also was seen for the "prenatal influence" category, but the difference was less pronounced. However, the percentage of females in whom the cause was "diabetes" was higher than the corresponding percentage for males, and this was most apparent among nonwhites. This sex difference may reflect the higher morbidity from diabetes for females in the general population. Females of both colors similarly exceeded males in the percentage who were reported to have senile degeneration as a cause. About 12 percent of all first additions to the register had causes "unknown to science," but this comprised almost 10 percent of whites and 22 percent of the nonwhite blind (26 percent male and 19 percent female). Glaucoma caused almost all of the "unknown to science" cases (543 of 586 persons). The cause was not reported in about one-seventh of all cases, regardless of sex or color. There were no other appreciable differences between whites and nonwhites according to major etiologic groups, although there was a somewhat larger percentage of whites than nonwhites in the senile degeneration category. The sum of this category and the "unknown to science" was almost uniformly 45 percent for both sexes and colors.

For persons under 45 years old, as expected, prenatal influence was by far the most frequently reported cause of blindness (Table A.12.5). Injuries and poisonings accounted for about 8 percent of all blindness in persons less than 45 years old. Diabetes was of particular etiologic significance in persons who were between 20 and 74 years old. For those 65 and older, the most common causes were "senile degeneration," and "unknown to science" (mostly glaucoma). Vascular disease as a cause remained at less than 5 percent, even in the elderly. Proportions "not reported" were little influenced by age except for decreases at the oldest ages.

In the etiologic categories of "injuries and poisonings" and "neoplasms," about one-fourth of the persons were reported as being totally blind (Table A.12.6). In the remaining etiologic groups, the largest percentages of those affected were classified as having 20/200 visual acuity.

The four major affection groups with highest frequencies were cataract, retinal degeneration, other retinal affections, and glaucoma, accounting for 63.3 percent of all affections. When these affection groups were analyzed by major etiologic groups, retinal degeneration and cataract were similarly distributed in relative etiologic frequency, and together most of them were associated with the etiologic group "senile degeneration" (Table 12.6). The diabetics in this series were mainly found in the "other retinal affections" group which for diabetes consisted essentially in retinopathies. Prenatal influence was manifested in all affection categories, the two largest being retinal degeneration and cataract. As stated previously, most of the cases classified as "unknown to science" were of glaucoma.

MRA Prevalence

The total blind on the register at any one time constitute, in effect, a reported prevalence which probably is understated (Table 12.7).

For all ages combined, the rates for end-of-1966 register totals for males and females were similar. For both sexes, the lowest rates were for those less than 5 years old, the rates increasing sharply thereafter with age. The age-specific rates for males were higher than those for females up to 75 years, above which age the rates for females exceeded those for males. In the MRA states as a whole, about 3 percent of the total population 85 or older was reported as being blind.

As in the case of reported incidence (Table 12.3), the end-of-year total on the register rate for nonwhites (all ages and both sexes combined) was about twice the corresponding rate for whites. When such comparison by color was further divided by sex, the approximate two-to-one ratio was maintained (Table 12.7).

Degree of vision for persons on the register at the end of the year was based on the results of the latest recorded examination for each registrant. Nonwhites appeared to have somewhat higher relative frequencies than whites in the groups with more severe visual loss (Table 12.8). This was also found in the data for all additions (Table 12.4) and may be a result of the greater reported incidence rates among nonwhites of such ocular disorders as glaucoma, which is associated with more severe visual loss.

The percentage of those on the register at the end of the year who were totally blind (absolute blindness) was about twice that of all additions to the register in a year (Tables 12.4 and 12.8). In every age group the percentage on the register who were totally blind was higher than that of the same age group of all additions (Tables 12.5 and A.12.7). The percentage of the blind with "unknown" extent of vision was relatively high in younger age groups and in those 85 or older, and this is probably indicative of the difficulty in obtaining valid examinations of persons in these age groups (Table A.12.7).

Table 12.6 Percentage distribution of first additions[a] to blindness register by selected major affection and cause groups: MRA[b] total, 1966

Major cause group[c]	Total	Major affection group[c]							(Number of first additions)
		Glaucoma, noncongenital	Cataract	Retinal degeneration	Other retinal affec.[d]	Optic nerve atrophy	Multiple affec.	All others	
Total	100.0	10.9	18.9	18.9	14.6	5.2	9.2	22.2	...
Diabetes	11.6	-	-	-	10.0	0.0	1.5	0.1	(577)
Senile degeneration	33.0	-	15.6	14.1	0.5	-	2.7	0.2	(1,640)
Prenatal influence[e]	13.7	-	2.1	3.8	0.4	0.8	-	6.6	(680)
Unknown to science	11.8	10.9	-	0.3	0.1	-	-	0.4	(586)
Not reported/determined	14.1	-	0.7	0.5	1.5	2.2	0.2	9.1	(700)
All others	15.8	-	0.5	0.1	2.2	2.2	4.9	5.8	(782)
(Number of first additions)	...	(543)	(938)	(936)	(727)	(259)	(459)	(1,103)	(4,965)

[a] Data limited to first additions examined by ophthalmologists or eye-ear-nose-and-throat specialists.
[b] Model Reporting Area for Blindness Statistics, United States. Includes data on first additions for 14 states in 1966. (See Table 12.2)
[c] Standard Classification of Causes of Severe Vision Impairment and Blindness, 1966 Revision.
[d] Includes retinitis, retinopathy, detachment of retina, retinitis pigmentosa, glioblastoma, hemangiomatosis, hypoplasia, neuroepithelioma, neurofibroma, neurofibromatosis, retinoblastoma, retinocytoma and retinal affection - unspecified.
[e] See Table 12.1 for description.

Table 12.7 Rates per 100,000 population for total on blindness register[a] (reported prevalence) by color, sex and age as of end of year: MRA[b] total, 1966

Age	Total			White			Nonwhite		
	Total	Male	Female	Total	Male	Female	Total	Male	Female
All ages	146.7	147.5	146.0	125.8	125.5	126.1	241.0	250.8	231.7
Under 5	8.2	8.4	8.0	c	c	c	c	c	c
5-19	52.6	58.4	46.6	47.9	52.7	43.0	55.0	63.0	46.9
20-44	73.9	88.2	60.1	63.5	76.9	50.3	137.5	160.2	117.5
45-64	204.9	230.8	180.5	156.0	179.0	134.2	567.7	621.9	518.4
65-74	418.2	437.6	402.3	330.7	343.9	319.5	1,110.1	1,152.6	1,073.7
75-84	955.6	901.6	995.2	857.7	808.0	893.7	1,723.9	1,576.2	1,848.0
85 & over	2,935.4	2,581.0	3,126.7	2,803.2	2,418.6	3,005.9	c	c	c

[a] See Table 12.8 for total number on register by color and Table A.12.7 for total number by age.

[b] Model Reporting Area for Blindness Statistics, United States. Includes data on persons on register for 15 states in 1966. (See Table 12.2)

[c] Rate not computed when estimated population was less than 25,000 or where percentage with unknown information, such as color, was 10 percent or more.

Table 12.8 Percentage distribution of total on blindness register as of end of year by degree of vision in better eye by color: MRA[a] total, 1966

Degree of vision	Total	White	Nonwhite
Total	100.0	100.0	100.0
Absolute blindness	11.7	10.6	16.1
Light perception	11.9	11.1	15.1
Light projection	1.1	1.0	1.3
Less than 5/200	15.7	15.1	18.7
5/200 to less than 10/200	9.5	9.9	8.3
10/200 to less than 20/200	14.5	15.5	10.9
20/200	20.8	22.1	16.5
Restricted field	5.5	5.2	6.8
Unknown	9.3	9.5	6.3
(Number on register)	(61,037[b])	(45,135)	(13,786)

[a] Model Reporting Area for Blindness Statistics, United States. Includes data on persons on register for 15 states in 1966. (See Table 12.2)

[b] Includes 2,116 persons of unknown color.

Value and Limitations of MRA Register Statistics

The production of blindness statistics by a reporting system, unlike that of a survey, results in continuing periodic reports. Data on trends by age, sex, race, ethnic group, and cause of blindness could help in defining the need and location of specific facilities and personnel for the care and training of blind children and adults. Uniform statistics on the number, distribution, and characteristics of the total number of blind persons are of utmost importance in evaluating the adequacy of community resources to meet this problem.

The value of register data is limited by (*a*) the degree to which all the blind are diagnosed and reported to the register, (*b*) the completeness and accuracy of the data reported for each registrant, and (*c*) the degree of completeness of periodic clearance from the registers (updating) of all who are not blind, not alive, or not residents of the state. The value of register data nationally is further limited by the number, location, and population composition of states that can furnish these statistics. Even though the total MRA population distributions by age, sex, and color (white and nonwhite) are close at present to those of the United States as a whole, the MRA is not geographically representative of the total United States. There is a disproportionately heavy concentration of MRA states on the East Coast. In two of the nine geographic census regions, there were no MRA states in 1966, and in several other geographic divisions MRA was meagerly represented.

Although the MRA cause data have limitations, they are based on a common definition of blindness and on the use of a standard classification of causes of blindness on a large segment of the United States population (19 percent of the total). The data are considered sufficiently reliable to provide meaningful insight into the causes of blindness.

Blindness Statistics in Other Countries

Incidence

We have used the "first additions" in the MRA data to define incidence rates for blindness as of date of addition to register, which is closer to date of diagnosis than to date of onset. Similar data are available for England and Wales, where the official definition of blindness is an acuity of 3/60 (10/200) or less, or 6/60 or less with markedly reduced fields.

Sorsby (1966) presented a comprehensive study of the incidence and causes of blindness in England and Wales from 1948 to 1962. For these years the rate of newly registered blind females for all ages combined was about 30 per 100,000, with little variation over the fifteen years. The rates for males were somewhat more variable during this period and averaged about 20 per 100,000. Both rates were notably higher than those seen in the 1966 MRA data in the United States. The rates for newly registered females up to age 50 appeared to be generally lower than those for males. However, after that age the rates for females were almost always higher than those for males. This is similar to the sex differentiation noted in the 1966 MRA data previously discussed.

During the fifteen years rates for both males and females decreased in most age groups. In children under 5, increases in particular years were caused by an increase in patients with retrolental fibroplasia. For persons 70 or older, the rate was essentially stationary, with some minor fluctuations. Sorsby (1966) pointed out that during the fifteen-year period the proportion of the newly registered having severe degrees of blindness has declined steadily. He attributes this to the increasing proportion of the elderly among the newly registered.

During 1948-62 the major changes according to Sorsby were as follows: (*a*) rates for cataract decreased markedly for those over age 60, compatible with more frequent surgery; (*b*) rates for senile macular degeneration increased greatly in these same age groups, reflecting largely the increasing proportion of the most elderly in the general population; (*c*) rates for glaucoma decreased moderately in the group 60-69 years old (perhaps related to treatment), but no clear pattern emerged for those 70 or older; (*d*) rates for myopic chorioretinal atrophy showed substantial decreases in the age group 30-59 years up to 1954, but since 1955 there has been little change; (*e*) rates for diabetic retinopathy increased sharply for all persons 50 or older to 1954, but since 1955 the rates have been reasonably steady. One might wonder about the reciprocal changes reported for the last two categories between 1948 and 1954. In general, the rates for glaucoma, optic atrophy, and congenital defect in males were consistently higher than those in females, while the reverse was true for cataract, myopic chorioretinal atrophy, and diabetic retinopathy.

Prevalence

According to a recent World Health Organization report (1966), there were about 7,700,000 blind persons known in various countries. Asia accounted for about 72 percent and Africa for about 15 percent of all the blind persons reported in this publication. Presented in Table A.12.8 is a summary of estimates of the prevalence of blindness available from countries throughout the world.

To facilitate comparison, we have grouped the studies according to the definition of blindness used. Thus all definitions indicating that the central visual acuity or visual acuity was 20/200 (6/60, 1/10, 0.1) or less, or less than 20/200, were combined (whether or not this acuity was for the better eye, either eye, or both eyes; with or without best correction; and whether or not there was a reduction of field of vision, and regardless of the amount of such reduction). Similarly, studies were grouped when the definitions referred to a visual acuity of (*a*) 10/200 (3/60, 1/20, 0.05) or less, or less than 10/200; (*b*) 3/200 (1/60 or equivalent) or less, or less than 3/200; and (*c*) total blindness (Table A.12.8). Many studies that were reviewed did not use definitions of blindness in terms of ophthalmic measurements. Some lacked any definition. Although the value of the latter studies is limited, they have been included.

Since there were several comprehensive reviews of the worldwide literature in the early 1950s (Sorsby 1950; World Health Organization 1953), it was decided to cover here only the latest data available. Accordingly, only studies published since 1940 have been reviewed. Table A.12.8 shows the latest blindness prevalence rates per 100,000 population derived either by census (C), estimate (E), registration (R), or survey (S), grouped by previous definition and by continent. It is obvious that, even with an attempt to standardize by definition, great variation in prevalence rates still exists among the various countries listed. Obviously, the method of securing information on prevalence must be a factor in determining to some degree the validity and completeness of the data and hence in contributing to the observed variation. Furthermore, the rates shown are crude and would require age-sex-race standardization to be more meaningful. Table A.12.8 reveals that, where definitions equivalent to 20/200 were used, the prevalence rates per 100,000 population varied from 57 in Bulgaria (based on census) to 214 in the United States (based on estimate).

MacDonald (1965) indicated that his survey of the register of the Canadian National Institute for the Blind is not a national survey of all blind persons in Canada, and that registration of blindness is not mandatory in Canada. Despite these limitations, the register is the most comprehensive of its kind in Canada.

No countries in Africa or Asia used so liberal a definition for blindness as 20/200. It would seem that where blindness is highly prevalent, particularly in such developing countries as Egypt or India, the definition is likely to be more restricted—that is, only those persons with very severe vision impairment are considered blind. It may be that, because of the great number of persons in these countries with visual disorders, restriction is related to the need to keep services or financial aid within the bounds of economic reality.

Countries using a 10/200 definition of blindness had rates that varied from 50-60 per 100,000 in the Netherlands to 1,050-1,150 in Kenya (both based on estimate). In general, the rates in African countries were highest, followed by those in Asian and then European countries. The low prevalence rate of blindness in Russia is attributed to the "rise in the material welfare of the people; the improvement of the sanitary and hygienic conditions of life" (Tatimov 1966).

With the more restrictive definition for blindness of 3/200, the rates per 100,000 varied from 56 in Spain (based on estimate) to 3,000 in northern Ghana (based on survey). No countries on the American continents were known to use so limited a definition. Rodger (1958) commented that the prevalence rate in Ghana is one of the highest in the world, and is largely a result of the ravages of onchocerciasis. As a result of his surveys of Africa, a general picture of blindness has emerged that is supported by figures from other parts of the world. He estimated that the prevalence rate per 100,000 in Europe is about 200. Where trachoma exists, as in some of the Middle East countries, the rate increases to about 500 or even higher. In heavily endemic onchocerciasis areas, the rate increases to more than 1,500. About 80 percent of the world's blind are found where trachoma, smallpox, leprosy, and onchocerciasis are found. He pointed out that in the four West African territories of Nigeria, Ghana, the Cameroons, and Gambia, the rate is approximately 1,000. All of these figures are based on a definition for blindness of 3/200.

A number of countries defined the blind as only those who suffer from absolute or total blindness. In these countries the rates per 100,000 varied from 91 in Syria (based on survey) to 4,000 in Yemen (based on estimate). The highest rates appeared to be in Asian countries. The rates in European countries were, in general, the lowest.

Some countries define blindness in nonophthalmic terms, such as the inability to move about in unfamiliar surroundings unaided (including use of the blind man's stick) or the inability to do any kind of work for which eyesight is essential. It would appear that these definitions lie somewhere between the 3/200 and the total blindness definitions. Kuwait and Zambia were the only countries using such definitions for which fairly recent data were available. The rate in Zambia (based on estimate) was 500 to 750 per 100,000 and varied markedly in different parts of the country. In Kuwait, the rate (based on census) was 230 per 100,000.

In the absence of a definition of blindness, it is difficult to interpret differences in rates. No doubt many countries in the group that failed to mention a definition in their published studies had used some definition.

In general, countries in Africa and Asia have the highest rates. To what extent these rates result from practically nonexistent medical care is difficult to determine. In Tanganyika, which is typical of a number of African countries, there is no eye clinic to serve the population of 9,500,000. Five hundred of every 100,000 persons were blind, and the figure increased to 1,000 or even 2,000 in some areas (Around the World 1963).

Age and Sex

The WHO publication for 1966 lists the number of blind and the rate per 100,000 population in fifty-six countries by age and sex, as determined by censuses, estimates, surveys, or registers. In addition to the sixty-five definitions used, there were no less than thirty-eight different types of age groupings employed.

In Table A.12.9, age-sex blindness prevalence rates are shown grouped by definition and continent. Controlling by type of definition, however, did not solve the problems of noncomparability introduced by the great variety of age groupings used by different countries. Because of this variation, it rarely was possible to make age-specific rate comparisons. It is unfortunate that data available in sufficient detail through census, register, or survey and secured at considerable cost, effort, and time are not published with groupings adequate for international comparisons. As seen in Table A.12.9, there was no appreciable difference between the overall rates for males and females, nor in general between the age-specific rates for the two sexes. Overall comparisons of the rates of the sexes should be made on an age-standardized basis, however, to rule out the effect of possible differences in age distributions of the sexes. As expected, the rates increased with age, and in most countries markedly so, starting at about age 40.

Surveys in Africa indicate that the proportion of younger blind people was much higher than that found in Europe or America; in a two-year survey in Kenya, about 12 percent of the blind were less than 15 years of age and 27 percent were in the age group 15-45 years (Greenslade 1956). This may be because of the high proportion of younger people in Africa and because trachoma has its highest incidence in the younger group. In Northern Rhodesia, where the average length of life is relatively short, only 12 percent of the blind were more than 60 years old. This situation is certain to change in both Asia and Africa as life expectancy increases (Wilson 1965).

In Iceland, for persons up to 60 years old, the rate of increase with age on the whole was similar to that observed in other countries but, for persons older than this, an extraordinarily rapid increase took place (Björnsson 1955). Thus, of the total number of blind, no less than 89 percent were 60 or older, a much higher percentage than that found elsewhere. There was also a considerable difference between the frequency of blindness in towns in contrast to rural districts, with a rate of 2.2 per 1,000 in towns and 4.3 in the rural districts. Reasons for this may be that it is more difficult for old people in the rural districts to get adequate treatment, and that the aged are more numerous in the rural districts.

Causes of Blindness

Comparisons by country of affection and cause responsible for blindness are likely to be misleading. In only one or two countries is it possible to state that most of the reported blind have been examined ophthalmologically, adequate diagnoses made, and reports sent to a centralized point for review, tabulation, and analysis.

The data on causes of blindness are most adequate for the British Isles (Sorsby 1950). Ophthalmologic reports on blind persons in England and Wales have been reviewed, classified, and coded by the ophthalmologic consultant to the British Ministry of Health. Detailed analyses of causes have been published by the Ministry since 1945. In Canada codification for topography (site and type of lesion causing blindness) and cause has been the responsibility of the consultant ophthalmologist to the Canadian National Institute for the Blind, who reviews each individual's record—a record that often includes reports of many medical examinations (MacDonald 1965).

In most countries the only diagnostic data available come from a few clinics, hospitals, institutions for the blind, or private physicians. The shortage of ophthalmologists in many countries often means that whatever cause data are gathered leave much to be desired. To show how acute these shortages have been, one report pointed out that in Ethiopia in 1957, where there were 15,000,000 inhabitants, there were three ophthalmologists, all located in the capital of Addis Ababa (Torgersruud 1957). In 1958, with a population of approximately 380,000,000 people, India had fewer than 500 members in the All-India Ophthalmological Society (Holmes 1958b). Without indication of the definition used, it has been estimated that India at that time had a blind population of about 2,000,000 (World Health Organization, Regional Office for South-East Asia 1962). In 1962, the estimate was 4,390,000 blind (Venkataswamy 1966). South Korea in 1958, with a population of approximately 23,000,000 people, had about 100 trained ophthalmologists. Half of these served in the Armed Forces, leaving 50 (mostly in urban areas) to treat the civilian population—a ratio of one ophthalmologist to 500,000 people (Holmes 1958a).

In Iceland in 1961 there were 22,507 inhabitants to each ophthalmologist (Björnsson 1967). With one exception, all the ophthalmologists resided in Reykjavik. There was no ophthalmic hospital in the country nor any special eye departments in the hospitals, which meant that ophthalmic patients were directed to the general hospitals. Finally, hospital outpatient eye clinics were nonexistent. In Iceland glaucoma causes 60 to 70 percent of blindness—blindness that is largely preventable. Björnsson (1955) has shown clearly that the districts where there was greatest difficulty of access to an ophthalmologist and where communications were poorer had the highest rate of blindness from glaucoma.

There were fewer than 50 practicing ophthalmologists and ophthalmologists-in-training in Indonesia among a population of 96,000,000 persons in 1963 (Oey-Khoenlian 1963). In the same year, all the ophthalmic surgeons in Western Australia, an area nearly half the size of Europe, were concentrated in the city of Perth (Mann 1963).

In some countries in which a register of the blind is kept, registration may be entirely voluntary, or may be voluntary for adults but compulsory for younger persons. For instance, in Denmark, blind persons under 30 must be reported by a practitioner in order for them to secure training and rehabilitation. This explains why the causes of blindness on the Danish register are dominated by congenital and hereditary conditions and diseases of the eye that develop early in life, whereas the causes of blindness in old age are not adequately represented (Vedel-Jensen 1962).

Generally, in studies made at clinics, hospitals, or institutions for the blind, no information is given as to the size and nature of the population from which the blind were drawn. There is therefore no assurance that the cases of blindness coming to the attention of these agencies are representative of the blind in their own communities, much less of the blind throughout the country.

Although comparison of rates by affection and cause among countries would be helpful, these comparisons require the availability of general population data by age, sex, and race for a specified time period and for specific countries. Frequently, such census data are not available. Finally, if the classifications by affection and cause, as well as the definitions of blindness, are not similar, then comparisons of rates or percentage distributions by affection and cause have little meaning.

The data presented in Table A.12.10 on percentage distribution of the site and type of affection in various countries should be used with caution, because they have many of the limitations previously mentioned. Some data are based on surveys of specific regions or towns, whereas other data are based on examinations of persons seen at certain institutions for the blind or registered as blind to secure benefits or services. No data before 1940 or based on fewer than 50 blind persons are included in this table. Also excluded are data presented for blind eyes only and not for blind persons, and data secured from institutions for blind students (because of the age limitation).

Considerable variation in percentage distribution of certain affections like glaucoma is shown even among countries on the same continent that use the same or similar definitions (Table A.12.10). Iceland, for instance, has one of the highest prevalence rates for glaucoma in the world. The Icelander Sveinsson (1959) asks,

What is the reason that blindness is so common in a country that does not have Trachoma, where Xerophthalmia is unknown, Venereal Disease is rare, and where there is little industry that would cause eye-injury? The main reason for this is the slowly progressing, painless, non-inflammatory glaucoma simplex which is very common in this country.

He further states:

Glaucoma has been studied extensively with reference to systemic diseases, refraction, hypertension, arteriosclerosis, endocrine disturbances, neurogenic and psychological factors, heredity, etc., but in spite of improved means for study such as gonioscopy and tonography, the cause of this disease is not fully known.

While an epidemiologic inquiry on glaucoma then is most desirable, it is unfortunate that lack of uniform diagnostic criteria, lack of distinction between narrow-angle and wide-angle glaucoma, incomplete information on the age distribution of persons examined, variations in the methods of examination, differences in collecting and recording statistics, and the influence of observer error all serve to prevent accurate comparisons (Holmes 1958*b*).

In general, the percentage of blindness resulting from cataract in African countries was as high as, or higher than, that in American, European, or Oceanic countries. This is somewhat difficult to interpret, since the most common cause of cataract in our western cultures is considered to be an ocular disorder closely associated with aging. In most, if not all, of the African countries, the life expectancy at birth and the proportion of aged in the population are lower than in countries on the American, European, and Oceanic continents. As expected, though, the percentage of cases involving the cornea (mostly as a result of trachoma) was considerably higher in African and Asiatic countries than in others.

The major purpose of Table A.12.10 is to show the dilemma in which the serious student of blindness finds himself, trying to interpret the data of the many studies that now find their way into the literature. There is urgent need for agreement on definition, standards of procedure, and so forth, so that it may be possible for uniformly collected statistics to serve preventive and control functions internationally.

The limitations on international comparisons of site and type of affection data mentioned for Table A.12.10, and the cautions to be observed in their interpretation, are equally valid for similar comparisons of data dealing with cause, as shown in Table A.12.11. This table is composed of the same sources listed in Table A.12.10. Despite the considerable variation, it appears that on the whole the African and Asian countries had the highest percentages of cases arising from infectious diseases, usually a combination of acute seasonal conjunctivitis and trachoma. These were followed by the Latin American, European, and Oceanic countries.

A report from a WHO European Conference on Trachoma stated:

In countries where virtually whole populations are affected with trachoma and seasonal conjunctivitis, it is not uncommon to find that more than one percent of adults are totally blind, and more than four percent are economically blind (i.e., unable to perform any useful work for which sight is essential). More than ten percent have serious impairment of vision and a much higher percentage have serious visual defects. With each successive age group, incidence of visual loss increases (World Health Organization, Regional Office for South-East Asia 1962).

In Morocco, Tunisia, and Egypt, as in all the countries of the North African coast and many parts of the Middle East, the combination of low socioeconomic status, overcrowding, poor sanitation, and a subtropical climate form an environment in which acute seasonal conjunctivitis and trachoma have become pandemic. A high proportion of all total blindness in these regions results from sequelae of corneal complications of seasonal conjunctivitis, while trachoma still remains the greatest single cause of serious reduction in vision short of blindness. There is a close epidemiologic connection between these two diseases. The evidence suggests that in most cases trachoma and acute conjunctivitis are transmitted together, and that the common fly is an important agent in spreading the infection from eye to eye. In these regions, the control of trachoma depends fundamentally on the control of seasonal conjunctivitis (Giaquinto and Lyons 1955). The statistics relating to these causes, however, are somewhat confusing in that, in apparently identical situations, some studies attribute the blindness to trachoma and others to keratoconjunctivitis.

There is considerable variation in percentage of blindness caused by accidents and poisonings, apparently independent of definition or continent. The same is true, more or less, concerning cause resulting from general diseases not elsewhere classified (such as diabetes), senile degeneration, and prenatal influence. Of great concern is the very sizable percentage in almost all countries of blindness from undetermined or unspecified cause.

It is difficult to determine whether the variation from study to study is a result of real differences among the populations in these studies, variations in environmental factors, variations in the collection of the data, definition used, sampling methods, classification employed, or a combination of all of these. One adherent to strict environmentalist philosophy states:

It is clear that since the statistics are influenced by numerous factors that vary from one country to another, there will also be substantial differences from one country to another. Furthermore, there may be very considerable differences not only among the various countries, but also even among the various cities of a given country, either as a result of the predominance of certain industries (mechanical or agricultural), or the presence of epidemic or endemic diseases, as in the characteristic case of trachoma, or differences in climate, or economic differences in the standard of living and variations in customs and usages characteristic of each locality, or (finally) as a consequence of wars (Maggiore 1951).

Summary and Conclusions

The United States, which in 1830 was the first nation to use the population census in an attempt to collect national statistics on blindness prevalence, is still without reliable national data. Although estimates are available, the errors of such estimates are unknown because of the limited base for projection and because of the lack of assurance of the representativeness of such base.

The Model Reporting Area (MRA) annual blindness prevalence rate for 1966 of about 150 per 100,000, while admittedly understated, is based on the most reliable data available to date on about one-fifth of the United States population. This rate is about ten times the annual incidence rate and would indicate that, on the average, a blind person remains on the register about ten years. The age-specific prevalence rates increased with age, rose sharply after age 45 until, in the age group 85 or older, 3 percent of that age group was registered as blind. Such increased rates in the aged reflect mainly the higher incidence of cataract, glaucoma, and retinal degeneration.

An explanation of why age-specific prevalence rates for males exceed rates for females until about age 75 may lie in the higher male rates (*a*) in infancy and childhood resulting from prenatal influence, (*b*) in childhood and youth resulting from injuries, presumably incurred in recreational pursuits, and (*c*) in adulthood resulting from greater exposure to toxins and occupational hazards. The reversal in rates after age 75 may be explained by (*a*) the greater female risk of having diabetes, and (*b*) the likelihood that females, as a result of their greater life expectancy, have a larger proportion of their members in higher ages in the open-end category, 85 years old or older. Age-specific incidence rates also rose with age, increasing sharply from age 45. Rates for males exceeded those for females up to age 65, when a reversal occurred.

Age-specific incidence and prevalence rates for nonwhites were always greater than for whites, sometimes by a wide margin. It is not known to what degree such differences result from racial susceptibility to specific blinding disorders or whether such differences derive mainly from environmental factors related to socioeconomic status, such as nutrition and availability of adequate medical care.

Blindness per se is not a disease but an impairment that may result from any of a number of diseases, injuries, or poisonings. In approximately 15 percent of all newly reported blindness the cause was not determined or reported by the ophthalmologist, and in another 10 percent (glaucoma, essentially) the cause has not been discovered to date. Conversely, in about 75 percent of newly reported blindness the cause is known.

Reliable statistics on eye diseases, as well as adequate care, depend on the availability of eye examiners. In the United States, there is one eye specialist for every 30,000 people; in northern Nigeria, there are four specialists for 30,000,000 people. Ironically, those countries that have the highest prevalence of blindness have the fewest resources in terms of ophthalmologic specialists.

Throughout the world, because of improved sanitation and living conditions and breakthroughs in medicine, an increasing proportion of the population is experiencing a lengthened life-span and reaching ages in which blindness has its highest incidence and prevalence. Thus there is a growing population at risk. Even if age-specific incidence rates do not increase, and even if trachoma is conquered, this portends, in the developing countries, an increasing number of blind individuals, most of whom will be older persons.

13 / HEARING DISORDERS
Jerome D. Schein

Deafness is a chronic reduction of sensitivity to sounds that may be accompanied by an impairment of the ability to correctly interpret meaningful sounds. The loss or impairment of hearing may be the result of illness, accident, or a genetic fault. Deafness, then, is the common expression of diverse causes. As such, it is not surprising to find a lack of agreement on terminology related to hearing impairment (Davis and Silverman 1970; Gregory 1964; Schein 1964).

The present chapter will be concerned primarily with hearing impairments in the frequencies from approximately 500 to 2,000 cycles per second—the "speech frequencies." These are the frequencies of importance in the comprehension of speech (Davis and Silverman 1970), although there is some disagreement about the precise limits for the range involved (Kryter et al. 1962). This focus on the speech range emphasizes the conception of hearing impairment as essentially a disorder affecting communication. Diseases in which the hearing impairment has a minor, usually nonhandicapping, role, such as Ménière's or Alport's syndrome (Cassady et al. 1965), are not considered.

In order to indicate the degree of impairment, three terms will be used: deafness, hard of hearing, and hearing impairment. *Deafness* will refer to losses of sensitivity to sound that range from severe to total. In general, a deaf person is considered to be one whose hearing level for speech is 70 dB or more beyond normal thresholds. However, such a level should be considered as a general reference point only. Persons with milder degrees of hearing impairment will be referred to as *hard of hearing*, a cumbersome term that has been chosen nonetheless because of its wide use. The term *hearing impairment* will be used to refer to all degrees of hearing loss, including both the hard of hearing and the deaf. In accordance with recommendations of the American Academy of Ophthalmology and Otolaryngology, 15 dB is considered the point above which the hearing is judged to be significantly impaired (Eagles 1964). Because the same difficulties apply to selecting the lower limits for hearing impairment as for deafness, this figure is approximate.

When reference is made in this chapter to hearing levels in decibels, the zero reference point is that established by the American Standards Association in 1951, and not the new sound pressures recommended in 1964 by the International Organization for Standardization. The reader is referred to the article by Davis and Kranz (1964) for a discussion of the standards.

As we shall use the term, hearing impairment refers to permanent bilateral decrease of auditory acuity. Insofar as can be determined, data on persons whose hearing loss is in one ear only will be excluded. Everberg (1960*a* and *b*) has summarized and added to the literature of unilateral loss of hearing. Deafness in one ear with the other normal was found in Danish schoolchildren at a rate of about 1 per 1,000. Rates for less-than-severe losses of hearing in only one ear, naturally, should be much higher, but such losses are also likely to be transient rather than chronic. Despite the substantial prevalence of unilateral losses, they will not be considered because impairment in one ear causes only a modest handicap and frequently is not even recognized.

Most of the studies of hearing impairment have based their estimates of prevalence on self-identification or on the report of a family member, rather than on audiologic assessment or examination by a physician. Comparisons between self-estimates of hearing and audiometric measures showed a high concurrence in the evaluation of the hearing scale used in the 1962-63 National Health Survey's special study of hearing ability (Schein et al. 1965). The scale appeared to be measuring hearing along a single dimension, as evidenced by the pattern of responses; that is, persons responding that they can hear at one level also indicated that they could hear at all levels requiring lesser degrees of hearing acuity. In the samples in which it was calculated, the correlation between scale responses and better-ear averages for pure tones in the speech range was 0.75, uncorrected for attenuation (Schein et al. 1965). Good results were also reported for the questions used in the 1935-36 National Health Survey; although the details of administration and precise wording of items were not reported, the study indicated that audiometric measurements and self-reports were in agreement (Beasley 1940).

Schein and his associates (1970) did additional work on the development of a hearing scale, in cooperation with the United States National Health Survey. Their earlier scale (1965) was effective in identifying severe hearing impairments but did not distinguish between impairments of lesser degree (that is, in the range of loss from 15 to 60 dB). For both clinical and field tests of the new scale, a set of questions could be devised to accomplish the desired objective with sufficient precision to warrant use of the scale in morbidity surveys. Again, the validity of self-reports of hearing status was supported.

But methods of inquiry that were found to be effective with one type of person at a given point in time may be less effective under other circumstances and at other times. De Reynier (1959) argued that deafness may be overestimated in Switzerland, where financial benefits accrue to the family having a deaf member. Others have given reasons for underestimation, such as feelings of shame or guilt on the part of respondents (Gregory 1964). Because both biases may be operating to mask the true prevalence, any rate must be considered in relation to its particular derivation.

Population Estimates

Incidence of Hearing Impairment

There have been only a few sporadic attempts to calculate the incidence of either hearing impairment or deafness. For the United States, Beasley arrived at a crude estimate of hearing impairment for persons 5 years old or older, basing his estimate on differences between successive age groups in the 1935-36 survey (Beasley 1940). It should be noted that incidence rates vary with both cause and type of impairment, but neither of these factors was considered by Beasley.

Trotter (1960) cited a rate for deafness as high as 1.2 to 1.7 per 1,000 births occurring from 1915 to 1922 in Switzerland. By 1925 the rate had decreased to 0.4 per 1,000, a level that Trotter believed was similar to that for other European countries.

Various studies have attempted to establish rates for the incidence of deafness after maternal rubella. Barr and Lundström (1961) estimated from their prospective investigation, begun during the rubella epidemic in Sweden in 1951, that the incidence of severe hearing impairment in the offspring of a mother infected during pregnancy was about 8 percent. They had estimated earlier that, based on a larger series, the incidence of hearing impairment was 4 percent for children whose mothers had rubella in the first four months of pregnancy. In the course of their investigation Barr and Lundström also determined the incidence of severe hearing impairment in the general Swedish population. From their enumeration of children in the schools for the deaf they concluded that the incidence was 70 per 100,000 births. Barton and his colleagues (1962) derived an identical estimate of incidence for Northumberland and Durham, England, for 1945-54.

The British study of maternal rubella also produced two estimates of hearing impairment, one for children whose mothers had been infected and the other for a control group (Annotation 1960 and 1961; Manson et al. 1961). Initially, the rubella group had an incidence rate of deafness of 3 percent, compared with 0.08 percent for the control group. An additional 3.6 percent of the rubella group were suspected of being deaf, while the corresponding figure for the controls was 0.4 percent. Only the rubella group was followed between 36 and 60 months of age. Follow-up revealed that 19 percent of the rubella group had suffered some loss of hearing. Almost without exception, the fetus was unaffected by rubella that occurred after the first trimester of pregnancy.

Lancaster (1951) has used registrations in schools for the deaf to support his hypothesis that epidemics of births of deaf children occurred in parts of Australia, some of which were associated with suspected epidemics of rubella. He did not calculate the incidence rates, however. From an extensive survey of the literature, Cockburn (1969) concluded that neither geographic nor temporal factors were associated with risk from maternal rubella. A similar conclusion was reached by White and his co-workers (1969). Thus estimates of the probable consequences of a rubella epidemic in one area can be inferred from the earlier experiences in other countries—a valuable fact with which to facilitate planning.

Recent studies aimed at developing new techniques for auditory screening of neonates give promise of producing more accurate determinations of the incidence of severe hearing impairments. The increased emphasis on early treatment for severe hearing losses in order to minimize their handicapping effect has prompted widespread efforts in the development of infant auditory screening. Because substantial numbers must be tested before one infant with hearing impairment is found, the suggestion has been made that such efforts be focused on infants who have a higher probability of deafness, that is, children whose mothers have suffered rubella or whose parents have impaired hearing. Davis (1965) noted, "The percentage of children who fail to pass the screening test in the three most extensive studies ranges from 0.1% to 2.0%. Careful consideration must be given to the value and economy of a screening program whose yield is so low." However, Campanelli and Schein (1969) believe that auditory screening of neonates can be so economically administered that it ought to be "as routinely administered as silver nitrate is put into the eyes of the neonate."

The finding of a failure on the screening tests, of course, is not the same as diagnosing a hearing loss. For diagnosis of a hearing loss, additional expense must be incurred in diagnostic examinations. The neonatal auditory screening program has not been conducted long enough to have produced adequate follow-up studies from which to calculate false-positive rates. It can be anticipated, however, that as such studies are published, improved information about the incidence of hearing impairment will become available.

Another approach to improvement of information about hearing impairment is the establishment of registers. Renwick (1967), in his discussion of the British Columbia Crippled Children's Registry, illustrated the difficulties of maintaining a voluntary system. He suggested that all rates derived from such registry data be accompanied by the qualifying term "minimum" to stress the likelihood of underestimation.

Under the auspices of the United States Office of Education, the Annual Survey of Hearing Impaired Children and Youth was inaugurated in May 1968 (Gentile and DiFrancesca 1969). It is a permanent center for statistical research on hearing impairment, having as its principal objectives the collection, processing, and dissemination of information on various characteristics of the entire population of hearing-impaired schoolchildren. The survey already has information on 22,000 students, representing 80 percent of known deaf schoolchildren. Reports emanating from this project will greatly enhance knowledge of deafness in the United States.

Prevalence of Prelingual Deafness

Census. To increase the degree of comparability, we have shown only data concerning those persons who suffered deafness in early childhood in Table 13.1. This syndrome provides more etiologic homogeneity, it being expected that a high proportion of cases are hereditary. Fraser (1964) has referred to this condition as "profound childhood deafness"; Brown (1967) prefers simply "childhood deafness." Both avoid "deaf-mute"—a term used in the United States until recently and still used in the European literature *(taubstummen, sourd-muet)*—because lack of speech is not a necessary consequence

Table 13.1 Prevalence rates per 100,000 population for prelingual deafness (deaf mutism) by sex: censuses of various countries, 1930-56

Country	Year	Total	Male	Female
Peru	1940	300.0	306.4	294.1
Honduras	1935	137.9	170.7	105.3
Finland	1950	130.7	---	---
Japan	1947	118.0[a]	129.6	106.9
Switzerland	1953	93.7	97.6	89.8
Sweden	1930	86.9	95.0	79.0
Iceland	1948	75.8	---	---
India	1931	66	76	55
Canada	1941	62.6	64.0	61.2
Egypt	1937	60	74	44
Belgium	1950	59.5	67.9	51.4
Norway	1930	53.0	60.9	45.5
Union of South Africa	1936	49.4[b]	55.1	43.5
France	1946	47	54	41
United States	1930	46.5	47.1	45.9
Northern Ireland	1956	45.0	48.1	41.6
Denmark	1940	43.4	46.6	40.3
West Germany	1950	43.1	---	---
Mexico	1940	39.1	45.0	33.5
Australia	1933	35.1	37.0	33.0

Source: Dirrecion Nacional de Estadistica 1943 (Peru); Lumio and Paljakka 1964 (Finland); De Reynier 1959 (Switzerland); Lindenov 1945 (Sweden, Norway, Denmark); United States Bureau of the Census 1931 (United States); Stevenson and Cheeseman 1956 (Northern Ireland); Matzker 1960 (West Germany); World Health Organization 1953 (all other countries).

[a] For ages 3-39 years only.
[b] European population only.

of early deafness. The child who is born deaf can be taught, and frequently is taught, by present methods to have some degree of speech. To retain the intent of many studies cited and at the same time not add to the mistaken belief that early deafness and lack of speech are caused by a common lesion, the name "prelingual deafness" has been adopted.

Each of the rates presented in Table 13.1 was obtained as part of a census or special attempt at total ascertainment in the country to which it pertains. In all instances the studies referred to persons considered to be prelingually deaf; that is, those unable to hear and speak. Since both of these abilities exist along a continuum, considerable variation was expected in the decisions of the enumerators as to who was to be so classified.

Prevalence. The highest rate was noted in Peru (Dirrecion Nacional de Estadistica 1943) at 300 per 100,000 population, which is two or three times the rates of the next six countries in order of prevalence. Even more striking is the variation within the Peruvian Republic. The 1940 census of that country showed that the Department of Amazonas had the highest rate, 843 per 100,000, and Callao the lowest, 30 per 100,000. In Peru, as in Argentina (Comision Nacional del Censo, Argentine Republic 1916) and Chile (Greenwald 1957), the rates for prelingual deafness tend to be strikingly lower in the plains than in the mountainous regions. The results of censuses in the latter two countries are not shown in Table 13.1 because they antedated 1930. In Argentina, moving from the eastern plains through the central provinces to those in the west and finally to those in the north, or most mountainous regions, the rates per 100,000 increased dramatically from 64 to 81 to 197 to 373. The earlier Argentina censuses of 1869 and 1895 gave the same geographic trends, though with much higher rates.

Even a relatively small country like Finland, which has the third highest rate, had markedly different rates among districts. Lumio and Paljakka (1964) noted proportionately higher rates for prelingual deafness in small isolated villages, three being on islands in the Gulf of Finland where there was much intermarriage. These two authors also presented evidence that suggests that the 1950 census was particularly complete in its enumeration of the deaf. In a substudy, the results of which may not be representative of the total population, the authors found that about 5 percent of those reported in the census to be "deaf and deaf-mutes" had lost their hearing after they were 5 years old. The over-5 segment of the population is not likely to be mute as well as deaf, since they will have lost their hearing considerably after the normal period for speech development. However, even with a reduction of 5 percent, this rate still was one of the highest.

The rate for Japan was based on a special census in 1947 (World Health Organization 1953). The study was limited to persons 3 to 39 years of age. The high rate obtained may have been caused by the instructions, which said that "deaf-mutes" were to be regarded as "those who cannot hear at all or can hear barely."

The Swiss data come from a special study conducted by De Reynier (1959) under the auspices of the federal government. The study made use of a list taken from the 1950 census of the population and supplemented by reference to registers maintained by agencies, under governmental auspices, providing services to the deaf. Without explanation as to why he chose the particular figures involved, De Reynier qualified his estimate with the following footnote (translated from the French): "If we desire to admit that 1,000 cases escaped our investigation, this number of 93.7 deaf-mutes per 100,000 habitants would be little changed, and then it would result in about 113 deaf-mutes per 100,000 inhabitants." The variation in rates ranged from 37.4 in the Canton of Neuchâtel to 262.9 in the Canton of Appenzell.

The data for India were questioned by the Commissioner of the Census, who thought that the number of female deaf persons was underreported and the number of aged persons excessive (World Health Organization 1953).

The definition used in the Canadian census of prelingual deafness was "any person who has been totally deaf from birth, in general persons who cannot hear or talk" (World Health Organization 1953). To the extent that enumerators took this definition to mean only persons whose hearing had been lost at birth, the rate for Canada can be expected to be a substantial underestimation compared to countries that used a less rigorous definition.

The 1930 census of Norway counted "all deaf persons who are unable to speak normally" (Lindenov 1945). The lack of precision of this instruction may have caused a number of cases of mental deficiency to be included and some cases of prelingual deafness to be excluded.

The data for the Union of South Africa applied only to the "European" (white) population in South Africa (World Health Organization 1953). This restriction of the reference population eliminated any opportunity to get much-needed information on presumed nonwhite-white differences in hearing impairment.

The last year that the United States Bureau of the Census (1931) attempted to enumerate persons with physical impairments in the decennial census was 1930. The bureau did not believe that it could obtain data of sufficient reliability to warrant continued collection in the censuses. Subsequent data on hearing impairment and deafness in the United States have been obtained by sample surveys and attempts at total ascertainment in various parts of the country.

The five countries with the lowest prevalence rates (Table 13.1) do not seem to share many characteristics. In the Northern Ireland study, great care seems to have been taken to eliminate cases in which deafness occurred after speech was acquired (Stevenson and Cheeseman 1956). None of the other censuses, however, appears to have been done more carefully than the others (World Health Organization 1953; Matzker 1960), so the substantial differences found in rates from various countries may reflect correctly a great geographic disparity in the prevalence of prelingual deafness.

The reasons for the differences are also likely to be diverse. Endemic thyroid dysfunction occurred more frequently in iodine-poor areas. However, the mountainous regions of South America, for example, were also generally less well off economically than were the lower regions, had climates more conducive to conditions like otitis media, and had many isolated communities where consanguineous marriages were likely to be more common. No doubt hosts of such factors contribute to the prevalence rates obtained from any given locale.

Special enumerations. Table 13.2 presents rates based on total ascertainments of prelingually deaf persons in metropolitan Washington, D.C. (Schein 1968), New York State (Rainer et al. 1963), and Georgia (*Georgia's Deaf* 1942). The first two studies were done within three years of each other and twenty-two years or more after the Georgia study; yet the prevalence rates established for each area are surprisingly close, ranging from 70.6 to 79.7 per 100,000. The highest estimate, that for New York, was for ages 12 and over. The Georgia rate, next highest, was for all ages. The Washington rate was for ages 18 to 65 years. Among other factors, these differences in age ranges may contribute substantially to the discrepancies in rates.

Table 13.2 Prevalence rates per 100,000 population for prelingual deafness by sex: United States, selected areas, various years, 1940-63

Area and year	Total	Male	Female
SMSA Washington, D.C., 1963[a]	70.6	69.4	71.8
New York State, 1960[b]	79.7	84.4	74.9
State of Georgia, 1940	75.5	77.8	73.3

[a] For ages 18-65 years.
[b] For ages 12 years old and older.

The fact that these three rates were all much greater than the 1930 estimate by the Bureau of the Census emphasizes its statements about underestimation. However, time was also a variable. Depressions, epidemics of infectious disease, and other events contributed to the prevalence rates; thus there is no one explanation for the differences between the 1930 estimate and the estimates for sections of the United States ten and thirty years later.

Because of the importance of recent, accurate demographic data to sound planning for any population, the United States Social and Rehabilitation Service (HEW) has recently awarded a grant to the National Association of the Deaf to conduct a National Census of the Deaf (Schein 1969). The term "census" in the grant award expresses the general nature of the study, but it is technically incorrect. Sample survey techniques were used to obtain the desired information, rather than a door-to-door canvass. The basic strategy to be followed is that used by Schein (1968) in Washington, D.C. An extensive list of names and addresses of deaf persons was gathered. Subsequently, samples were drawn from the list to obtain detailed information on social, educational, medical, and other characteristics of the deaf population (Schein 1971). Results of this four-year study will be available in late 1973 from the Social and Rehabilitation Service.

Prevalence of Hearing Impairment in School-Age Children

School registers. The number of schoolchildren known to be deaf or known to have a hearing impairment can be determined, but finding suitable denominators with which to calculate prevalence rates and interpreting such rates once they have been established present great difficulties. Not all children, and especially not all handicapped children, are enrolled in schools, nor have all handicapped children in school been identified as such. Countries differ widely as to the age ranges for compulsory education—if, in fact, they even have a system of compulsory education. Also, there is bound to be considerable variation in the care with which registers of handicapped children are maintained. Finally and inevitably, the definitions of terms for the classification of hearing-impaired children differ widely (Taylor and Taylor 1960; Ancona and Tomaino 1964; Doctor 1964).

In order to prepare Table 13.3, which shows available prevalence rates for school-age children, a number of estimates and adjustments had to be made. The highest prevalence rate for deafness shown in Table 13.3 was that for the Chicago public schools (Powers 1964). Very likely, hard-of-hearing children were included in the special classes for the deaf, which led to inflation of the rate. In addition, parents who cannot find services for their handicapped children in the area where they are living frequently move to a location where such services are satisfactory, usually into metropolitan areas like Chicago (Chalfant 1965). The much lower figure for the Chicago parochial schools illustrates another problem in using school enrollments to establish general prevalence rates. It is very likely that this estimate, the lowest in the table, is a result of the number of deaf

Table 13.3 Prevalence rates per 100,000 children for deafness based on children enrolled in school and children of school age: various countries, 1957-58

Country	Rate based on –	
	School enrollment[a]	Children of school age[b]
Austria	---	78
Belgium		
Public schools	70	---
Public and parochial	101	---
Denmark	---	91
England and Wales	47	---
France	---	38
Germany	---	52
Ireland	87	78
Luxembourg	55	---
Netherlands	---	67
Poland	93	89
Sweden	111	---
United States	59	---
Chicago Public Schools	144	---
Chicago Parochial Schools	33	---
Illinois, all schools	59	71
SMSA Minneapolis – St. Paul, Minnesota	80[c]	---

Source: Schein and Bushnaq 1962 (United States); Powers 1964 (Chicago); Doctor 1964 (Illinois); Educational Research and Development Council of the Twin Cities Metropolitan Area, Inc. 1964 (Minnesota); Taylor and Taylor 1960 (all other areas).

[a]Basis of calculation is estimated number of children enrolled in school.

[b]Basis of calculation is estimated number of children of compulsory school age.

[c]Rate shown is for 1960-61.

children attending nonparochial schools or not attending schools at all, because of a lack of facilities at the time in the parochial school system. Available staff and space, and not the number of deaf children alone, affected the size of enrollments.

The data for the State of Illinois were based on the information published in the *American Annals of the Deaf* (Doctor 1964), which obtained the information from questionnaires sent to each school and class for the deaf known to its staff. For the same year a survey in which each teacher, principal, and superintendent in turn, was asked to list any handicapped children known to him, regardless of whether or not the child was in school, showed that the prevalence rate for hearing impairment was 4.8 per 1,000 enrollment (Illinois Census of Exceptional Children 1959). Equally interesting, 245 children with hearing impairment were found for whom no special services were being provided. Although this number was small in proportion to the total number of children receiving special services for the hearing impaired, it is no doubt indicative of the probabilities of underestimation that arise when school enrollment figures are used as the bases for calculating prevalence rates. In that regard, the prevalence rate of 59 per 100,000 for the United States (Schein and Bushnaq 1962) must be considered a minimum in view of the known underreporting of deaf children.

As in Table 13.1, an interesting feature in Table 13.3 is the wide range of rates, although the differences between the highest and lowest prevalences are not so great as in Table 13.1. It is difficult to know the extent that these rates reflected educational policy, methodology, or the actual proportion of deaf children. Table 13.3 serves to caution against the interpretation of rates based on school data without first considering the denominator being used.

Audiometric school surveys. Many school systems in this country and abroad regularly administer audiologic tests to schoolchildren, providing what may at first seem to be an ideal source of data on the hearing deficit of children in attendance. There are several difficulties, however. First of all, the quality of the screening examination is frequently very poor (Eagles et al. 1963). Table 13.4 presents data only from studies in which children who failed screening were given a follow-up otologic or audiologic examination. The importance of doing this is attested to by the findings of Guyot (1963), who reported that only about one in six of those who initially failed screening had a chronic bilateral loss. Such high false-positive rates

Table 13.4 Prevalence rates per 100,000 population for hearing impairments among children in schools as determined by audiologic surveys: various areas and years, 1951-63

Survey area	Years	Rate
Baden-Württemberg, Germany	1960	3,120
Ferrarra, Italy	1959-63	1,790
Pittsburgh, Pennsylvania	1958-60	1,700
Canton of Geneva, Switzerland	1956-62	1,100
Jerusalem, Israel	1951-58	1,572
Canberra, Australia	1951-52	830

Source: Brendle et al. 1961 (Germany); Ancona and Tomaino 1964 (Italy); Eagles et al. 1963 (Pennsylvania); Guyot 1963 (Switzerland); Feinmesser et al. 1959 (Israel); Farrant 1958 (Australia).

do not result from poor technique and inadequate apparatus alone, but are usually an intentional feature of the screening programs. The encouragement of such a high rate of false positives is perhaps satisfactory in many cases, but not in those for whom no effort is made beyond informing parents that their child may have a hearing loss. Frequently, no means were provided for determining whether or not the child who failed the screening test received further examination and, when indicated, treatment. Most often, no record was kept of follow-up examinations when they did occur. Thus gross rates, such as the one frequently quoted from the study by Wishik and Kramm (1953), may substantially comprise acute unilateral hearing losses and false positives.

The prevalence rates in all but the German study (Brendle et al. 1961) in Table 13.4 probably underestimate hearing impairment. Deaf children are not usually in the regular school system; the Pittsburgh studies specifically excluded such children (Eagles et al. 1963). Very ill children are the ones most likely to be missing from school on the days when testing is done, and their absences are seldom taken into account. The Baden-Württemberg study (Brendle et al. 1961) apparently included children with severe hearing impairments who might otherwise have been in the school for the deaf. Since the testing was done during the winter months, it is also possible that some of the children may have been suffering acute conditions persisting to the time of the follow-up examination; thus the rate shown may be overestimated.

Prevalence of Hearing Impairment from General Population Surveys in the United States

In 1956 the National Health Survey was established as an ongoing activity of the National Center for Health Statistics, with the responsibility for providing continuing data on the health of the United States population. To save confusion with the ad hoc National Health Survey of 1935-36, and to differentiate between two separate programs within the ongoing National Health Survey, data from each of the divisions will be referred to by the division name alone. The Division of Health Examination Statistics conducts physical examinations of probability samples of the population, including audiometric testing. The Division of Health Interview Statistics conducts interviews with members of probability samples of households in the United States. These two programs provide the most extensive and most recent data on hearing impairments. The two approaches to determining prevalence complement each other.

To date the *Health Examination Survey* (Glorig and Roberts 1965) has reported only on the hearing of persons 18 to 79 years of age: 73 per 1,000 persons in this age group were estimated to have hearing levels for speech at or beyond 16 dB. If deafness is defined as loss of hearing in excess of 65 dB, then 415 per 100,000 would be so considered from the findings of this study (Table 13.5). Such a figure is far above the 71-80 per 100,000 reported for prelingual deafness found in Washington, D.C., New York State, and Georgia (Table 13.2), but the Health Examination estimate is for deafness of onset at any age.

The degree of hearing impairment for subjects of the *Health Interview Survey* (Gentile et al. 1967) was determined by a questionnaire mailed to each person indicated in the household interviews to have an impairment of hearing. The total bilateral impairment rate for all ages was estimated as 2,230 per 100,000. For a number of reasons this rate cannot be directly compared to that found in the Health Examination Survey. Because of the high positive correlation between age and loss of hearing, the two samples must be equated for age. Also, the interview estimate of ability to hear and understand speech must be related to the average hearing level for the speech frequencies. The lower limit of the audiometric level at which frequent difficulty with normal speech would be encountered is approximately 30 dB. If that is accepted as the point at and beyond which a person has hearing impairment—and there is some evidence to support this assumption in the pilot studies done for the Health

Table 13.5 Prevalence rates per 100,000 population for ability to hear at specified levels for speech[a] in the better ear among persons 18 to 79 years of age by age and sex: United States, 1960-62

Sex and age	Better-ear average in decibels						
	16-25	26-35	36-45	46-55	56-65	66-75	76+
Total							
18-79	3,981	1,445	813	426	230	250	165
18-24	276	84	283	-	-	-	129
25-34	830	79	223	-	-	65	88
35-44	1,751	418	266	262	46	89	38
45-54	2,474	885	505	287	131	-	73
55-64	6,389	1,970	1,234	179	115	333	128
65-74	15,210	5,079	2,678	2,562	1,317	600	770
75-79	20,167	15,594	5,294	1,324	1,846	4,319	488
Male							
18-79	3,800	1,500	1,100	600	200	300	100
18-24	400	-	500	-	-	-	300
25-34	800	100	500	-	-	-	-
35-44	2,400	200	300	500	-	200	100
45-54	2,400	700	600	100	300	-	-
55-64	5,600	2,600	1,500	400	200	-	300
65-74	13,800	7,000	4,100	3,300	1,500	400	400
75-79	18,900	11,700	5,900	2,600	900	8,700	-
Female							
18-79	4,200	1,400	600	300	200	200	200
18-24	100	200	100	-	-	-	-
25-34	900	100	-	-	-	100	200
35-44	1,200	600	300	-	100	-	-
45-54	2,600	1,100	400	400	-	-	100
55-64	7,100	1,400	1,000	-	-	600	-
65-74	16,300	3,500	1,500	1,900	1,200	800	1,000
75-79	21,400	17,500	4,700	-	2,800	-	1,000

Source: Glorig and Roberts 1965.

[a] Arithmetic average of thresholds for pure tones at 500, 1,000 and 2,000 cycles per second.

Interview Survey—then the two estimates for the age range 18 to 79 are identical. Both studies estimate that 27 per 1,000 persons in this age range often have trouble understanding what is said in a normal tone of voice. The coincidence of these two rates, obtained under different circumstances with different samples, though at approximately the same time, provides a strong likelihood that the true prevalence rate of hearing impairment of a handicapping degree is not far from a rate of 27 per 1,000 adults in the United States.

Age. As with most chronic impairments, the prevalence of hearing loss increases dramatically with age. In the Health Interview Survey (Table 13.6), the proportion of persons with binaural hearing loss increased from 350 per 100,000 for persons less than 17 years of age to 13,200 per 100,000 for persons 65 or older. The Health Examination Survey found a similar effect at each frequency from 500 to 6,000 cycles per second (cps). It would appear that the higher the auditory tone, the more pronounced is the decrement in average threshold for increasing age. At 500 cps, the median hearing levels were −5 dB for 20-year-olds and 13 dB for 75-year-olds. At 6,000 cps, 20-year-olds have a median threshold of 5 dB, compared to 55 dB for 75-year-olds. These figures are for the better ear of men, but the results for women follow the same trend. The higher the frequency, the more hearing sensitivity tends to decline with age.

Sex. Most studies have reported higher prevalence rates of hearing impairment for males than for females. The significant excess of males who are prelingually deaf has been repeatedly noted. Some of the excess of males appears to be a result of sex-linked recessive deafness, the prevalence rate of which was estimated by Fraser (1964) to be about 3 per 100,000 males. The genetic basis for preponderance of males, then, is small in relation to that from acquired causes. Brown (1967) in his review agreed that even in the hereditary group as a whole, the sex ratio is at most only slightly high. Considering a number of large series from several countries, Fraser (1964) concluded that the ratio of males to females for acquired prelingual deafness may be as high as 1.5 to 1. Whether this results from a less trauma-resistant auditory apparatus in the male or to superior recovery from potentially ototoxic diseases in the female has not been determined. Indeed, the findings may require several explanations. Nonetheless, it is clear that the greater prevalence rate for deafness in males is largely caused by exogenous factors.

Table 13.6 Prevalence rates per 100,000 population for hearing impairment by estimated degree of loss,[a] sex and age: United States, 1962-63

Sex and age	Bilateral and unilateral hearing impairment	Bilateral hearing impairment only			
		Total[b]	Can hear most spoken words	Can hear a few spoken words	Cannot hear spoken words
Total					
All ages	4,370	2,230	1,330	400	470
Under 17	810	350	210	60[c]	80
17-44	2,460	840	500	170	170
45-64	6,460	2,940	1,750	540	610
65 & over	20,780	13,200	7,920	2,310	2,780
Male					
All ages	4,970	2,550	1,630	430	470
Under 17	850	370	220	50[c]	80[c]
17-44	2,980	950	600	180	170
45-64	7,990	3,840	2,450	700	650
65 & over	23,910	15,510	9,970	2,400	2,970
Female					
All ages	3,810	1,930	1,050	380	460
Under 17	780	330	190	60[c]	80[c]
17-44	1,990	750	400	170	170
45-64	5,030	2,100	1,090	390	580
65 & over	18,270	11,340	6,260	2,240	2,630

Source: Gentile et al. 1967.

[a] Without the use of a hearing aid.

[b] Includes persons whose functional degree of impairment was unknown.

[c] Figure does not meet standards of reliability or precision.

When hearing impairment was determined audiometrically, as in the Health Examination Survey, the relation of (partial) hearing loss to sex was less clear than in the case of deafness. The median thresholds for each sex differed very little at 500, 1,000, and 2,000 cps, although women had substantially better hearing. The two sexes did not differ in the proportions having better-ear averages beyond 15 dB. This finding for the adult group, which included some persons likely to have suffered a hearing loss in childhood, was at variance with the results of studies of prelingual deafness.

That the lack of male excess in the Health Examination Survey may be caused by sampling variation appears likely from the findings of the Health Interview Survey, where the sex ratio for hearing impairments was 132 males to 100 females. Surprisingly, the difference was far greater for the milder than for the more severe impairments reported. Males and females almost equally reported an inability to understand even a few words without the use of a hearing aid. For those with hearing impairment who said that they could hear and understand most spoken words without the use of a hearing aid, there were nearly 1.5 times more males than females. Perhaps a greater exposure by males to acoustic trauma explains these results.

A condition that produces hearing loss in later life is otosclerosis. Larsson (1962) noted that females are affected twice as often as males with clinical otosclerosis. In their clinical series, Joseph and Frazer (1964) found nearly half again as many females as males. Larsson argued, however, that a greater proportion of females seek medical advice for otosclerosis, since he has found no significant sex difference among "unselected" cases. Should further research substantiate his contention, then the finding of hearing impairment in more males than females would hold for all but otosclerosis and some rare genetic syndromes.

Color. Higher prevalence rates for hearing impairment were consistently found for white than for nonwhite persons. The Health Interview Survey found nearly 1.5 times more white persons who reported a binaural hearing impairment, the overall rates being 23.3 per 1,000 for whites and 15.1 per 1,000 for nonwhites. Post (1964) reviewed five studies of mild hearing losses in samples of whites contrasted with Negroes. The adult whites appeared to have more hearing loss at the higher frequencies than did the adult Negroes, especially among males. Negroes appeared to have a higher rate of loss than whites in lower frequencies (below 2,000 cps). In the Pittsburgh study of schoolchildren (Eagles et al. 1963), no difference by color was found in the age group 5-14 years.

Tato et al. (1961) compared four Argentine Indian tribes with whites. The Indian tribes had less otosclerosis and appreciably less hearing loss than had been noted in whites. In their series, Joseph and Frazer (1964) found that otosclerosis was 2.1 times more frequent in Caucasian patients than in Japanese patients. Hinchcliffe (1964), however, found that among a representative sample of Jamaican Negro women 65-74 years of age, a higher proportion had hearing impairment than a similar group of Scottish women. The Jamaican male sample showed no significant difference from the Scottish males. This interesting discrepancy from the other studies deserves follow-up with larger samples and careful audiometry.

Among the prelingually deaf, the rates were consistently much higher for white than nonwhite persons. Without exception in the decennials of 1830-1930, the rates for prelingual deafness have been higher for whites than for nonwhites in the United States (United States Bureau of the Census 1931). The most disparate rates were seen in the census of 1920: 42.5 deaf whites per 100,000 compared to 18 per 100,000 nonwhites. In 1930, the rates were closest, being 46.5 per 100,000 for whites and 35.2 per 100,000 for nonwhites. The enumeration of the deaf in Georgia (*Georgia's Deaf* 1942), in 1940, yielded a substantial difference: 83.5 for whites and 60.6 for nonwhites. Similarly, the study of the Washington, D.C. area (Schein 1968) showed a far higher rate for whites, 73.7 per 100,000, than for nonwhites, 33.5 per 100,000, when only those who reported their loss of hearing as occurring before the age of 6 were considered.

The Health Examination Survey (Roberts and Bayliss 1967) found that better-than-normal hearing (defined as thresholds 5 dB or more below audiometric zero) was more prevalent among nonwhite than white adults. Conversely, hearing impairments were more prevalent among the white than the nonwhite samples. Figure 13.1 illustrates

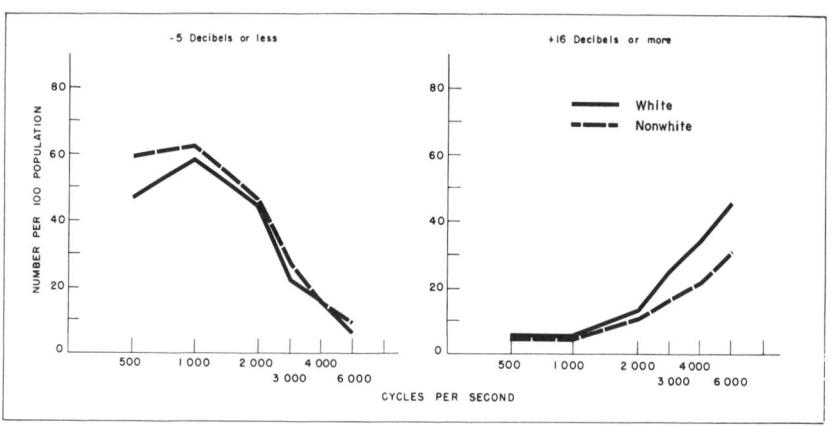

Figure 13.1 Number of persons per 100 adult population having hearing levels (in decibels, reference to audiometric zero) (*a*) better than "normal," and (*b*) with some hearing handicap in the better ear, at specified cycles per second, by color (Source: Roberts and Bayliss 1967.)

the comparison. Except for a reversal at 6,000 cps for those with excellent hearing, the nonwhite sample (predominantly Negro) consistently had greater proportions with superior hearing.

In explaining these observed differences, the tendency has been to avoid genetic arguments in favor of methodologic and economic ones. There is a strong possibility of underestimation of the nonwhite deaf, because they fall into the group most difficult to enumerate, that of low socioeconomic status. Schein (1968) found that nonwhite deaf persons had higher rates of unemployment and much lower average incomes than did white deaf persons, the latter having incomes averaging slightly above the median for all persons. Another reason for the comparatively lower rates is that nonwhites often receive less adequate medical care, so that they succumb to diseases which in whites lead to hearing impairments. Meningitis, particularly, has been suggested in this regard. The physiologic explanation offered by Rosen and his associates (1964) must also be considered, along with Post's differential-selection hypothesis (1964). As with the other observations discussed, the basis for this finding is likely to be complex, representing the resultant of a number of factors.

Geographic distribution. According to the findings of the Health Interview Survey, binaural hearing impairment was more prevalent in rural than in urban areas. This was true for all age groups. Hearing impairment occurred more frequently in rural farm residents, except for persons 65 years old or older. Beyond age 65, the prevalence rate was greatest for rural nonfarm residents.

The rate reported for hearing impairment was lowest in the Northeast section of the United States and highest in the South, with some minor variations by degree of impairment and age. The West had the next highest rate of hearing impairment, followed by the North Central region. Similar results were obtained in the Health Examination Survey (Roberts and Bayliss 1967). In the census of 1930, the North Central had the highest proportion of prelingually deaf persons, followed by the South, the West, and the Northeast, in that order. In view of the high residential mobility of the population, it is difficult to know what these shifts in prevalence may mean in epidemiologic terms.

Economic conditions. As income increases, the prevalence of most chronic impairments tends to decrease, a relationship that holds also for hearing loss. The data from the Health Interview Survey shown in Fig. 13.2 need to be corrected for family size, at least; yet despite the crude form of the information, the figure clearly illustrates the relation between income and hearing loss. With some exceptions probably caused by sampling error, the rates of binaural hearing impairment were higher for those with lower incomes and lower for those with the higher incomes. Except for the group under 45 years of age, the same held true for educational attainment, a factor strongly correlated with income. Compared to the figures for the general population, persons with binaural hearing loss tended to be overrepresented among those with less than nine years of completed schooling and underrepresented among those with thirteen years or more of completed schooling. The results of the Health Examination Survey (Roberts and Cohrssen 1968) agreed with these trends.

Feinmesser and his associates (1959) compared the results of screening audiometry in two groups of schoolchildren, one from a relatively high socioeconomic background and the other from a relatively low one. Of the children from the low group, 3.5 percent failed the screening test versus 2.1 percent from the high group.

As already noted, the pattern of low income-high prevalence does not hold for the whites who are prelingually deaf, although incidence may well maintain the relationship. Lunde and Bigman (1959) gathered income data from 10,000 deaf adults. Their median individual income was $3,465, compared to the general population median for persons 14 or older of $2,818. Similarly, in metropolitan Washington, D.C. (Schein 1968), the white deaf males had a median income of $6,473 compared to $5,514 for males in general; white deaf females averaged $3,542 as against $2,972 for females in general. The figures for the nonwhite deaf reverse this picture in the Washington study. The Lunde-Bigman study unfortunately had too few nonwhites to justify analysis by color; in fact, the authors did not believe that their sample, though large, was representative of deaf persons in the United States. Nonetheless, the data from these various studies do suggest that early deafness need not be economically handicapping.

Etiology of Hearing Impairments

Fraser (1964), after an extensive review of the literature, concluded that the causes of prelingual deafness were genetic (51.5 percent), adventitious (46.0 percent), and congenital malformations

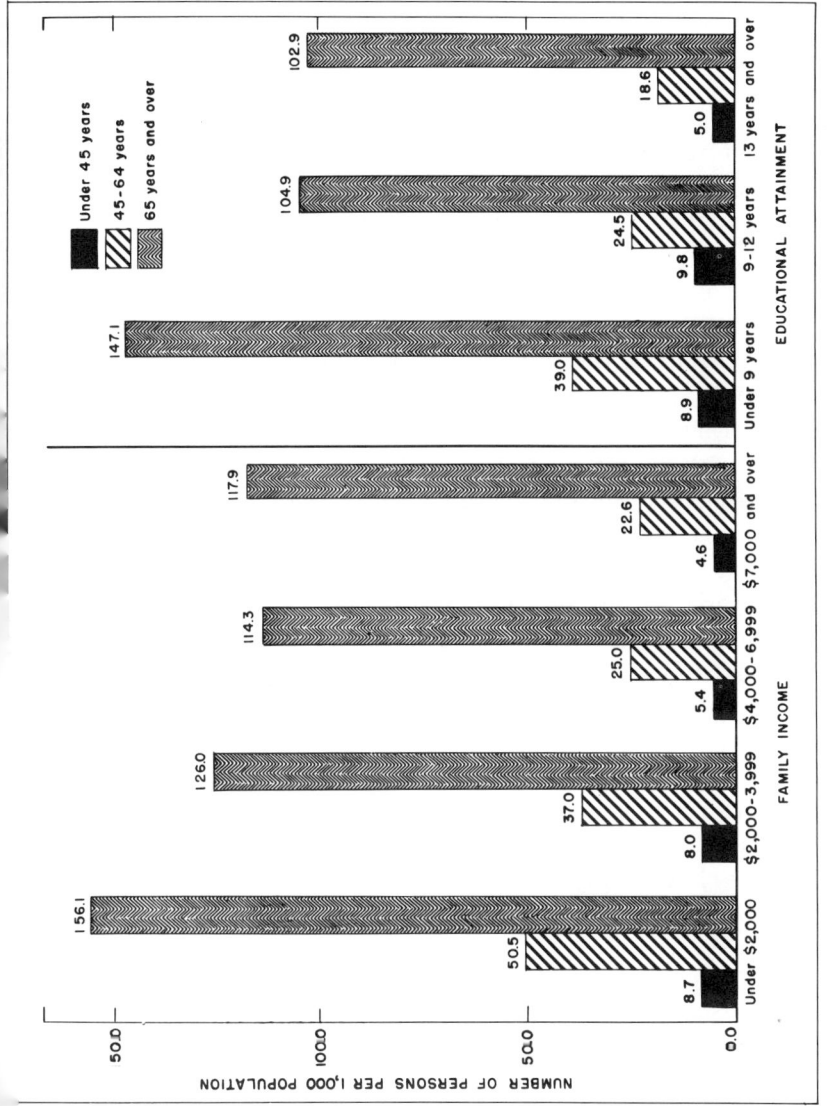

Figure 13.2 Number of persons per 1,000 population with binaural hearing loss by family income, educational attainment of individual, and age (Source: Gentile et al. 1967)

(2.5 percent). Because he accepted an overall prevalence rate of 1.0 per 1,000 births, Fraser points out that these percentages also can be read as numbers per 100,000 births. However, the figures will be markedly altered by local conditions. Brown's analysis (1967) of results from three sizable cohorts of prelingually deaf children confirms in broad terms the previously mentioned attribution of causes.

The Health Interview Survey data on cause must be considered with respect to the source, that of reports by laymen. Nearly 40 percent said they did not know the cause of their hearing loss. This response tendency increased with age at onset, from 19.3 percent of those whose onset was prior to 6 years of age to 54.1 percent of those whose onset was at or after age 65. Those with the severest impairments gave the lowest proportion of "don't know" answers. About 21 percent of the total group gave illness as the cause of loss, 13.5 percent accidents, 4.9 percent presbycusis, and 4 percent congenital or hereditary.

Hearing losses are associated with various chronic conditions. Webb and his colleagues (1966) reviewed studies of hearing losses in mental retardates. A loss of 30 dB at one or more frequencies has been found in from 19 to 42 percent of institutionalized retardates. With such wide variation in rates, the necessity for separate data by age, race, and sex seems apparent (Rigrodsky et al. 1961). Furthermore, follow-up examinations are essential. Pantelakos (1963) found that only 3 percent of his sample had severe impairments when examined thoroughly.

Many children with cerebral palsy also have hearing impairment. Hatchuel (1962) estimated that 5 percent have handicapping losses.

Ear disease, often accompanied by hearing loss, is greater than usual among children with cleft palates (Mesolella and Laurini 1961). Fahey (1965) urged audiologic examinations of all children with this condition.

Allergies frequently cause some disturbance of hearing sensitivity, but not necessarily a chronic or handicapping loss. Szanton and Szanton (1961) reported that 22 percent of their patients who were 9 or older and 56 percent of those under 9 had some audiometrically demonstrable loss of hearing. However, the losses were usually small and transient, though worthy of note.

The number of persons who have lost some or all hearing as a result of antibiotic therapy is difficult to determine. Dihydrostreptomycin was found to be so ototoxic that it was withdrawn from the market. Furthermore, hearing impairment may occur and grow progressively worse weeks after cessation of neomycin therapy (Kelly et al. 1969). Kanamycin and, to a lesser extent, neomycin also have been shown to be severely damaging, specifically to the hair cells on the basal membrane. The possibilities of cochlear damage from other drugs has not been established, although such a possibility has been long suspected—for example, in the cases of quinine and aspirin. It must be pointed out, however, that the size and duration of dosage are important factors in determining hearing loss (Tsuiki 1963).

Freeman and Freeman (1960) contended that the frequency of serous otitis media is increasing. Phillips and Lehman (1961) presented evidence from Alaska that favors this view. Waggoner (1964) noted that 73 of a series of 200 patients with adenoid-tonsillectomy had serous otitis media. Left untreated, this condition leads to a chronic impairment of hearing, characterized by a flat loss of 25 to 40 dB.

Yassin and Taha (1963) pointed to vitamin B deficiency as a cause of hearing impairment in Egypt. They found that 7 of their 25 patients with pellagra had moderate bilateral losses. Nicotinic acid injections produced some improvement. The fact that war prisoners frequently had a similar loss was also discussed in relation to the prevalence of such losses in Egypt.

The relation between goiter and deafness has been noted for a long time (Greenwald 1957). When thyroid dysfunction and deafness are found together, the question arises as to whether they result from common genetic or environmental causes (Gusic 1964; Thould and Scowen 1964). Nilsson and his fellow-workers (1964) estimated that nonendemic goiter and deafness occurred in a minimum of 2 per 100,000 Swedish schoolchildren. Trotter (1960) reviewed the Swiss studies and concluded that about 80 cases of deafness per 100,000 births were a result of iodine deficiency. Fraser (1964) estimated that Pendred's syndrome (sporadic goiter and congenital deafness) probably occurs in 7.5 per 100,000 births in the British Isles. Because Pendred's syndrome is far more difficult to diagnose than cretinism, a trend in the incidence of Pendred's syndrome has not even been guessed at, despite the fact that the condition was described more than seventy years ago (Pendred 1896). The rate for cretinism, however, is declining (Batsakis and Nishiyama 1962).

Probably the commonest accidental cause of hearing loss is prolonged exposure to intensive noise. Although numerous rates have been calculated for specific industrial groups, no overall figure for the general population is available. Rosen and his colleagues (1964) found an African tribe, the Mabaans, whose elderly do not have the characteristic presbycusis found in Western cities. But the Mabaans also have less cardiovascular disease. It may be that the latter condition, rather than the pervading quiet of their environment, spares the Mabaans from presbycusis.

Maternal rubella occurring in the first trimester of pregnancy frequently leads to defects of the ears, eyes and heart. Lundström's prospective study (1962) and analysis of other research led him to estimate the risk of such defects after maternal rubella as between 7.1 and 17.0 percent of live births. Earlier series had suggested rates between 8.9 and 27.3 percent. Monif and his associates (1966) reported on a series they studied after the 1964 rubella epidemic in Baltimore: "When maternal rubella occurred in the first trimester, in excess of 50 percent of the liveborn infants, in a limited series had defects compatible with the rubella syndrome." When hearing loss occurs it is often unilateral, with deafness infrequently occurring (Murray 1949; Jackson 1963). The differences in estimates of the incidence rate for deafness as a result of maternal rubella have been attributed to diagnostic problems—both in the early detection of hearing impairment and the determination of rubella in the mother— and to the severity of the viral infection, among other possible explanations. However, the evidence of the risk of defects which rubella epidemics create has been sufficient to convince public health authorities of the need for preventive measures, especially immunization against the disease to hold down the spread of infection and eventually to lessen the number of cases of deafness arising from this cause.

Otosclerosis is among the most common causes of hearing loss (Altmann 1962). Glorig and Gallo (1962), however, do not believe that it accounts for more than 5 percent of persons with impaired hearing. Larsson (1962) distinguished between clinical and histologic otosclerosis. The latter occurred in about 8 percent of the general population, but in only about 1 percent of nonwhites. Joseph and Frazer (1964) also found a lower prevalence rate for their Oriental patients. Because of the increased effectiveness of surgical treatment, proper diagnosis of otosclerosis has become more important. In turn, the prevalence of this condition may also decrease.

Treatment

Since the stapes mobilization operation was reintroduced with considerable refinement in 1955, many persons with hearing losses caused by otosclerosis and other diseases that affect the middle ear have had their hearing restored. Although the long-term effects of this operation are not known, the number of persons who have received immediate benefit from such surgery is large. The increasing expertise in middle-ear surgery promises to reduce the future prevalence of hearing impairments.

Even when middle-ear surgery is able to bring about some gain in hearing, a hearing aid may still be required to increase sensitivity to a socially acceptable level. The improvements in electronic amplification, like those in middle-ear surgery, are also likely to have their effect on estimates of the prevalence of hearing impairment. Persons who may have once considered themselves "deaf" may be able to hear sufficiently well with a hearing aid to think of themselves as being without handicap. Thus persons who would have reported a severe impairment of hearing without a hearing aid may report no hearing loss once the hearing aid provides them with enough gain in usable hearing (Schein et al. 1965).

Some evidence from a study of Australian schoolchildren (Macrae 1968) warns that use of high-powered hearing aids may cause some deterioration in residual hearing over time. The loss seems to occur regardless of the cause of the original deficit. Interestingly, children with sensorineural losses tend to lose acuity in the unaided ear as well. The possibilities of alternative explantions of these findings (progressive decline in hearing unassociated with hearing aid use and differences in pretesting and posttesting techniques) should prevent unqualified opposition to the hearing aid as a therapeutic device. As with surgery, it is likely, but not damning, that use of a hearing aid entails some risk.

The association of these two treatments with economic status should not be overlooked. Both surgery and hearing aids are expensive. The hearing aid, in addition, involves continuing expenditure for batteries and other maintenance. The benefits that can now be obtained for those who have a hearing impairment are likely to be provided in direct ratio to economic circumstances (Gentile et al. 1967).

Trend of Hearing Impairments

If the hundred years of census data for the United States, are considered as in Table 13.7, the impression emerges that there has been little change in the prevalence rate for prelingual deafness,

Table 13.7 Prevalence rates per 100,000 population for prelingual deafness: United States, 1830-1930

Year	Rate	Year	Rate
1930	46.5	1870	42.0
1920	42.5	1860	40.8
1910	48.6	1850	42.3
1900	32.1	1840	45.0
1890	64.8	1830	47.5
1880	67.5		

Source: United States Bureau of the Census 1931.

except as the estimates of its prevalence fluctuated with obvious methodologic changes. The United States Bureau of the Census itself, however, decided that such an inference would not be warranted (1931). In fact, 1930 was the last year that the bureau included an attempt to ascertain the prevalence of chronic conditions in the general population. Beginning in 1957, the task of gathering such information about the health of the nation belonged to the National Health Survey. Unfortunately, because the size of its sample relative to the frequency of hearing impairment was too small and because the means of gathering and of processing data have changed from time to time, its estimates of hearing impairment and of deafness for successive years cannot be compared without considerable qualification.

Prevalence data from Switzerland, however, appear to have been gathered with sufficient uniformity to make possible some inferences with regard to trends in the prevalence rate for prelingual deafness in that country (De Reynier 1959). Switzerland has maintained registers of deaf persons since 1880; these lists in turn have been updated by total ascertainments in 1930 and 1953. For these three points in time, the rates of prelingual deafness per 100,000 have declined from 254 in 1880 to 179 in 1930, and to 93.7 in 1953. Trotter (1960) has critically examined incidence data calculated from enrollments in Swiss schools for the deaf arranged by year and place of birth. He noted the correlation between iodine prophylaxis and the decline of prelingual deafness in that country. He cautioned, however, that a

Table 13.8 Rate of enrollments in schools and classes for the deaf per 100,000 total school enrollments: United States, 1900-60

Year	Rate	Year	Rate
1960	60.0	1920	60.0
1950	69.0	1910	63.0
1940	69.0	1900	60.0
1930	63.0		

number of other factors may be at work and that some cyclic variations which have been previously noted may have coincided to produce the overall reduction in prevalence.

Schein and Bushnaq (1962) compared enrollments in United States schools for the deaf to figures for all children enrolled in schools (Table 13.8). Although many more factors contribute to enrollments in schools for the deaf than the presence of deaf children, particularly the availability of facilities to accommodate such children, the figures nevertheless indicate relatively minor variation in prevalence rate over sixty years. Such observations must be viewed in light of other factors than hearing loss which influence school enrollments (Doctor 1964); for example, policies on age at admission and dismissal, availability of facilities, variations between schools in hearing levels of children admitted, and other policies of exclusion, such as skin color. In the absence of other evidence, a conclusion that the prevalence rate of deafness in the United States has remained fairly constant over the last six decades appears warranted. Deafness in some other countries, however, definitely appears to be declining. Reductions in Argentina and Switzerland seemed to be related to iodine therapy for the prevention of goiter. The increase of prevalence of deafness in Peru has not been explained but may in part be associated with thyroid dysfunction.

Because the data from earlier years are suspect, the trends with regard to the number of deaf and hard-of-hearing persons cannot be certain. For the United States the evidence suggests that the prevalence rate of deafness has remained fairly stable, while for some countries it has declined. The prevalence rate of hearing impairment, however, will probably increase because of the increase in the aged population. The added tendency of the population to move into urban areas, with the attendant increase in exposure to acoustic trauma, is also likely to result in proportionally more hard-of-hearing persons. Taken together, then, the findings lead to the prediction that in the United States hearing impairment will continue to be a major public health problem.

14 / NEUROEPIDEMIOLOGY A SUMMATION

John F. Kurtzke
Leonard T. Kurland

The analysis of special mortality data of the United States for 1959-61 has provided the basis for our consideration of the population characteristics of many disorders of the nervous system, including the better defined and more common neuromuscular disorders. Cerebrovascular diseases (Moriyama et al. 1971), brain tumors (Lilienfeld et al. 1972), and a majority of the infectious neurologic diseases have not been covered here because they are presented in other volumes of this series. However, in this summation we have provided estimates on the frequency of cerebrovascular diseases and brain tumors based on special sources available to us.

Despite the doubts and pitfalls in the analysis of mortality statistics, they are readily available for large and diverse populations and, if interpreted with care, can be of value in learning about disease. As an example, we cite the experience with multiple sclerosis. The mortality rates for this disorder suggested a north-south variation, which has now been confirmed by intensive morbidity studies. In the course of analysis of new mortality data for this report, we evaluated the residence at birth and at death, and these results, along with morbidity data on migrating populations, have provided evidence of a geographic risk factor that is effective around the adolescent years. Although we may still be far from identifying this etiologic factor, the available information has provided a reasonable basis for further laboratory and epidemiologic studies.

Mortality data also suggest that nonwhites may be more likely to develop myasthenia gravis and less likely to develop parkinsonism, Down's syndrome, and multiple sclerosis than their white compatriots. Here too the need for morbidity comparisons by race is emphasized since the results currently available for these disorders are either inadequate or inconsistent.

Because adequate nationwide statistics on chronic neurologic diseases are presently unavailable, except for death data, the identification of new etiologic clues related to geographic distribution and population selectivity will continue to rest largely on death certification. The validity of mortality statistics is primarily dependent on the practicing physician who provides the information on which these tables and figures depend. If he can be convinced that knowledge of mortality rates, distributions, and survivorship are of value in the decision-making involved in diagnosis and care of his patients, then statistics in which we can have a greater degree of confidence will become available.

Accordingly, then, we think the medical practitioner should be cognizant of the present volume and, indeed, it has been written with him in mind. If he does find it of value in his practice, then we will have achieved one goal at least in this work.

The International Statistical Classification of Diseases was not designed as a Baedecker's guide to the nomenclature of diseases, and this concept is expressed in the introduction to the classification (National Center for Health Statistics 1968a). Each succeeding revision of the classification, however, has tended more toward medical utility. In neurology, many disease entities previously placed together in a single category have been assigned distinct rubrics in the recently adopted Eighth Revision. However, some, such as primary lateral sclerosis, still seem to be misplaced; and others, as in the coding of cerebrovascular diseases in the Eighth Revision, result in categories that are no longer mutually exclusive and can be utilized in their full panoply only when patients have had exhaustive diagnostic evaluations. Despite such problems there is a need to familiarize the physician with the ISC, even though ideally this should have been done as part of his early medical education.

Summary by Chapters

We now present in brief summation the major points covered in the preceding chapters of this monograph.

Chapter 1

This book was designed as one of a series of Vital and Health Statistics monographs based on 1959-61 mortality data in the United States. We have taken advantage of the opportunity to provide a more extensive survey of the epidemiology of selected neurologic and sense organ disorders. As stated, stroke, tumor, and infection were not within our purview.

Epidemiology is concerned with the distribution of human disease over time in terms of geography, race, age, sex, and so forth, and the explanation of the pattern of distribution in terms of causal factors (MacMahon and Pugh 1970). Essential to all epidemiologic inquiry is the diagnosis of the disorder in question, which is ordinarily the function of the physician in contact with his patient. For most neurologic disorders, such diagnoses are principally based on clinical impression and thus subject to appreciable variations in different times and places. Most of our prior information as to the natural history of neurologic disease has arisen from case series of various clinics or hospitals, and as such often reflects the bias of case selection and incomplete ascertainment.

In order to approach comparability among different series, it is important to relate the cases to the population from which they were drawn. The population-based rates in common use are *incidence, prevalence,* and *mortality rates.* The incidence or attack rate is the number of new cases per unit of population over a given time, ordinarily expressed as cases per 100,000 per year. Mortality or death rates in like fashion refer to deaths per 100,000 per year and usually are limited to those coded as the underlying (primary) cause of death. Prevalence rates refer to the number of cases present in the population at a given time, again expressed per unit of population.

Prevalence and incidence rates are usually derived from community surveys of illnesses, and are therefore available for but few diseases and places. Mortality data are provided by death certificates encoded (for the present data) according to the Seventh Revision of the International Statistical Classification of Diseases, Injuries and Causes of Death (ISC). Questions as to diagnostic and coding accuracy for this last need be considered, as well as the case-fatality ratio (the proportion of those affected who die) for the disease under discussion.

Chapter 2

Although "epilepsy" is a single rubric for death coding, the clinical definitions for *convulsive disorders* are varied. The case-fatality ratio for epilepsy is very low; deaths so classified will represent but a fraction of the cases, and almost certainly this fraction is not representative of all cases. The death rate for epilepsy was about 1 per 100,000 in the United States in 1959-61. Age-specific death rates showed bimodal peaks at about age 40 and in the oldest age group. Nonwhite males had the highest rates and white females the lowest. Among whites, there was little noteworthy geographic variation.

A number of prevalence studies of epilepsy have been accomplished in England, Scandinavia, and Rochester, Minnesota, among others. The majority indicate a prevalence of about 4 to 6 cases per 1,000 population. Primary grand mal and petit mal are disorders with incidence rates that decline from their peak in infancy. Secondary seizures are found to begin throughout life, but more often at either extreme of the age spectrum.

Febrile convulsions are disorders of early life, with a peak age at onset of about 18 months and with almost all beginning by 4 years of age. Although recurrent febrile fits are found in one-fourth to one-half of the cases, *afebrile* seizures subsequently develop in only about 1 in 40 of those with febrile convulsions.

An increased familial frequency of fits is present with primary and secondary seizure disorders, but the evidence is insufficient to define a precise genetic mechanism for the predisposition.

Chapter 3

Deaths from *parkinsonism* are recorded at nearly 2 per 100,000 population in the United States for 1959-61. From prevalence studies, an annual incidence of about 20 per 100,000 and a prevalence of nearly 200 per 100,000 are reported. This is a disorder of the elderly, with the age-specific incidence rates increasing steeply to a maximum at about age 75, and the death rates similarly rising until about age 80. The best available evidence is that parkinsonism at present is the "idiopathic" disorder described first in 1817 and that new cases of the postencephalitic disorder that followed the influenza pandemic after World War I have not recurred. Only few instances of the disease are attributable to toxins or focal cerebral lesions, and a separate category for an arteriosclerotic form seems superfluous. There is a notably increased familial frequency of this disorder, in a pattern compatible with inheritance as an autosomal dominant trait with reduced penetrance.

Although international mortality comparisons show wide variations in reported death rates, the available prevalence studies are actually in reasonable accord. Within the United States, deaths from parkinsonism were reported somewhat less often from the southern states. The death rates for males slightly exceeded those for females, and whites had four times the deaths of nonwhites, per capita.

Chapter 4

There has been more work on the epidemiology of *multiple sclerosis* than on any other chronic neurologic disease. Despite the intensive efforts of neural scientists of all persuasions, it seems to us that thus far the major leads for the ultimate deciphering of this enigmatic disorder have come from epidemiologic investigations. The most tantalizing clue for perhaps half a century has been the curious geographic distribution, with MS preponderance in northern Europe and northern North America and its virtual absence in the tropics and in Asia.

There is no valid evidence that the incidence of MS has changed appreciably during the twentieth century in those few areas where reliable data are available. The mortality rate has shown a modest decline in the United States, and reported prevalence rates have tended to move upward. This would suggest a longer survival in recent years, and current evidence indicates a median duration of about thirty-five years from clinical onset to death, a much more optimistic view than has been generally held.

Studies of migration patterns in MS have led to the hypothesis that the disorder is acquired long before clinical onset, perhaps at about the age of puberty, and that it remains clinically silent or latent for a number of years before the symptoms become manifest. It seems to make little difference what one's geographic locale is after the middle of the second decade of life, with regard to the presence, type, severity, or course of symptomatology.

The migration studies, together with the presence of clusters or foci of the disease in parts of Europe, suggest analogies with the "slow, latent, or temperate" virus disorders of the nervous system, and this hypothesis as to cause has been favored by some over the concept of MS as an autoimmune disorder. Early exposure to such an agent may be a better explanation for the increased familial frequency of the disease that has been reported than a simple genetic mechanism.

As to the disorder itself, both prevalence and mortality data indicate that there is a female preponderance at perhaps 0.7 to 1, male to female. Age-specific incidence rates rise rapidly from essentially 0 at age 10 to reach a maximum from about ages 20-40, and return to near 0 by about age 60. Age-specific death rates are maximal from about ages 50 to 70, and in prevalence surveys, the large majority of patients are between 25 and 70 years of age.

Chapter 5

The *motor neuron diseases* include amyotrophic lateral sclerosis and the variants of anterior-horn-cell degeneration called progressive myelopathic (spinal) muscular atrophy and progressive bulbar palsy. In the opinion of some, including one of us (LTK), these are all one disease; others prefer to retain the differentiations. In addition to these disorders, there is a familial form of ALS, which accounts for 5 to 10 percent of cases, and the curious "Mariana Islands" form of ALS, which is prevalent on Guam and neighboring islands as well as on the Kii Peninsula of Japan.

Motor neuron disease appears to occur in all countries where data are available and with the exception of the Mariana Islands has an even international geographic distribution of death rates at about 1 per 100,000. Population studies suggest an annual incidence rate between 1 and 2 per 100,000, and a prevalence of about 5 per 100,000. The distribution of this disorder seems so uniform that case ratios of other neurologic disorders to ALS may provide a useful estimate of prevalence rates for the former where direct data are unavailable.

Within the United States, death rates were reasonably uniform. A slight decrease in the southern United States is explicable on the basis of incomplete ascertainment; a reported preponderance for whites also may reflect such inadequacies. The available population studies are not pertinent to this point because they are essentially limited to whites. In both the death data and the prevalence studies, though, a male excess in the order of 1.7 to 1 has been found. The mean age at death for ALS in the United States was 61, which implies a mean age at onset of about 57.

Although a combination of genetic predisposition and some widely distributed exogenous factor that is concentrated in the immediate environment of the people of the Marianas has been proposed, no specific agent has been identified. The elucidation of the western Pacific foci or the identification of other populations with an unusual incidence of ALS hopefully will result in some etiologic breakthrough of this uniformly fatal disease.

Chapter 6

The *muscular dystrophies* are included under the Seventh Revision ISC rubric 744.1, called "inborn defect of muscle." The Duchenne type is a disorder of childhood transmitted as a sex-linked recessive and affects males. This variety is probably responsible for the peak in adolescence for the age-specific death rates, and for the male predominance in all deaths so coded. The other major types—facioscapulohumeral and limb-girdle—are found in either sex, because the former is transmitted as an autosomal dominant and the latter chiefly as an autosomal recessive trait.

Death rates for "inborn defect of muscle" have been about 0.3 per 100,000, and there is no demonstrable variation of importance from this rate either within the United States or among the several nations for which data are available—although again data are limited to whites. In the various studies, prevalence rates among the nations have ranged from 4 to 9 per 100,000, none of which differs significantly from the others.

Myotonic dystrophy is included in the ISC rubric previously mentioned. Prevalence studies have ranged from 1 to 10 per 100,000, based on small numbers. In Guam a phenomenal rate of 76 per 100,000 was noted, with 29 patients. This disorder is transmitted as an autosomal dominant trait.

Polymyositis is an acquired myopathy that has been recognized as a clinical entity sui generis only in the past decade or two. When the disorder is not part of a more widespread collagen disease, its recognition may be difficult. When the disorder is acute, a misdiagnosis of anterior poliomyelitis or the Guillain-Barré syndrome is possible. In its more chronic varieties, the illness may be misclassified as muscular dystrophy or progressive myelopathic muscular atrophy. Polymyositis is a disorder of all ages, reported from all continents and in all races. There is a female preponderance among recognized cases. Prevalence is currently considered to be about 6 per 100,000, with an annual incidence rate of less than 1 per 100,000; but both figures may prove to be underestimates as the disorder becomes more widely recognized.

Chapter 7

Myasthenia gravis is a rare disease, accounting for only 1 death a year per 1,000,000 population in the United States. Rates for nonwhites were found to be about twice as high as those for whites, and females were affected slightly more often than males. From several surveys, the incidence rate was about 3 or 4 per 1,000,000, with prevalence rates about ten times as high. Although a familial excess has been reported in some clinical reports, evidence seems insufficient to postulate a genetic mechanism. With the small numbers available, there is no evidence of notable geographic variation. It would appear that new approaches, particularly those utilizing new immunologic data, are needed to shed light on the etiology of this disorder.

Chapter 8

Down's syndrome occurs predominantly as a sporadic chromosomal aberration which causes a typical appearance and mental retardation associated with a number of somatic changes. About 95 percent of cases are characterized by trisomy 21 (Denver system). Death rates in the United States for 1959-61 were about 0.2 per 100,000 population, and the rate for those less than 1 year of age was more than 4 per 100,000. Three-fifths of the deaths were recorded in the first year of life. It is evident, though, that only a small proportion of those affected with Down's syndrome have this disorder recorded as the primary cause of death on which the mortality rates were based.

The disorder seems to affect males and females equally, but death rates for nonwhites were about half those for whites in the United States. With small numbers, there was no evidence of differences by color from births in hospitals in the Republic of South Africa; results in the United States were contradictory. The WHO survey of nearly half a million births in twenty-four centers throughout the world indicates a paucity of births with Down's syndrome for all regions of Asia, including Chinese, Indians, and Malaysians. However, limitation of attention to hospital births and the early postnatal period and, perhaps too, diagnostic difficulties, lead to caution in accepting such differences at present. For the remainder of the centers, from Australia, South America, Africa, and Europe, the rates seemed reasonably uniform. Other studies from Europe and the United States are within the same range as the WHO survey, and the incidence rate tends to center at 1 per 1,000 births or slightly higher. Within the United States, the death rates for Down's syndrome seemed to reflect only chance variation among the states, and there was no evidence of an urban-rural difference.

Down's syndrome only rarely is familial. Most monozygous twins are concordant, and most dizygous twins are discordant for this abnormality. There is a striking correlation of frequency with maternal age; in the WHO survey, the rate per 1,000 births was nearly 17 for mothers age 45 or older at parturition.

Chapter 9

The principal categories of *congenital malformations* affecting the nervous system are anencephaly, spina bifida, and hydrocephalus. Spina bifida is often found together with anencephaly or with hydrocephalus. Microcephaly comprises a much smaller portion of these malformations, but still an appreciable one, and this often occurs together with spina bifida. Death data were coded as monstrosity (code 750), spina bifida (code 751), congenital hydrocephalus (code 752), and other (essentially neurologic) malformations (code 753). The sum of these four categories would represent deaths caused by congenital malformations of the nervous system as the underlying cause of death. Admixtures of spina bifida and hydrocephalus were variably coded to either 751 or 752. When listed on death certificates, malformations of the nervous system were coded as the primary or underlying cause in virtually all deaths in the category of monstrosity, three-fifths to four-fifths of spina bifida, one-half to nine-tenths of hydrocephalus, and two-thirds to three-fourths of other malformations.

International comparisons for deaths in the 1950s provided average annual death rates of about 2 to 4 per 100,000 population, all ages, for neurologic malformations (codes 750 through 753). Scotland and Ireland had rates of 6 and 7, respectively. The range among the various nations was modest for monstrosity and other malformations, not much greater for hydrocephalus, but large for spina bifida, from 0.2 to 3.4 per 100,000. Highest rates were found for Ireland and Scotland for each of the three specific categories of malformation, and England-Wales was high for spina bifida. Northern Ireland, too, was high for spina bifida, the only category for which data were available.

From 1950 to 1967, mortality rates (all ages) for neural malformations in the United States declined by half because of approximately equal decrements in the rates for spina bifida and for hydrocephalus. Only part of the decline can be attributed to a decreasing birth rate in this interval.

In the United States for 1959-61, death rates per 100,000 population, all ages, summed to 2.7 for this category: 0.6 for monstrosity, 0.7 for deaths allocated to spina bifida, 0.9 for those coded to hydrocephalus, and 0.5 for other neural malformations. Because most of the deaths occurred under 1 year of age, the death rates per 100,000 population less than 1 year old provide the best basis for comparison. These totaled 94, with the respective rates for the four constituents in the same order at 27, 27, 27, and 13.

From studies in various lands, rates per 1,000 births were between 2 and 8 for neural malformations, mostly about 4. The range was small for hydrocephalus, near 1 per 1,000 births, and notably wider for anencephaly and spina bifida. Again Northern Ireland, South Wales, several (but not all) parts of England, and probably Scotland had the highest rates for spina bifida and for anencephaly.

Based on the data of the WHO study, about 39 percent of congenital neural malformations were anencephaly (34 percent alone and 5 percent with spina bifida). Hydrocephalus comprised 33 percent (23 percent alone and 10 percent with spina bifida), and spina bifida alone was 21 percent (36 percent total). All other neural malformations totaled 7 percent of the cases.

Morbidity data show many more females than males are affected by spina bifida and anencephaly; but in mortality data the female preponderance with spina bifida and monstrosity is smaller. Although anencephaly is probably the largest single component of monstrosity, the proportion of anencephaly within the latter category is unknown. Most anencephalics are stillborn and thus are not counted in the mortality data for the population as a whole.

For hydrocephalus, morbidity data and most of the international mortality statistics, including that of the United States, 1962-67, reveal a slight male preponderance. The United States mortality rates for the years 1959-61, however, showed no difference by sex. Admixture with spina bifida deaths in these years may explain this discrepancy.

Geographic variation in the United States for 1959-61 was small and scattered for other neural malformations (code 753), small but concentrated in the Southeast for hydrocephalus (code 752), and noteworthy for spina bifida (code 751) and monstrosity (code 750). Higher death rates for monstrosity (code 750) clustered in the Northeast, and those for spina bifida (code 751) were higher in the eastern half of the country. The spina bifida and monstrosity rates by state showed a highly significant positive correlation, but no pair of the other combinations showed any significant relationship. When rates for births from the WHO study of twenty-four international centers were compared in a like manner, the highest positive correlation was for anencephaly and spina bifida, although the rates for hydrocephalus and spina bifida or anencephaly also showed statistically significant correlations.

Color differences were apparent in the United States mortality data for 1959-61, with about a two-to-one white-nonwhite ratio for monstrosity and spina bifida. Hydrocephalus rates were virtually equal by color. Other malformations somewhat predominated in whites (1.4 to 1). Limited morbidity data from South Africa did not support a color difference for any type of malformation of the nervous system.

From a number of studies, remarkable changes with time within a given region have been noted in birth rates for anencephaly (and spina bifida). There is, however, no consistency in either time or locality that we can decipher for these truly dramatic changes.

Chapter 10

This is our potpourri of neurologic disorders which do not have separate ISC rubrics as cause of death, *or* which very rarely are fatal. Accordingly, the special mortality investigations underlying this monograph series are not relevant here.

Syringomyelia: Prevalence rates ranged from 3 to 9 per 100,000, and the annual incidence has been estimated at about 3 per 1,000,000 from several population surveys.

Dorsolateral sclerosis: Most instances of this disorder are attributable to pernicious anemia, which has a high familial frequency. Average annual incidence of dorsolateral sclerosis is 2 to 3 per 100,000 population, and prevalence is about ten times as high. Most patients are elderly, the average age at onset in Rochester, Minnesota, being 60 years. Despite the common clinical impression that males are more often affected, there was no sex difference in the population studies.

A peculiar neuromyelopathy with gastrointestinal disorders has been described in Japan, with 752 cases in Nagoya from 1956 to 1969. The clinical features are predominantly those of dorsolateral sclerosis, but also with other signs including optic neuropathy. It appears to affect females almost twice as often as males and to be common throughout adult life, but it has not been reported in childhood. The excessive use of hydroxyquinolines recently has been suggested as a cause of this illness, which is also called SMON (subacute myelo-optico-neuropathy).

Bell's palsy: The annual incidence, based on various population surveys, ranges from 10 to 30 per 100,000. The disorder is infrequently seen in those less than 20 years old. In Iceland there was a male-female ratio of 0.5 to 1, but in other series the sexes were equally affected. Age-specific incidence rates throughout adult life were rather uniform. Several recent studies have raised the question as to whether there is a familial predisposition in Bell's palsy; at present, however, the presumption of a genetic factor seems premature.

Trigeminal neuralgia: This disorder is found more often in later adult life. An incidence rate of about 4 per 100,000 population seems likely. No difference by sex is apparent.

Herpes zoster: Also known as "shingles," this is a condition more common in the elderly. Attack rates have varied widely in the few population surveys available from 1 to almost 5 per 1,000 per year. Age-specific incidence rates rise steadily with age from 0 in early childhood to about 10 per 1,000 at the oldest ages. It is possible but not proved that there are real geographic or temporal differences. Among the several surveys, there is no consistent seasonal variation. Postherpetic neuralgia occurred in about 3 percent of the cases ascertained in the population surveys, a proportion considerably less than hospital series have suggested. The clinical impression of a relation of herpes zoster to underlying malignancy, particularly of the lymphoid system, has been reinforced by the results of the survey from Rochester, Minnesota.

The *Guillain-Barré syndrome* or infectious neuronitis: Annual incidence rates are about 1 per 100,000 population. There may be a male preponderance but no age predilection, the disorder being found in infants as well as in those more than 80 years of age. Seasonal variation has been described in some surveys.

Huntington's chorea: This is a classic example of an autosomal dominant illness with high penetrance; the symptoms begin in adults who are generally near 40 years old, and the disease progresses inexorably to death. The reported death rate in Canada in 1951 was 0.2 per 100,000. Prevalence in Europe, Australia, and the United States generally has been about 6 per 100,000, and the annual incidence is calculated at about 0.5 per 100,000.

Wilson's disease: Presumably caused by an inherited deficiency of ceruloplasmin, a copper-binding protein, the disease is associated with symptoms that usually begin in adolescence or early adult life. Transmission is probably as an autosomal recessive trait. The death rate in Canada in 1951 was 0.3 per 1,000,000 and the incidence in Iceland was 0.2 per 100,000 based on 3 patients, all of whom were related.

Hereditary ataxias: This group of cerebellar-system disorders is not satisfactorily delineated. One type is Friedreich's ataxia, which in Iceland had a prevalence of about 1 per 100,000. There are only fragmentary data, and a prevalence of about 5 per 100,000 could be estimated for this group of diseases.

Charcot-Marie-Tooth peroneal muscular atrophy: Various patterns of genetic transmission have been described. Prevalence seems to be between 2 and 5 per 100,000, although on Guam a rate of 24 per 100,000 was recorded.

Dystonia musculorum deformans: This is a basal-ganglion disease, usually of childhood, with mental deterioration in its later stages. In one geographic isolate in Sweden, the mean age at onset was 37. Although traditionally classified as autosomal dominant, an autosomal recessive form recently has been identified. Prevalence rates based on systematic surveys are unavailable, but Eldridge (1970) has estimated that the prevalence rate was about 0.3 per 100,000 in the United States. He considered that in this country the rate was particularly high among Jews (2.5) and low among Negroes (0.03).

Chapter 11

Cerebral palsy (CP) is a category of neurologic dysfunction of varied and multiple causes. Deaths before 28 days of life are coded to what we have called neonatal CP (ISC code 760) and those occurring after this age to infantile CP (ISC code 351). Since 1949 there has been a steady decline in NCP death rates in the United States to about one-third of the early value by 1967. However, ICP deaths in this same interval showed little change. NCP death rates were greater for males and for nonwhites. Little geographic variation was found in the United States. For ICP also there was a male preponderance, but the difference by color was not present. Age-specific death rates for ICP were maximal under age 1 year, dropped sharply between ages 1 and 5, then declined slowly thereafter to a plateau at about age 40. The ICP rates were perhaps somewhat high in the southern United States in comparison with other parts of the country.

For morbidity data, the artificial separation into neonatal and infantile forms is not required. Reported incidence per 1,000 births is about 2; the prevalence among children is about 2 per 1,000, and prevalence per 1,000 population (all ages) varies between 0.3 and 1.2. Age-specific prevalence is low beyond age 30, a reflection of the poor survival of these handicapped persons.

Chapter 12

Another category of dysfunction considered in this monograph was *blindness*. Much of the information available in the United States as to this disability has arisen from the Model Reporting Area for Blindness Statistics (MRA), which comprises the NINDB evaluations and collations of data supplied by fifteen states that agreed to participate. The MRA blindness prevalence rate for 1966 based on these fifteen statewide registers was about 125 per 100,000 for whites and about 240 per 100,000 for nonwhites. Age-specific prevalence rates increased almost geometrically with age to about 3 percent of the population age 85 or older. Incidence rates for 1966 were about 15 per 100,000 (13 for whites and 22 for nonwhites). Age-specific incidence at 4 to 5 per 100,000 changed little up to age 45, but then increased from 19 (age 45-64) to about 340 (age 85 or older) per 100,000. Blindness as noted here refers to maximal acuity of 20/200 or less, or visual field of 20 degrees or less in diameter, in the better eye.

The major known etiologic categories in the MRA project were senile degeneration, prenatal influence, and diabetes. The major categories of affection were cataract and retinal degeneration. Glaucoma provides about 10 percent of all cases of blindness.

International comparisons are presented. Rates for blindness in the tropics and subtropics greatly exceed those in our advanced western cultures. The major causes in these lands are onchocerciasis, trachoma, and seasonal conjunctivitis—all potentially preventable. Rates for cataract were similar throughout the world.

Chapter 13

The last category of disability we have considered is that of *hearing disorders*. The National Center for Health Statistics has provided information by means of the Health Interview Survey in which a questionnaire was sent to each person identified as claiming an impairment of hearing at interviews of probability samples of households in the United States. No confirmation of the reported complaints was made. Bilateral hearing impairment was recorded in this manner for about 2 percent of the population. Rates increased with age and were greater for males. The rate of 15 per 1,000 for nonwhites was much lower than that for whites (23 per 1,000).

In the Health Interview Survey, rural rates exceeded the urban, and rates were highest in the southern and lowest in the northeastern United States.

From school surveys of various countries, a prevalence of somewhat less than 1 per 1,000 children seems likely for prelingual deafness—the preferred term for "deaf-mutism." Audiologic surveys of schoolchildren have indicated that about 1 to 3 percent have impaired hearing.

When hearing impairment was determined audiometrically in the Health Examination Survey, there was no notable variation by sex, although the increasing frequencies with age were striking. Audiometric deficits of a loss of 16 dB or more were found in about 7 percent of the population 18-79 years of age—lower than this below age 55, and increasingly more frequent at older ages.

Only limited population-based data from large and representative samples are available for specific causes of hearing impairment. Much of the excess in the elderly population is probably attributable to presbycusis, otosclerosis, and perhaps acoustic trauma (noise). Prelingual deafness has many causes, including maternal rubella, hypothyroidism, otitis media, hereditary disease, and various congenital malformations. Deafness is excessively prevalent among the mentally retarded and those with cerebral palsy.

Distribution of Neurologic Disorders

We now provide the reader with summary tables on mortality, incidence, and prevalence rates. Because the data must be considered in the context of a number of provisos, the reader is referred to the appropriate chapter for interpretation of these values. Data will be presented as rather arbitrary "best estimates," taking into account those studies that seem to be the most accurate or representative. For a few entities there is only a single rate or estimate, based on potentially sound data, and this perforce is presented.

Rates are all cited in cases or deaths per 100,000 population. Translation of the rates relevant to a given community or country is readily made by multiplying the rates by the appropriate population factor. For example, expected numbers in the United States at present can be approximated by multiplying the cited rate by 2,000.

Thus a rate of 10 per 100,000 represents 20,000 cases in the United States. Similar factors for the United Kingdom at this time would be about 500, for Denmark about 50, and for Canada about 200.

The rates given, of course, refer to the population of all ages, even though the disorder is manifest in but a portion of the age spectrum (for example, amyotrophic lateral sclerosis among adults and Werdnig-Hoffman disease or progressive muscular atrophy among infants). Accordingly, a meaningful consideration of the rates once again requires a review of the appropriate chapter or source.

Many of these rates vary considerably in different studies or are based on few cases, so that most of the numbers are presented to one significant figure. Thus a rate of 20 means probably less than 25 and more than 14. Only when we subdivide an entity, such as cerebrovascular disease or epilepsy, will more than one figure be used in order to keep to the total provided.

Mortality Rates

In Table 14.1 are approximate annual mortality rates per 100,000 population that one might expect at the present time for various neurologic ills. They are given for both sexes combined, even for diseases with some predilection for either sex. Further, they should be considered as reflecting rates for white populations such as those of the United States, Canada, and northern Europe. Later, we shall briefly discuss variations by color and sex in the United States.

The data for cerebrovascular disease as a whole come from death rates as published (Kurtzke 1969b; Kurtzke and Kurland 1970), but the subdivisions are cited for what the first author believes might be the "true" frequencies, as the reported rates vary widely (Kurtzke 1969b). The rates for brain tumor are taken from a separate review of this entity (Kurland 1972); the remainder are from this volume. All rates refer to the disorder when coded as the underlying (primary) cause of death and do not include those for secondary causes or associated conditions.

Of these illnesses, the only ones for which a geographic pattern has been documented are motor neuron diseases (uniform distribution except for Mariana Islands and Kii Peninsula foci) and multiple sclerosis. Rates for MS in this and succeeding tables refer to the "high-risk" areas of northern United States, Canada, and northern Europe; they are considerably lower in the southern United States and southern Europe.

Table 14.1 Approximate annual death rates[a] per 100,000 population for various neurologic disorders reported as underlying cause of death among white populations: selected areas in the western hemisphere, about 1960

Disorder	Death rate	
Cerebrovascular disease[b]	100	
Subarachnoid hemorrhage		10
Cerebral hemorrhage		30
Cerebral thromboembolism		50
Other cerebrovascular disease		10
Primary brain tumor[c]	5	
Malformations of nervous system	3	
Monstrosity		0.6
Spina bifida		0.7
Hydrocephalus		0.9
Other		0.5
Cerebral palsy	2	
Parkinsonism	2	
Epilepsy	1	
Multiple sclerosis[d]	1	
Motor neuron disease	1	
Muscular dystrophy	0.3	
Down's syndrome	0.2	
Huntington's chorea	0.2	
Myasthenia gravis	0.1	
Wilson's disease	0.03	

[a] All rates are best available estimates rounded to one significant figure based on data referable to the period near 1960.

[b] Kurtzke 1969b.

[c] Kurland 1972.

[d] Northern regions (northerly United States, Canada, northerly Europe).

Incidence Rates

Average annual incidence rates per 100,000 population are presented in Table 14.2. Reported rates for herpes zoster vary widely, but 400 seems to be a reasonable estimate overall. Again, the rates for cerebrovascular disease are based on estimates, but this time they are drawn from averages for population surveys (Kurtzke 1969b; Kurtzke and Kurland 1970; Whisnant et al. 1971). The rate for polymyositis may be an underestimate. Huntington's chorea can be expected to vary by chance with the earlier migrations of affected persons, particularly to sparsely settled areas. The rate for Wilson's disease is based solely on a survey from Iceland (Gudmundsson 1969).

When disorders of infancy are considered, it is more appropriate to use the birth incidence rate (Table 14.3). For comparison, we include not only the neural defects but also a rate for all significant congenital malformations recognized at birth. The neurologic defects account for about one-third of the total. Among infants, 1 in 500 will die of a neurologic disorder before his first birthday (see Table 14.6 below). As discussed elsewhere, neural tube defects seem to vary in frequency, both temporally and geographically.

Prevalence Rates

The estimated number of cases in a community at a given time is provided by the data of Table 14.4. The rate for dorsolateral sclerosis may prove to be an overestimate since, with appropriate therapy, many cases should be preventable by early treatment of pernicious anemia. The rate offered for MS again refers to the northern regions of North America and Europe. The rates for epilepsy are a conservative average for the major population surveys cited in Chapter 2. Prevalence for stroke in Rochester, Minnesota, was 547 per 100,000 (Whisnant et al. 1971). Most of those who survive stroke have had cerebral thrombosis rather than hemorrhage.

The reported prevalence rate for blindness was 126 per 100,000 among whites in the Model Reporting Area project, and that for binaural hearing impairment was 2,300 per 100,000 according to the Health Interview Survey questionnaire. Note that this last rate is based on subjects interviewed and is without medical documentation.

Excluding the rates for auditory and visual disorders, the sum of the rates from Table 14.4 is approximately 1,500 per 100,000. This translates to about 3,000,000 persons affected in the United States.

Table 14.2 Approximate annual incidence rates[a] per 100,000 population for various neurologic and sensory disorders from surveys of white populations: selected areas in the western hemisphere, about 1960

Disorder	Incidence rate	
Herpes zoster	400	
Cerebrovascular disease[b]	200	
Subarachnoid hemorrhage		20
Cerebral hemorrhage		30
Cerebral thrombosis		120
Cerebral embolism		10
Other cerebrovascular disease		20
Convulsive disorders	40	
Primary grand mal		12
Petit mal alone		3
Secondary seizures		25
Bell's palsy	20	
Parkinsonism	20	
Blindness[c]	10	
Primary brain tumor[d]	10	
Trigeminal neuralgia	4	
Dorsolateral sclerosis	3	
Multiple sclerosis[e]	2	
Guillain-Barré syndrome	1	
Motor neuron disease	1	
Polymyositis	0.5	
Huntington's chorea	0.5	
Myasthenia gravis	0.4	
Syringomyelia	0.3	
Wilson's disease	0.2	

[a]All rates are best available estimates rounded to one significant figure for each category of disease, based on data referable to the period near 1960.

[b]Kurtzke 1969b; Kurtzke and Kurland 1970.

[c]National Institute of Neurological Diseases and Blindness 1969.

[d]Kurland 1972.

[e]Northern regions (northerly United States, Canada, northerly Europe).

Table 14.3 Approximate annual incidence rates[a] per 1,000 births for various disorders of infancy: selected areas, about 1960

Disorder	Incidence rate
All congenital malformations	13[b]
All congenital malformations	11[c]
Neural tube birth defects	4[b]
Hydrocephalus	1[b]
Spina bifida	2[b]
Anencephaly	1[b]
Cerebral palsy	2[c]
Down's syndrome	1[c]

[a]All rates are best available estimates rounded to whole numbers, based on data referable to the period near 1960.

[b]Rate per 1,000 total births, including stillbirths in numerator and denominator.

[c]Rate per 1,000 live births.

In other words, at any given time 1 person in 70 in the general population may be expected to have one of these disorders of the nervous system. If we add patients suspected clinically of these disorders and those with neurologic ills not considered here—such as peripheral neuropathies, radiculopathies, and headache problems—then the great impact of neurologic dysfunction on the population may be appreciated, as well as the need for physicians trained in neurology.

Rate Variations by Sex

Some comments as to differences in these rates according to sex are warranted. In Table 14.5 we have summarized the death rates for

Table 14.4 Approximate point prevalence rates[a] per 100,000 population for various neurologic and sensory disorders from surveys of white populations: selected areas in the western hemisphere, about 1960

Disorder	Prevalence rate
Binaural hearing impairment[b]	2,000
Cerebrovascular disease[c]	500
Convulsive disorders	500
Parkinsonism	200
Blindness[d]	100
Cerebral palsy	60
Multiple sclerosis[e]	50
Brain tumor[f]	40
Dorsolateral sclerosis	20
Syringoymelia	8
Muscular dystrophy	6
Polymyositis	6
Huntington's chorea	6
Motor neuron disease	5
Myasthenia gravis	4
Myotonic dystrophy	2
Charcot-Marie-Tooth disease	2
Friedreich's ataxia	1
Wilson's disease	1

[a]All rates are best available estimates rounded to one significant figure, based on data referable to the period near 1960.

[b]Gentile et al. 1967.

[c]Kurtzke and Kurland 1970.

[d]National Institute of Neurological Diseases and Blindness 1969.

[e]Northern regions (northerly United States, Canada, northerly Europe).

[f]Kurland 1972.

Table 14.5 Average annual age-adjusted and crude death rates per 100,000 population for various neurologic disorders by color, sex and type of disorder: United States, 1959-61

(ISC codes 345, 350, 351, 353, 356.1, 744.0, 744.1, 760)

Disorder (ISC code)	Death rate	Total			White			Nonwhite		
		Total	Male	Female	Total	Male	Female	Total	Male	Female
Epilepsy (353)	Age-adj.	1.2	1.4	0.9	1.0	1.2	0.8	2.8	3.9	1.7
	Crude	1.1	1.4	0.9	0.9	1.1	0.8	2.5	3.4	1.6
Parkinsonism (350)	Age-adj.	1.2	1.5	1.0*	1.3	1.5	1.1*	0.4*	0.5*	0.3*
	Crude	1.6	1.8	1.5	1.8	1.9	1.6	0.4	0.5	0.3
Multiple sclerosis (345)	Age-adj.	0.8	0.7	0.8	0.8	0.7	0.9	0.5*	0.4*	0.6*
	Crude	0.8	0.7	0.9	0.8	0.7	0.9	0.4	0.4	0.5
Amyotrophic lateral sclerosis (356.1)	Age-adj.	0.5	0.7	0.4*	0.5	0.7	0.4*	0.3*	0.4*	0.2*
	Crude	0.6	0.8	0.4	0.6	0.8	0.4	0.3	0.3	0.2
Inborn defect of muscle (744.1)	Age-adj.	0.3	0.4	0.2	0.3	0.5	0.2	0.2*	0.3*	0.1*
	Crude	0.3	0.4	0.2	0.3	0.5	0.2	0.2	0.3	0.1
Myasthenia gravis (744.0)	Age-adj.	0.1	0.1*	0.1	0.1	0.1*	0.1	0.2*	0.1*	0.3*
	Crude	0.1	0.1	0.1	0.1	0.1	0.1	0.2	0.1	0.2
Infantile cerebral palsy (351)	Age-adj.	0.4	0.4	0.3	0.4	0.4	0.3	0.4*	0.5*	0.3*
	Crude	0.4	0.5	0.3	0.4	0.4	0.3	0.5	0.6	0.4
Neonatal cerebral palsy (760)[a]	Crude	1.8	2.3	1.3	1.6	2.0	1.1	3.6	4.5	2.8

[a] Only crude rates are shown for neonatal cerebral palsy (all deaths occurred under 28 days of age).

the United States, as discussed in previous chapters, according to color and sex. In Table 14.6 are similarly cited the infantile death rates for the appropriate disorders.

There is a male predominance in reported mortality rates for epilepsy, ALS, muscular dystrophy, and cerebral palsy. There is a female preponderance for monstrosity (anencephaly) and spina bifida. A slight male excess is present for parkinsonism, and a slight female preponderance is found for MS.

For epilepsy, from the population surveys and clinical data considered, we concluded that males were in excess for secondary seizure disorders, perhaps because of greater exposure to trauma and toxins, whereas there was little difference by sex for primary fits (idiopathic grand mal, petit mal).

The male preponderance in ALS and muscular dystrophy found in death data is well supported by prevalence studies and clinical experience. An explanation for the imbalance in ALS is unavailable, but that in muscular dystrophy is explicable on the basis of the sex-linked Duchenne type of dystrophy.

Males outnumbered females for both infantile (ISC code 351) and neonatal (ISC code 760) cerebral palsy—and by appreciable amounts. Again, this feature would seem worthy of further study, as we do not see any ready explanation.

The female excess in spina bifida and anencephaly is recorded from all studies. Here too an explanation is wanting.

For parkinsonism, a slight male preponderance was noted in the prevalence studies of Rochester and Iceland as well as in the United States mortality data.

A female preponderance for MS seems borne out in recent prevalence studies as well as in the death data. However, most studies before 1950 reported essentially equal rates or even a male preponderance, although the study in Rochester revealed a higher rate for females over several decades.

In myasthenia gravis, there has long been the clinical impression that females were more often affected. The difference in death rates by sex is not apparent in Table 14.5; but the male-female ratio was 0.6 to 1 for the respective rates of 0.9 and 1.4 per 1,000,000. The population studies support a female preponderance.

Table 14.5 does not include data for blindness or deafness. While incidence varies slightly, prevalence rates for blindness were equal for the two sexes in the MRA project that provided data from fifteen states. For 1966 the rates for whites were 126 for both males and

Table 14.6 Average annual death rates per 100,000 population under 1 year of age for various neurologic disorders present at or near birth by color, sex and type of disorder: United States, 1959-61

(ISC codes 325.4, 351, 750, 751, 752, 753, 760)

Disorder (ISC code)	Total			White			Nonwhite		
	Total	Male	Female	Total	Male	Female	Total	Male	Female
Total listed	179.0	190.1	167.0	177.4	186.1	168.1	187.5	214.1	161.1
Down's syndrome (325.4)	4.3	4.3	4.2	4.6	4.6	4.5	2.6	2.7	2.5
Neural malformations (750-753)	93.5	84.9	102.2	99.3	89.0	109.9	60.2	61.4	59.1
Monstrosity (750)	26.5	21.2	31.8	29.0	23.1	35.1	12.0	10.2	13.8
Spina bifida (751)[a]	27.1	23.2	31.1	29.4	24.7	34.2	14.0	14.6	13.4
Hydrocephalus (752)[a]	26.9	26.7	27.1	27.4	26.9	27.8	24.3	25.7	23.0
Other neural malformations (753)	13.0	13.8	12.2	13.5	14.3	12.8	9.9	10.9	8.9
Neonatal cerebral palsy (760)[b]	78.1	97.6	57.8	70.6	89.4	51.0	120.8	145.6	96.1
Infantile cerebral palsy (351)	3.1	3.3	2.8	2.9	3.1	2.7	3.9	4.4	3.4

[a] Concurrent spina bifida and hydrocephalus were variably included in code 751 or code 752.

[b] All deaths occurred under 28 days of age.

females; for nonwhites, 251 for males and 232 for females; and they were 148 for all males and 146 for all females. Bilateral hearing impairment reported by respondents—without medical confirmation—was appreciably more common in males (2.6 percent vs 1.9 for females, according to the Health Interview Survey).

Rate Variations by Color

In the United States about 95 percent of those listed as nonwhites are classified as Negro, with the major remaining classes being the American Indian and the Oriental groups. Accordingly, data for nonwhites must be considered as referring basically to Negroes. In Chapters 1 and 2, we discussed the validity of death data for Negroes, pointing out not only the lesser availability and utilization of medical care that are likely to be found but also the greater uncertainty of the population counts used as denominators. The extent to which underreporting for the numerator balances undercounting for the denominator is conjectural. Keeping in mind the tenuous nature of these rates, let us then look at mortality data by color in the United States (Tables 14.5 and 14.6).

Whites are reported in excess for parkinsonism, MS, ALS, Down's syndrome, monstrosity, spina bifida, and muscular dystrophy. Nonwhites (hence Negroes) are in excess for seizure disorders, myasthenia gravis, and cerebral palsy.

The differences for parkinsonism are in the order of four to one (white to nonwhite), which is the largest variation encountered. This difference is noted in all census regions and for metropolitan as well as nonmetropolitan counties. The only prevalence study available which includes an appreciable nonwhite population is that of Kessler in Baltimore, and it indicated a lower rate for Negroes than for whites. Although it is still possible that this reflects lower utilization of medical care facilities or underdiagnosis for other reasons in Negroes, the magnitude of the difference warrants careful study in other appropriate populations as to the reality and nature of the discrepancy.

Whether the deficit of nonwhites for the other disorders in which whites predominated is real or an artifact of ascertainment also remains uncertain. Scattered data for Down's syndrome and neural tube defects do not support a difference by color, but are not conclusive.

The color difference for MS rates has been discussed in Chapter 4;

controversy continues as to whether that difference is artifactual or valid. The mortality data could be dismissed as a confounding of geography and color (rates are low in the southern United States, where Negroes predominate). Still, it does have support in the survey of United States Army men with MS reported by Beebe and his associates (1967). The reason for this is as elusive as the cause of the disorder.

All the ills in which nonwhites predominated in the death data could be dismissed as color differences in case-fatality rates or diagnostic accuracy consequent to variations in available treatment. Such a facile explanation might serve for the convulsive disorders but does not seem likely for the cerebral palsies or myasthenia gravis. Our standard prevalence surveys fail us here, too, because nonwhites are sparsely represented in the subject works. Yet an illness such as myasthenia gravis is generally diagnosed in specialty facilities and, when identified, patients are usually kept under supervision through these facilities for further management. The point is that such a "sophisticated" illness should, if anything, be underdiagnosed in Negroes. Here then is another clue of potential etiologic importance worthy of better definition.

Reported prevalence of blindness in the MRA project was twice as high for nonwhites as for whites. The difference between whites and nonwhites was less for those under age 20 than for those above 20, but was found for all age groups and for both sexes. Some of this difference by color may be artifact because reporting to the blindness registers, on which the MRA data were based, may have been more complete for low-income groups (welfare and rehabilitation agencies were major reporting sources). Nevertheless, a detailed study of causes of blindness would seem indicated to determine the reasons for the variations between whites and nonwhites.

On the other hand, bilateral hearing impairment was reported more frequently for whites in the Health Interview Survey, at 2.3 versus 1.5 percent of the population. A true difference does seem likely, according to examination data. Again, however, rates for specific causes of deafness need to be ascertained for interpretation.

Geographic Variations

In the United States the only broad-based information on the geographic distribution of the neurologic disorders is that available from mortality statistics. We shall not consider further the intriguing aspects of the distribution of multiple sclerosis (see Chapter 4).

Prevalence studies for entities other than MS are mostly "spot surveys" of small discrete regions.

Death rates for convulsive disorders were irregularly high in the eastern half of the country. This was in part the consequence of higher death rates for nonwhites in the Southeast. With one exception, rates for whites by census region were reasonably uniform. In New England death rates for epilepsy were high for white as well as for nonwhite males. Even here, though, the female rates were in accord with those for the rest of the country. On the whole, there is little evidence for geographic variation distinct from color and sex differences in epilepsy deaths.

For parkinsonism and ALS, there were slightly higher death rates north of about 37 degrees north latitude than were reported in the southern states. The difference may stem from reporting artifact as a reflection of a decreased availability of general and specialty medical facilities in the southern (especially the southeast) United States.

Cerebral palsy, especially the infantile form, showed some degree of preponderance in the southeastern United States for both sexes and colors. The neonatal CP death rates were reasonably uniform.

With the small numbers available, deaths from muscular dystrophy and myasthenia gravis showed no major variations in geographic distribution.

The variations for Down's syndrome are minimal, except for a reported paucity of cases from Asia in the WHO survey. As discussed previously, a proper study including nonhospital births and community-wide examinations for those beyond the neonatal period would be required to validate this finding.

Variations in neural tube defects are appreciable, even though hydrocephalus seems reasonably uniform in time and space. Anencephaly and spina bifida show striking variations. Highest rates are recorded for the Irish and for much of the rest of the British Isles. In the United States monstrosity and spina bifida deaths are concentrated in the eastern part of the country. Dramatic variations with time have occurred in birth rates from anencephaly and spina bifida in both Europe and the United States, but without a common pattern that we were able to delineate. This would seem a topic well worth further investigation.

Concluding Remarks

In the introductory chapter, we mentioned some of the difficulties in obtaining valid data concerning the natural history of neurologic diseases. In subsequent parts, we have presented that material which is now available. It is safe to say that by and large more questions have been raised than solved.

We will not recapitulate the problems of diagnostic criteria and case ascertainment that underlie all the data considered. Certainly, the value of mortality statistics in the epidemiologic inquiry into neurologic disease needs no further support, and the necessity of properly selected prevalence studies also would seem readily apparent. But under all these numbers and labels lies the physician in contact with his patient. In the United States in the past, neurology has not occupied a major role in many medical schools. Accordingly, the average practitioner is often ill equipped to provide the specific diagnoses required in these studies. Further, the number of neurologists in practice has been small, so that referrals for specialty evaluation are often delayed or nonexistent. It is true that there has been an almost geometric increase in the number of neurologists since World War II, but the base then was so small that there are still many population centers without a neurologist.

It is not only to attach proper labels to esoteric entities that we need more neurologists. We have pointed out that, at any one time, 1 in 70 of the general population has a major neurologic disorder in need of diagnosis and treatment. Who has been taking care of these people? Who will? Besides neurologists, this burden also reflects a need for such specialists as neurosurgeons, physiatrists, ophthalmologists, and otolaryngologists, with all the paramedical skills and facilities and the clinics and hospitals that this entails.

This same entourage is required for the management of disorders of vision or hearing—perhaps 1 person in 50 of the general population has binaural hearing loss. Only a small proportion of these are consequent to the neurologic ills we have discussed, so there is little overlap. Accordingly, about 1 person in 30 of the general population at any given time will have one of the disorders in question in this volume—or about 7 million persons in the United States!

The practicing physician's responsibility to statistical and epidemiologic analysis ends with his proper definition of the case or death. However, the encoding of these ills is still unsatisfactory. Each entity should have a specific code number under the International Classification. Perhaps (from the neurologic viewpoint) there should be senior neurologists on the panels which revise this classification. The potential value of a properly encoded—and codable—roster of neurologic diseases and deaths is enormous for the inquiry into the natural history of neurologic and sense organ disorders.

APPENDIX TABLES
REFERENCES
INDEX

APPENDIX A

Table A.2.1 Definition of convulsive disorders by clinical forms, ILAE,[a] and modification used in Rochester, Minnesota, study

Clinical forms	Preliminary ILAE[b]	Final ILAE[c]	Rochester modification[d]
Grand mal	2B	II6 (plus II4, 5, 8)	IId, e
Petit mal	2A	IIIa, IIIb	IIa, b
Focal or focal onset	1A, 1C, 3	IA, IC, III	Ia, b, c, d, e, III, IV
Psychomotor	1B, 1C	IB, IC	If, g, h
Other or unclassified	5	IV (plus II2, 3, 7, if not in above)	Others

[a] ILAE - International League Against Epilepsy.
[b] Commission on Terminology 1964.
[c] Gastaut 1969.
[d] Hauser et al., unpublished data.

Table A.2.2 Deaths and average annual death rates per 100,000 population for epilepsy by age, color and sex: United States, 1959-61
(ISC code 353)

Age	Total			White			Nonwhite		
	Total	Male	Female	Total	Male	Female	Total	Male	Female
	Number of deaths								
All ages	5,961	3,640	2,321	4,443	2,622	1,821	1,518	1,018	500
Under 1	65	42	23	54	36	18	11	6	5
1-4	271	147	124	205	114	91	66	33	33
5-14	509	307	202	372	226	146	137	81	56
15-24	844	512	332	628	376	252	216	136	80
25-34	971	607	364	689	430	259	282	177	105
35-44	1,180	747	433	843	496	347	337	251	86
45-54	889	568	321	650	393	257	239	175	64
55-64	598	365	233	470	272	198	128	93	35
65-74	389	222	167	307	167	140	82	55	27
75-84	180	90	90	167	84	83	13	6	7
85 & over	60	31	29	53	26	27	7	5	2
Unknown	5	2	3	5	2	3	-	-	-
	Death rate								
All ages	1.1	1.4	0.9	0.9	1.1	0.8	2.5	3.4	1.6
Under 1	0.5	0.7	0.4	0.5	0.7	0.4*	0.6*	0.7*	0.5*
1-4	0.6	0.6	0.5	0.5	0.5	0.4	0.9	0.9	0.9
5-14	0.5	0.6	0.4	0.4	0.5	0.3	1.0	1.1	0.8
15-24	1.2	1.4	0.9	1.0	1.2	0.8	2.4	3.2	1.8
25-34	1.4	1.8	1.0	1.1	1.4	0.8	3.5	4.8	2.4
35-44	1.6	2.1	1.2	1.3	1.6	1.1	4.5	7.0	2.2
45-54	1.4	1.9	1.0	1.2	1.4	0.9	4.0	6.0	2.1
55-64	1.3	1.6	1.0	1.1	1.3	0.9	3.1	4.5	1.6
65-74	1.2	1.4	0.9	1.0	1.2	0.9	3.2	4.4	2.0
75-84	1.3	1.5	1.1	1.3	1.5	1.1	1.4*	1.3*	1.4*
85 & over	2.2	2.9	1.7	2.1	2.6	1.7	3.3*	5.3*	1.7*

Table A.2.3 Deaths and average annual age-adjusted death rates per 100,000 population for epilepsy, all ages: United States and each state, 1959-61
(ISC code 353)

State	Deaths	Rate	State	Deaths	Rate
United States	5,961	1.2	Arkansas	59	1.2*
			Maryland	108	1.2*
Nevada	3	0.3*	Missouri	151	1.2*
Minnesota	65	0.7*	New Mexico	34	1.2*
California	354	0.8	Ohio	325	1.2
Oklahoma	56	0.8*			
Oregon	42	0.8*	Pennsylvania	409	1.2
			South Dakota	24	1.2*
Alaska	6	0.9*	Tennessee	128	1.2*
Connecticut	75	0.9*	Florida	183	1.3*
Indiana	115	0.9*	Nebraska	50	1.3*
Texas	249	0.9*			
Washington	78	0.9*	New York	622	1.3
			Rhode Island	33	1.3*
Arizona	37	1.0*	Utah	31	1.3*
Idaho	17	1.0*	Virginia	151	1.3*
Illinois	285	1.0	Louisiana	124	1.4*
Iowa	78	1.0*			
Michigan	239	1.0*	New Hampshire	25	1.5*
			North Carolina	183	1.5*
Montana	19	1.0*	South Carolina	100	1.5*
New Jersey	179	1.0*	Alabama	145	1.6*
West Virginia	55	1.0*	Delaware	21	1.6*
Colorado	60	1.1*			
Hawaiian Islands	20	1.1*	Maine	45	1.6*
			Massachusetts	253	1.6
Kansas	67	1.1*	Kentucky	149	1.7*
Mississippi	68	1.1*	Georgia	195	1.8
North Dakota	22	1.1*	Wyoming	20	2.2*
Vermont	13	1.1*	Dist. of Col.	64	2.7*
Wisconsin	127	1.1*			

Table A.2.4 Average annual age-adjusted death rates per 100,000 population for epilepsy by color, sex and type of county: United States and census regions, 1959-61
(ISC code 353)

Region and color	Metropolitan counties			Nonmetropolitan counties		
	Total	Male	Female	Total	Male	Female
United States	1.1	1.4	0.8	1.3	1.6	1.0
Region						
New England	1.4	2.0*	0.9*	1.4*	1.8*	1.0*
Middle Atlantic	1.2	1.6	0.9	1.1*	1.4*	0.9*
East North Central	1.0	1.2	0.8	1.2	1.4	0.9*
West North Central	0.9*	1.0*	0.7*	1.2	1.4*	0.9*
South Atlantic	1.4	1.9	1.0*	1.5	1.9	1.1*
East South Central	1.5*	1.9*	1.2*	1.4	1.6*	1.2*
West South Central	0.8*	1.0*	0.7*	1.3	1.5*	1.0*
Mountain	0.8*	1.0*	0.6*	1.4*	1.6*	1.2*
Pacific	0.8	0.9*	0.6*	1.0*	1.1*	0.8*
Color						
White	0.9	1.1	0.7	1.1	1.3	0.8
Nonwhite	2.6	3.9	1.5	3.1	4.0	2.2

	Metropolitan counties					
	With central city			Without central city		
	Total	Male	Female	Total	Male	Female
United States	1.1	1.5	0.8	0.8	0.9	0.7*
Region						
New England	1.4	2.1*	0.8*	1.2*	1.6*	0.9*
Middle Atlantic	1.4	1.9	1.0	0.8*	1.0*	0.7*
East North Central	1.0	1.3	0.7*	0.9*	1.0*	0.9*
West North Central	0.9*	1.1*	0.8*	0.7*	0.6*	0.7*
South Atlantic	1.7	2.3*	1.1*	0.7*	0.9*	0.5*
East South Central	1.6*	2.0*	1.2*	0.8*	0.7*	0.9*
West South Central	0.9*	1.0*	0.7*	0.8*	1.2*	0.4*
Mountain	0.8*	1.0*	0.6*	0.8*	1.0*	0.6*
Pacific	0.8	1.0*	0.7*	0.4*	0.5*	0.4*

Table A.2.5 Deaths and average annual age-adjusted death rates per 100,000 population for epilepsy by age, sex and marital status: United States, 1959-61 (ISC code 353)

Age & sex	Single	Married	Widowed	Divorced
	\multicolumn{4}{c}{Number of deaths}			
15 & over				
Total	2,679	1,541	472	342
Male	1,843	824	181	231
Female	836	717	291	111
15-64				
Total	2,531	1,349	229	305
Male	1,749	695	92	205
Female	782	654	137	100
65 & over				
Total	148	192	243	37
Male	94	129	89	26
Female	54	63	154	11
	\multicolumn{4}{c}{Death rate}			
15 & over				
Total	6.5	0.6	2.1	3.1
Male	8.3	0.6	4.4*	4.6*
Female	4.5	0.5	1.6*	2.0*
15-64				
Total	6.8	0.5	2.2	3.1
Male	8.5	0.5	4.6*	4.6
Female	4.7	0.5	1.6*	2.0*
65 & over				
Total	3.8	0.8	1.3	3.5*
Male	5.6*	0.9	2.2*	5.0*
Female	2.3*	0.6*	1.1	2.0*

Table A.2.6 Average annual age-adjusted death rates per 100,000 population for epilepsy, white persons, by sex and nativity: United States and census regions, 1959-61
(ISC code 353)

Region	Native born			Foreign born		
	Total	Male	Female	Total	Male	Female
United States	1.0	1.2	0.8	0.6*	0.8*	0.5*
New England	1.4	1.9	0.9*	0.6*	0.9*	0.2*
Middle Atlantic	1.0	1.3	0.8	0.6*	0.6*	0.6*
East North Central	1.0	1.2	0.8	0.8*	1.0*	0.5*
West North Central	0.9	1.2*	0.8*	1.1*	2.2*	0.3*
South Atlantic	0.9	1.1	0.7*	0.6*	0.5*	0.6*
East South Central	1.0	1.1*	1.0*	0.1*	-	0.3*
West South Central	0.7	0.9*	0.6*	1.1*	1.5*	0.9*
Mountain	1.0*	1.2*	0.9*	1.0*	1.4*	0.7*
Pacific	0.8	0.9*	0.7*	0.4*	0.5*	0.3*

Table A.2.7 Average annual age-adjusted[a] death rates per 100,000 population for epilepsy by sex: selected countries, various years, 1951-58

(ISC code 353)

Country	Years	Death rate		M:F ratio
		Male	Female	
Australia	1954-58	1.8	1.5	1.2
Austria	1953-57	2.5	1.9	1.3
Belgium	1954-58	2.2	1.7	1.3
Canada[b]	1953-57	1.8	1.4	1.3
Colombia	1957	4.8	4.5	1.1
Denmark	1953-57	1.3	0.8	1.6
England-Wales	1953-57	1.8	1.5	1.2
Finland	1954-58	2.8	2.0	1.4
France	1953-57	1.7	1.0	1.7
Iceland	1951-55	2.3	0.9	2.6
Ireland	1954-58	2.6	2.3	1.1
Israel (Jewish)	1956-58	1.0	1.3	0.8
Italy	1953-57	2.2	1.6	1.4
Japan	1953-57	2.2	1.6	1.4
Mexico	1952-56	3.8	3.3	1.2
Netherlands	1953-57	1.5	1.3	1.2
New Zealand (Maoris)	1952-56	5.1	3.9	1.3
New Zealand (European)	1952-56	2.9	1.7	1.7
Northern Ireland	1951-55	2.0	1.7	1.2
Norway	1953-57	2.5	1.7	1.5
Philippines	1956-57	1.6	1.1	1.4
Poland	1954-57	1.3	1.0	1.3
Portugal	1955-58	5.3	3.3	1.6
Scotland	1951-55	2.5	2.0	1.2
Sweden	1953-57	1.4	0.9	1.6
Switzerland	1953-57	1.8	1.2	1.5
Union of South Africa (white)	1953-57	2.4	2.2	1.1
United States (white)	1953-57	1.4	0.9	1.6
United States (nonwhite)	1953-57	4.1	1.9	2.2
United States (total)	1953-57	1.6	1.0	1.6
Uruguay	1955-57	2.5	1.8	1.4
West Germany	1953-57	2.1	1.5	1.4

[a] Adjusted to the 1950 census population of the United States.
[b] Yukon and Northwest Territories included only in 1956-57.

Table A.3.1 Deaths and average annual age-adjusted death rates per 100,000 population for parkinsonism: United States and each state, 1959-61 (ISC code 350)

State	Number of deaths, all ages	Rate 65 & over	Rate 65 & over (white)	Rate All ages	State	Number of deaths, all ages	Rate 65 & over	Rate 65 & over (white)	Rate All ages
United States	8,674	14.1	15.0	1.2					
Mississippi	43	5.9*	8.9*	0.5*	Indiana	252	14.6	15.1	1.3*
Louisiana	61	6.5	7.9*	0.6*	Maryland	129	14.8	16.5	1.3*
Arkansas	53	7.2*	8.7*	0.7*	New Jersey	324	14.9	15.2	1.4*
Alabama	75	7.6	10.1	0.7*	Connecticut	137	15.3	15.3	1.3*
Arizona	27	7.8*	8.0*	0.7*	Pennsylvania	647	15.4	16.0	1.4*
Hawaii	11	8.1*	9.3*	0.8*	California	770	15.6	16.0	1.3*
South Carolina	53	9.1	13.0*	0.8*	Massachusetts	332	15.6	15.9	1.3*
Delaware	12	9.2*	9.1*	0.8*	Missouri	297	16.4	17.2	1.4*
Florida	183	9.3	9.9	0.8*	Maine	68	16.6	16.6	1.5*
Georgia	107	9.3	12.1	0.9*	Ohio	553	16.9	17.5	1.4*
North Carolina	117	9.6	11.2	0.9*	Michigan	389	17.3	17.9	1.4*
Tennessee	114	9.8	11.1	0.8*	Utah	41	18.0*	18.3*	1.6*
Texas	303	10.6	11.6	0.9*	Montana	43	18.2*	18.1*	1.6*
West Virginia	72	10.8	11.1	1.0*	Nebraska	104	18.3	18.5	1.5*
Illinois	441	12.1	12.5	1.1*	Washington	198	18.5	18.2	1.6*
Nevada	9	12.4*	13.0*	1.1*	South Dakota	53	18.8*	19.1*	1.8*
Dist. of Col.	29	12.5*	17.1*	1.0*	North Dakota	37	19.6*	19.2*	1.4*
Kentucky	142	12.8	13.6	1.1*	Minnesota	241	19.7	19.8	1.6*
Virginia	139	12.8	14.1	1.1*	Wyoming	16	19.7*	20.0*	1.5*
Colorado	72	13.7	13.5	1.0*	Kansas	171	19.8	20.2	1.6*
Rhode Island	47	13.8*	13.7*	1.3*	Idaho	42	19.8*	20.0*	1.7*
Oklahoma	128	13.9	15.0	1.2*	Oregon	128	19.9	20.0	1.6*
New Mexico	27	14.0*	14.9*	1.2*	Vermont	37	20.5*	20.5*	1.8*
New York	905	14.1	14.3	1.3*	Iowa	241	21.0	21.1	1.7*
New Hampshire	34	14.3*	14.3*	1.2*	Alaska	5	23.5*	25.0*	1.9*
Wisconsin	215	14.5	14.6	1.2*					

Table A.3.2 Average annual age-adjusted[a] death rates per 100,000 population for parkinsonism by sex: selected countries, **various years, 1951-58**
(ISC code 350)

Country	Years	Male	Female	M:F ratio[b]
Australia	1954-58	4.7	3.1	1.5
Belgium	1954-58	3.8	3.1	1.3
Canada[c]	1953-57	2.2	1.8	1.3
Chile	1956, 1958	1.3	1.1	1.3
Czechoslovakia	1953-57	0.5		---
Denmark	1953-57	1.6	1.1	1.6
England and Wales	1953-57	2.7	2.3	1.2
Finland	1954-58	1.5	1.1	1.4
France	1953-57	3.2	2.3	1.4
Iceland	1951-55	0.6	1.3	0.5
Ireland	1954-58	3.2	2.6	1.2
Israel[d]	1956-58	4.2	3.2	1.3
Italy	1953-57	2.4	1.5	1.6
Japan	1953-57	0.6	0.5	1.3
Mexico	1956	0.5	0.4	1.2
Netherlands	1953-57	3.4	2.8	1.2
New Zealand[e]	1952-56	3.2	2.8	1.1
Norway	1953-57	1.9	1.5	1.2
Scotland	1951-55	2.9	2.6	1.1
Sweden	1953-57	1.3	1.1	1.3
Switzerland	1953-57	2.7	2.3	1.2
Union of South Africa[f]	1953-57	2.3	1.8	1.3
United States	1953-57	1.7	1.2	1.4
Uruguay	1955-57	3.5	2.8	1.3

[a] Adjusted to the 1950 census population of the United States.

[b] Sex ratio is computed from rates available to two decimal places.

[c] Yukon and Northwest Territories are included for 1956 and 1957 only.

[d] Jewish population only.

[e] Excludes Maori population.

[f] White population only.

Table A.4.1 Average annual age-adjusted[a] death rates per 100,000 population for multiple sclerosis with male-to-female ratios: selected countries, various years, 1951-58
(ISC code 345)

Country	Years	Rate	M:F ratio
Australia	1954-58	0.7	0.8
Austria	1953-57	1.9	0.7
Belgium	1954-58	2.0	1.1
Canada[b]	1953-57	1.2	1.0
Chile	1956,1958	0.3	1.8
Colombia	1957	0.2	1.8
Czechoslovakia	1953-57	2.0	---
Denmark	1953-57	2.0	0.9
England and Wales	1953-57	1.6	0.7
Finland	1954-58	0.9	1.3
France	1953-57	2.7	1.4
Greece	1956-57	0.3	---
Iceland	1951-55	0.3	1.0
Ireland	1954-58	2.9	0.9
Israel[c]	1956-58	0.5	1.4
Italy	1953-57	0.7	1.1
Japan	1953-57	0.1	1.4
Mexico	1952-56	0.2	1.0
Netherlands	1953-57	2.0	0.8
New Zealand[d]	1952-56	1.2	0.7
Northern Ireland	1951-55	3.3	0.8
Norway	1953-57	1.5	1.1
Philippines	1956-57	0.02	0.3
Portugal	1955-58	1.2	1.8
Scotland	1951-55	3.0	0.8
Sweden	1953-57	1.0	0.9
Switzerland	1953-57	2.2	0.6
Union of South Africa[e]	1953-57	0.1	0.4
United States (white)	1953-57	0.9	0.9
United States (total)	1953-57	0.9	0.9
Uruguay	1955-57	0.6	1.1
West Germany	1953-57	2.1	0.8

Source: Goldberg and Kurland (1962; unpublished data).

[a] Adjusted to the 1950 census population of the United States.

[b] Yukon and N.W. Terr. included for 1956 and 1957 only.

[c] Jewish population only.

[d] Excludes Maori population.

[e] White population only.

Table A.4.2 Deaths and average annual death rates per 100,000 population for multiple sclerosis by age, color and sex: United States, 1959-61
(ISC code 345)

Age	Total			White			Nonwhite		
	Total	Male	Female	Total	Male	Female	Total	Male	Female
	Number of deaths								
All ages	4,305	1,862	2,443	4,044	1,756	2,288	261	106	155
Under 15	14	8	6	13	8	5	1	-	1
15-24	64	21	43	54	19	35	10	2	8
25-34	312	124	188	270	103	167	42	21	21
35-44	898	329	569	822	297	525	76	32	44
45-54	1,200	499	701	1,138	478	660	62	21	41
55-64	950	437	513	903	419	484	47	18	29
65-74	639	326	313	623	317	306	16	9	7
75-84	204	104	100	197	101	96	7	3	4
85 & over	23	14	9	23	14	9	-	-	-
Unknown	1	-	1	1	-	1	-	-	-
	Crude death rate								
All ages	0.8	0.7	0.9	0.8	0.7	0.9	0.4	0.4	0.5
Under 15	0.0*	0.0*	0.0*	0.0*	0.0*	0.0*	0.0*	-	0.0*
15-24	0.1	0.1	0.1	0.1	0.1	0.1	0.1*	0.0*	0.2*
25-34	0.5	0.4	0.5	0.4	0.3	0.5	0.5	0.6	0.5
35-44	1.2	0.9	1.5	1.3	0.9	1.6	1.0	0.9	1.1
45-54	2.0	1.6	2.2	2.1	1.7	2.3	1.0	0.7	1.3
55-64	2.0	1.9	2.1	2.1	2.0	2.2	1.1	0.9*	1.4
65-74	1.9	2.1	1.8	2.0	2.2	1.9	0.6*	0.7*	0.5*
75-84	1.5	1.7	1.3	1.5	1.8	1.3	0.7*	0.7*	0.8*
85 & over	0.8	1.3*	0.5*	0.9	1.4*	0.6*	-	-	-
	Age-adjusted death rate								
All ages	0.8	0.7	0.8	0.8	0.7	0.9	0.5*	0.4*	0.6*
65 & over	1.8	2.0	1.6	1.8	2.1	1.7	0.6*	0.7*	0.6*

Table A.4.3 Average annual death rates per 100,000 population for multiple sclerosis among native born by state of birth and color: United States and each state, 1959-61

(ISC code 345)

State	Total	White	Nonwhite	State	Total	White	Nonwhite
United States	0.8	0.8	0.4				
New England				East North Central			
Maine	1.1	1.1	-	Ohio	1.0	1.0	0.9*
New Hampshire	0.8*	0.8*	-	Michigan	0.8	0.9	0.3*
Vermont	1.5	1.5	-	Indiana	0.8	0.8	0.4*
Massachusetts	1.1	1.2	0.5*	Illinois	1.2	1.2	0.1*
Rhode Island	1.1	1.1	2.2*	Wisconsin	1.2	1.2	-
Connecticut	1.2	1.2	1.3*	West North Central			
Middle Atlantic				Minnesota	1.2	1.2	1.1*
New York	0.9	0.9	0.6*	Iowa	1.2	1.2	-
New Jersey	0.8	0.9	0.7*	North Dakota	1.4	1.4	-
Pennsylvania	1.1	1.1	0.7*	South Dakota	1.4	1.4	-
South Atlantic				Nebraska	1.4	1.4	-
Delaware	1.0*	0.8*	2.1*	Missouri	0.8	0.8	0.1*
Maryland	0.7	0.7	0.6*	Kansas	1.1	1.1	1.2*
Dist. of Col.	0.6*	0.5*	0.7*	Mountain			
Virginia	0.7	0.7	0.5*	Montana	1.2	1.2	-
West Virginia	0.9	0.9	0.9*	Wyoming	1.2*	1.2*	-
North Carolina	0.6	0.6	0.6	Colorado	0.7	0.7	-
South Carolina	0.5	0.5	0.6	New Mexico	0.2*	0.2*	-
Georgia	0.5	0.5	0.4	Idaho	1.0	1.1	-
Florida	0.2*	0.1*	0.3*	Utah	0.9	0.9	-
East South Central				Arizona	0.2*	0.2*	-
Kentucky	0.5	0.5	0.6*	Nevada	0.7*	0.8*	-
Tennessee	0.6	0.6	0.8*	Pacific			
Alabama	0.4	0.5	0.4*	Washington	1.0	1.0	0.6*
Mississippi	0.4	0.5	0.4*	Oregon	1.0	1.0	-
West South Central				California	0.4	0.4	-
Louisiana	0.3	0.3*	0.2*	Alaska	-	-	-
Texas	0.4	0.4	0.3*	Hawaii	0.2*	0.5*	0.1*
Arkansas	0.4	0.4	0.4*				
Oklahoma	0.4	0.5	0.1*				

Table A.4.4 Average annual age-adjusted death rates per 100,000 population, all ages and 65 and over, for multiple sclerosis by color: United States and census regions, 1959-61

(ISC code 345)

Region of residence at death	Total		White		Nonwhite	
	All ages	65 & over	All ages	65 & over	All ages	65 & over
United States	0.8	1.8	0.8	1.8	0.5*	0.6*
New England	1.0	1.8*	1.0	1.9*	1.0*	-
Middle Atlantic	0.9	1.7	0.9	1.7	0.8*	0.9*
East North Central	0.9	2.1	1.0	2.1	0.5*	0.9*
West North Central	0.9	2.5	0.9	2.6	0.6*	1.4*
South Atlantic	0.6	1.3*	0.6*	1.4*	0.5*	0.5*
East South Central	0.5*	1.0*	0.5*	1.0*	0.5*	0.9*
West South Central	0.4*	1.1*	0.4*	1.2*	0.4*	0.1*
Mountain	0.9*	2.5*	0.9*	2.6*	0.2*	-
Pacific	0.8	1.9	0.8	2.1	0.2*	0.4*

Table A.4.5 Average annual crude death rates per 100,000 population for multiple sclerosis by region of birth and death, native born: United States and census regions, 1959-61 (ISC code 345)

Region of death	Total, death regions	Region of birth								
		NE	MA	ENC	WNC	SA	ESC	WSC	M	P
Total (birth regions)	0.8	1.1	1.0	1.0	1.1	0.6	0.5	0.4	0.7	0.5
New England (NE)	1.1	1.1	1.4	0.7*	0.6*	1.1*	-	-	-	0.8*
Mid. Atlantic (MA)	0.9	1.6	1.0	1.6	2.5*	0.8	1.2*	0.5*	1.4*	0.3*
E. No. Central (ENC)	0.9	1.0*	1.1	1.0	1.4	1.0	0.5	0.3*	2.2*	2.0*
W. No. Central (WNC)	0.9	2.4*	1.2*	1.7	0.9	0.9*	0.6*	0.5*	0.9*	0.8*
So. Atlantic (SA)	0.6	1.4*	0.8	1.3	0.5*	0.5	0.5*	0.5*	1.4*	0.7*
E. So. Central (ESC)	0.5	-	0.3*	0.7*	0.7*	0.5	0.5	0.1*	-	-
W. So. Central (WSC)	0.4	0.6*	0.2*	0.6*	0.9*	0.5*	0.9*	0.3	-	0.2*
Mountain (M)	0.8	1.2*	0.9*	1.7	1.7	0.6*	1.2*	0.6*	0.6	0.6*
Pacific (P)	0.8	1.2*	1.0	1.4	1.6	0.4*	0.6*	0.6	1.0	0.5

Table A.4.6 Deaths from multiple sclerosis, 1959-61, among native born by region of birth and region of death, and 3-year total populations (in thousands) in each region by birthplace based on 1960 census: United States and census regions
(ISC code 345)

	Region of birth						
	Northern tier				Southern tier		
Region of death	NE	MA	ENC	WNC	SA	ESC	WSC
Northern tier							
New England							
Deaths	265	24	3	1	6	-	-
Population (000's)	23,962	1,725	402	172	556	129	121
Middle Atlantic							
Deaths	24	738	25	13	36	8	2
Population (000's)	1,540	77,619	1,585	511	4,372	683	380
East North Central							
Deaths	5	34	774	45	32	32	5
Population (000's)	492	3,069	81,382	3,206	3,114	6,234	1,617
West North Central							
Deaths	3	5	41	356	3	4	7
Population (000's)	126	403	2,359	37,776	339	705	1,461
Southern tier							
South Atlantic							
Deaths	14	31	36	4	328	16	4
Population (000's)	1,035	4,059	2,686	875	60,983	2,953	801
East South Central							
Deaths	-	1	6	2	7	146	1
Population (000's)	84	286	857	273	1,292	31,730	689
West South Central							
Deaths	1	1	7	15	4	17	139
Population (000's)	166	531	1,097	1,691	792	1,921	41,367

Table A.4.7 Average annual age-adjusted death rates per 100,000 population for multiple sclerosis by sex and type of county: United States and census regions, 1959-61
(ISC code 345)

	Metropolitan counties			Nonmetropolitan counties		
Region	Total	Male	Female	Total	Male	Female
United States	0.8	0.7	0.9	0.8	0.6	0.8
New England	1.0*	1.0*	1.1*	0.9*	0.7*	1.1*
Middle Atlantic	0.9	0.8*	0.9*	1.0*	0.9*	1.2*
East North Central	0.9	0.8*	1.1*	0.9*	0.8*	1.0*
West North Central	0.8*	0.7*	0.9*	1.0*	0.8*	1.1*
South Atlantic	0.6*	0.5*	0.7*	0.6*	0.6*	0.6*
East South Central	0.4*	0.4*	0.5*	0.5*	0.5*	0.5*
West South Central	0.3*	0.4*	0.4*	0.4*	0.4*	0.4*
Mountain	0.9*	0.7*	1.1*	0.9*	0.9*	0.9*
Pacific	0.8*	0.7*	0.8*	0.7*	0.5*	0.9*

Table A.4.8 Deaths and average annual crude death rates per 100,000 population for multiple sclerosis, foreign-born white residents, by country of birth: United States, 1959-61
(ISC code 345)

Place of birth	Deaths	Rate		
		Total	Male	Female
Total foreign born, nativity known	349[a]	1.3	1.4	1.1
Ireland	29	2.9	4.4*	1.8*
Austria	21	2.3	2.6*	2.0*
Rumania	5	2.0*	1.6*	2.4*
Portugal	3	1.8*	1.1*	2.6*
Norway	8	1.7*	1.7*	1.9*
Sweden	11	1.7*	1.8*	1.6*
Germany	47	1.6	1.8	1.4
Lithuania	6	1.6*	1.1*	2.1*
Canada	46	1.6	2.1	1.3
France	5	1.5*	2.4*	1.0*
Czechoslovakia	10	1.5*	2.2*	0.8*
USSR	27	1.3	0.9*	1.7*
United Kingdom	30	1.2	1.4*	1.0*
Denmark	3	1.2*	2.1*	-
Poland	28	1.2	1.4*	1.1*
Finland	2	1.0*	1.1*	0.9*
Italy	36	1.0	1.1	0.8*
Greece	3	0.6*	0.7*	0.6*
Switzerland	1	0.5*	-	1.1*
Hungary	4	0.5*	0.6*	0.5*
Mexico	8	0.5*	0.5*	0.4*
Netherlands	1	0.3*	0.5*	-
Yugoslavia	-	-	-	-
Other Europe	5	0.8*	0.6*	1.1*
Asia	5	0.8*	0.9*	0.7*
South-Central America	1[b]	0.1*	-	0.3*
All other	4	1.8*	1.8*	1.4*

[a] Excludes three nonwhites (rate 0.2; total rate = 1.2).

[b] Excludes three nonwhites (1.0); total (white plus nonwhite) crude rate of 0.4 with 0.2 male and 0.6 female.

Table A.5.1 Average annual age-adjusted[a] death rates per 100,000 population for motor neuron disease by sex: selected countries, various years, 1951-58
(ISC code 356)

Country	Years	Male	Female	M:F ratio[b]
Australia	1954-58	1.2	0.7	1.8
Belgium	1954-58	0.8	0.4	1.9
Canada[c]	1953-57	0.9	0.5	1.7
Chile	1956,1958	0.3	0.2	1.5
Denmark	1953-57	1.1	0.7	1.5
England-Wales	1953-57	1.2	0.7	1.8
Finland	1954-58	0.8	0.4	1.9
France	1953-57	0.6	0.4	1.4
Iceland	1951-55	1.2	0.9	1.4
Ireland	1954-58	1.3	0.4	2.9
Israel[d]	1956-58	0.5	0.2	2.0
Italy	1953-57	1.3	0.6	2.1
Japan	1953-57	1.0	0.5	2.0
Mexico	1956	0.1	0.1	1.2
Netherlands	1953-57	1.5	0.9	1.6
New Zealand[e]	1952-56	1.2	0.9	1.3
Norway	1953-57	1.2	0.9	1.4
Scotland	1951-55	1.4	0.6	2.3
Sweden	1953-57	1.1	0.5	2.1
Switzerland	1953-57	1.3	1.0	1.4
Union of South Africa[f]	1953-57	0.3	0.3	1.4
United States (white)	1953-57	0.8	0.5	1.7
United States (nonwhite)	1953-57	0.6	0.3	1.9
United States (total)	1953-57	0.8	0.5	1.7
Uruguay	1955-57	0.6	0.4	1.5

[a]Adjusted to the 1950 census population of the United States.

[b]Sex ratio is computed from rates available to two decimal places.

[c]Yukon and Northwest Territories were included in 1956 and 1957 only.

[d]Jewish population only.

[e]Excludes Maori population.

[f]White population only.

Table A.5.2 Death rates per 100,000 population for amyotrophic lateral sclerosis and for progressive muscular atrophy by color and sex: United States, selected years, 1949-64

(ISC codes 356.1 and 356.0)

Cause of death and year	Total	White		Nonwhite	
		Male	Female	Male	Female
ALS + PMA[a]					
1949	0.7	0.9	0.6	0.3	0.3
1954	0.6	0.8	0.5	0.4	0.2*
1959	0.7	0.9	0.5	0.4	0.2
1964	0.7	0.8	0.6	0.5	0.4
ALS (356.1)					
1949	0.4	0.6	0.3	0.2*	0.1*
1954	0.5	0.6	0.4	0.2*	0.1*
1959	0.6	0.8	0.4	0.3	0.2
1964	0.6	0.8	0.5	0.4	0.3
PMA (356.0)					
1949	0.2	0.3	0.2	0.1*	0.2*
1954	0.2	0.2	0.1	0.2*	0.1*
1959	0.1	0.1	0.1	0.1*	0.0*
1964	0.1	0.1	0.1	0.0*	0.0*

[a]The rates shown for this combined category do not always agree with the sum of the individual rates for ALS and PMA due to rounding. The total rates for all motor neuron disease (ISC code 356) are essentially the same as those for this combined category.

Table A.5.3 Deaths and average annual death rates per 100,000 population for amyotrophic lateral sclerosis by age, color and sex: United States, 1959-61

(ISC code 356.1)

Age	Total			White			Nonwhite		
	Total	Male	Female	Total	Male	Female	Total	Male	Female
Number of deaths									
All ages	3,149	2,007	1,142	2,987	1,904	1,083	162	103	59
Under 15	2	-	2	2	-	2	-	-	-
15-24	8	5	3	7	5	2	1	-	1
25-34	39	28	11	33	24	9	6	4	2
35-44	199	143	56	178	132	46	21	11	10
45-54	612	391	221	569	364	205	43	27	16
55-64	1,038	647	391	990	617	373	48	30	18
65-74	989	627	362	955	603	352	34	24	10
75-84	248	155	93	240	149	91	8	6	2
85 & over	14	11	3	13	10	3	1	1	-
Death rate									
All ages	0.6	0.8	0.4	0.6	0.8	0.4	0.3	0.3	0.2
Under 15	0.0*	-	0.0*	0.0*	-	0.0*	-	-	-
15-24	0.0*	0.0*	0.0*	0.0*	0.0*	0.0*	0.0*	-	0.0*
25-34	0.1	0.1	0.0*	0.1	0.1	0.0*	0.1*	0.1*	0.0*
35-44	0.3	0.4	0.2	0.3	0.4	0.1	0.3	0.3*	0.3*
45-54	1.0	1.3	0.7	1.0	1.3	0.7	0.7	0.9	0.5*
55-64	2.2	2.9	1.6	2.3	3.0	1.7	1.1	1.5	0.8*
65-74	3.0	4.1	2.1	3.1	4.3	2.2	1.3	1.9	0.7*
75-84	1.8	2.6	1.2	1.9	2.6	1.2	0.8*	1.3*	0.4*
85 & over	0.5*	1.0*	0.2*	0.5*	1.0*	0.2*	0.5*	1.1*	-

APPENDIX / 353

Table A.5.4 Deaths and average annual age-adjusted death rates per 100,000 population, all ages and age 65 and over, for amyotrophic lateral sclerosis: United States and each state, 1959-61 (ISC code 356.1)

State	65 and over Deaths	65 and over Rate	All ages Deaths	All ages Rate	State	65 and over Deaths	65 and over Rate	All ages Deaths	All ages Rate
United States	1,251	2.6	3,149	0.5					
Alaska	-	-	1	0.3*	Washington	21	2.5*	53	0.6*
Alabama	7	0.9*	34	0.4*	Arizona	7	2.6*	18	0.5*
South Carolina	5	1.1*	26	0.4*	Kentucky	22	2.6*	46	0.4*
Georgia	10	1.2*	39	0.4*	Pennsylvania	85	2.6*	194	0.5*
Mississippi	8	1.4*	24	0.4*	New York	137	2.7	342	0.5*
Tennessee	13	1.5*	50	0.4*	Missouri	41	2.8*	92	0.6*
Louisiana	11	1.6*	33	0.4*	Ohio	75	2.8	190	0.6*
Arkansas	9	1.6*	22	0.4*	Utah	5	2.9*	12	0.5*
Rhode Island	4	1.6*	17	0.6*	Kansas	21	3.0*	40	0.5*
Maryland	11	1.7*	40	0.4*	Oregon	16	3.0*	40	0.6*
North Carolina	17	1.8*	61	0.5*	Connecticut	22	3.1*	47	0.5*
West Virginia	9	1.8*	19	0.3*	Massachusetts	51	3.1*	101	0.5*
Nebraska	9	1.9*	33	0.7*	Michigan	60	3.2*	149	0.6*
Idaho	3	1.9*	7	0.4*	Minnesota	33	3.2	89	0.7*
South Dakota	4	2.0*	13	0.6*	Montana	6	3.2*	14	0.6*
New Mexico	3	2.1*	10	0.4*	New Jersey	53	3.2*	123	0.6*
Florida	36	2.2*	83	0.5*	Dist. of Col.	7	3.5*	12	0.4*
Texas	48	2.2*	130	0.4*	Vermont	4	3.5*	9	0.7*
North Dakota	4	2.3*	9	0.4*	Wisconsin	42	3.6*	93	0.6*
Maine	7	2.3*	20	0.6*	Nevada	2	3.7*	4	0.5*
Illinois	69	2.4*	191	0.5*	Iowa	36	3.9*	87	0.9*
Virginia	20	2.4*	52	0.5*	Colorado	22	4.7*	36	0.6*
California	102	2.5*	276	0.5*	Wyoming	4	5.4*	10	1.0*
Indiana	32	2.5*	82	0.5*	Hawaii	5	5.9*	13	0.9*
New Hampshire	5	2.5*	10	0.4*	Delaware	9	8.7*	12	0.8*
Oklahoma	19	2.5*	41	0.5*					

Table A.5.5 Deaths and average annual death rates per 100,000 population for motor neuron disease by place of birth for foreign-born residents by sex, with male-female ratio of rates: United States, 1959-61
(ISC code 356)

Place of birth	Deaths[a]			Rate			M:F ratio
	Total	Male	Female	Total	Male	Female	
All foreign born	516	335	181	1.8	2.3	1.2	1.9
United Kingdom	41	27	14	1.6	2.5	1.0*	2.5
Ireland	21	10	11	2.1	2.5*	1.8*	1.4
Norway	19	15	4	4.1*	6.2*	1.9*	3.3
Sweden	20	13	7	3.1	3.9*	2.3*	1.7
Denmark	3	1	2	1.2*	0.7*	1.8*	0.4
Netherlands	7	3	4	2.0*	1.6*	2.5*	0.6
Switzerland	2	1	1	1.1*	1.1*	1.1*	1.0
France	2	-	2	0.6*	-	1.0*	-
Germany	47	29	18	1.6	2.2	1.1*	2.0
Poland	54	36	18	2.4	3.3	1.6*	2.1
Czechoslovakia	19	13	6	2.8*	4.1*	1.6*	2.6
Austria	20	14	6	2.2	3.3*	1.2*	2.8
Hungary	6	4	2	0.8*	1.1*	0.5*	2.2
Yugoslavia	10	8	2	2.0*	2.9*	0.9*	3.2
USSR	58	40	18	2.8	3.9	1.7*	2.3
Lithuania	5	2	3	1.4*	1.1*	1.6*	0.7
Finland	4	-	4	2.0*	-	3.5*	-
Rumania	3	2	1	1.2*	1.6*	0.8*	2.0
Greece	9	7	2	1.9*	2.4*	1.1*	2.2
Italy	75	55	20	2.0	2.7	1.2	2.3
Portugal	2	2	-	1.2*	2.1*	-	-
Other Europe	9	5	4	1.5*	1.6*	1.4*	1.1
Asia	19	14	5	1.3*	1.6*	0.8*	2.0
Canada	42	21	21	1.5	1.7	1.3	1.3
Mexico	10	8	2	0.6*	0.9*	0.2*	4.5
Other America	5	2	3	0.5*	0.4*	0.6*	0.7
All other	4	3	1	1.6*	2.7*	0.7*	3.9
Unknown	18	11	7	-	-	-	-

[a] Only 16 of these deaths refer to nonwhites (12 Asians, 3 other American, and 1 all other), and in 1, nativity was unknown.

APPENDIX / 355

Table A.7.1 Deaths and average annual death rates for myasthenia gravis per 1,000,000 population by age, color and sex: United States, 1959-61
(ISC code 744.0)

Age	Total			White			Nonwhite		
	Total	Male	Female	Total	Male	Female	Total	Male	Female
				Number of deaths					
All ages	675	269	406	567	234	333	108	35	73
Under 1	7	6	1	7	6	1	-	-	-
1-4	4	2	2	2	2	-	2	-	2
5-14	18	4	14	12	3	9	6	1	5
15-24	33	7	26	22	2	20	11	5	6
25-34	55	15	40	30	7	23	25	8	17
35-44	72	21	51	50	15	35	22	6	16
45-54	84	22	62	70	19	51	14	3	11
55-64	135	61	74	118	54	64	17	7	10
65-74	163	77	86	157	75	82	6	2	4
75-84	89	48	41	86	46	40	3	2	1
85 & over	15	6	9	13	5	8	2	1	1
				Death rate					
All ages	1.3	1.0	1.5	1.2	1.0	1.4	1.8	1.2	2.3
Under 1	0.6*	1.0*	0.2*	0.7*	1.1*	0.2*	-	-	-
1-4	0.1*	0.1*	0.1*	0.0*	0.1*	-	0.3*	-	0.6*
5-14	0.2*	0.1*	0.3*	0.1*	0.1*	0.2*	0.4*	0.1*	0.7*
15-24	0.5	0.2*	0.7	0.3	0.1*	0.6	1.2*	1.2*	1.3*
25-34	0.8	0.4*	1.1	0.5	0.2*	0.8	3.1	2.2*	4.0*
35-44	1.0	0.6	1.4	0.8	0.5*	1.1	2.9	1.7*	4.0*
45-54	1.4	0.7	2.0	1.3	0.7*	1.8	2.3*	1.0*	3.6*
55-64	2.9	2.7	3.0	2.8	2.6	2.9	4.1*	3.4*	4.7*
65-74	4.9	5.0	4.9	5.2	5.3	5.0	2.3*	1.6*	2.9*
75-84	6.4	7.9	5.2	6.6	8.2	5.5	3.1*	4.4*	2.0*
85 & over	5.4*	5.5*	5.3*	5.1*	5.0*	5.1*	9.3*	10.6*	8.3*

Table A.7.2 Average annual age-adjusted death rates per 1,000,000 population for myasthenia gravis by color, sex and type of county: United States and census regions, 1959-61
(ISC code 744.0)

Region and color	Metropolitan counties			Nonmetropolitan counties		
	Total	Male	Female	Total	Male	Female
United States	1.1	0.9*	1.4	1.2*	1.0*	1.4*
Region						
New England	1.1*	1.0*	1.2*	1.5*	1.1*	1.9*
Middle Atlantic	1.2*	0.7*	1.7*	1.1*	0.9*	1.4*
East North Central	1.2*	1.0*	1.5*	1.1*	1.0*	1.2*
West North Central	1.1*	1.2*	1.0*	1.2*	1.0*	1.4*
South Atlantic	1.0*	0.8*	1.1*	1.2*	1.2*	1.3*
East South Central	1.6*	1.5*	1.8*	1.0*	0.9*	1.2*
West South Central	1.1*	0.8*	1.4*	1.3*	0.9*	1.6*
Mountain	0.6*	0.5*	0.7*	0.9*	0.4*	1.3*
Pacific	1.0*	0.8*	1.2*	1.2*	1.0*	1.5*
Color						
White	1.0*	0.8*	1.2*	1.1*	0.9*	1.3*
Nonwhite	2.2*	1.4*	2.9*	1.7*	1.5*	1.9*

Table A.7.3 Average annual age-adjusted death rates per 1,000,000 population age 65 and over for myasthenia gravis by color, sex and type of county: United States and census regions, 1959-61
(ISC code 744.0)

Region and color	Metropolitan counties			Nonmetropolitan counties		
	Total	Male	Female	Total	Male	Female
United States	4.6	5.0	4.2	6.5	6.8	6.2*
Region						
New England	5.1*	5.5*	4.9*	6.8*	11.9*	2.7*
Middle Atlantic	4.3*	4.2*	4.4*	5.8*	4.7*	6.7*
East North Central	4.7*	5.9*	3.8*	7.0*	8.6*	5.6*
West North Central	5.8*	7.4*	4.5*	8.6*	7.2*	10.0*
South Atlantic	3.3*	5.2*	1.8*	5.6*	6.6*	4.6*
East South Central	7.1*	9.5*	5.4*	6.7*	7.3*	6.3*
West South Central	6.3*	3.6*	8.5*	5.8*	5.4*	6.2*
Mountain	-	-	-	5.6*	6.5*	4.7*
Pacific	4.7*	4.7*	4.6*	3.8*	2.7*	5.0*
Color						
White	4.7	5.3	4.2	6.9	7.1	6.8*
Nonwhite	3.7*	2.0*	5.1*	1.5*	3.2*	-

Table A.8.1 Deaths and average annual death rates per 100,000 population for Down's syndrome by age, color and sex: United States, 1959-61 (ISC code 325.4)

Age	Total			White			Nonwhite		
	Total	Male	Female	Total	Male	Female	Total	Male	Female
	Number of deaths								
All ages	871	454	417	801	415	386	70	39	31
Under 1	528	272	256	480	247	233	48	25	23
1-4	178	90	88	164	81	83	14	9	5
5-14	63	38	25	58	35	23	5	3	2
15-24	20	14	6	19	13	6	1	1	-
25-34	25	11	14	23	10	13	2	1	1
35-44	19	9	10	19	9	10	-	-	-
45-54	20	10	10	20	10	10	-	-	-
55-64	13	7	6	13	7	6	-	-	-
65-74	4	2	2	4	2	2	-	-	-
75-84	1	1	-	1	1	-	-	-	-
85 & over	-	-	-	-	-	-	-	-	-
	Death rate								
All ages									
Crude	0.2	0.2	0.2	0.2	0.2	0.2	0.1	0.1	0.1
Age adjusted	0.1	0.1*	0.1*	0.1*	0.1*	0.1*	0.1*	0.1*	0.1*
Under 1	4.3	4.3	4.2	4.6	4.6	4.5	2.6	2.7	2.5
1-4	0.4	0.4	0.4	0.4	0.4	0.4	0.2*	0.3*	0.1*
5-14	0.1	0.1	0.0	0.1	0.1	0.1	0.0*	0.0*	0.0*
15 & over	0.0	0.0	0.0	0.0	0.0	0.0	0.0*	0.0*	0.0*

Table A.8.2 Deaths from Down's syndrome by age, color and sex: each census region, United States, 1959-61
(ISC code 325.4)

Census region and age	Total			White			Nonwhite		
	Total	Male	Female	Total	Male	Female	Total	Male	Female
New England									
All ages	62	35	27	61	34	27	1	1	-
Under 1	32	19	13	32	19	13	-	-	-
Under 15	51	28	23	50	27	23	1	1	-
Middle Atlantic									
All ages	163	85	78	150	76	74	13	9	4
Under 1	103	53	50	95	47	48	8	6	2
Under 15	145	73	72	132	64	68	13	9	4
East North Central									
All ages	186	103	83	176	96	80	10	7	3
Under 1	109	53	56	103	49	54	6	4	2
Under 15	160	87	73	151	81	70	9	6	3
West North Central									
All ages	95	51	44	94	50	44	1	1	-
Under 1	46	29	17	45	28	17	1	1	-
Under 15	77	43	34	76	42	34	1	1	-
South Atlantic									
All ages	121	59	62	98	51	47	23	8	15
Under 1	76	39	37	60	34	26	16	5	11
Under 15	108	53	55	87	46	41	21	7	14
East South Central									
All ages	54	22	32	50	18	32	4	4	-
Under 1	34	13	21	31	10	21	3	3	-
Under 15	54	22	32	50	18	32	4	4	-
West South Central									
All ages	80	38	42	67	31	36	13	7	6
Under 1	54	25	29	44	20	24	10	5	5
Under 15	74	37	37	61	30	31	13	7	6
Mountain									
All ages	32	17	15	31	17	14	1	-	1
Under 1	21	11	10	20	11	9	1	-	1
Under 15	29	16	13	28	16	12	1	-	1
Pacific									
All ages	78	44	34	74	42	32	4	2	2
Under 1	53	30	23	50	29	21	3	1	2
Under 15	71	41	30	67	39	28	4	2	2

Table A.8.3 Deaths and average annual death rates per 100,000 population under one year of age and deaths all ages for Down's syndrome: United States and each state, 1959-61
(ISC code 325.4)

State	Deaths All ages	Deaths Under one year	Rate under one year	State	Deaths All ages	Deaths Under one year	Rate under one year
United States	871	528	4.3				
Nevada	3	3	14.5*	Wyoming	1	1	4.0*
South Dakota	6	5	9.7*	Colorado	6	5	3.9*
Kentucky	24	18	8.6*	Arizona	7	4	3.9*
Wisconsin	41	22	7.6	Vermont	2	1	3.7*
West Virginia	15	8	6.9*	Florida	20	12	3.6*
Minnesota	41	17	6.6*	Rhode Island	7	2	3.6*
Virginia	20	17	6.1*	Pennsylvania	45	25	3.5
Maine	5	4	6.0*	Missouri	16	10	3.5*
Maryland	20	13	5.9*	Oklahoma	9	5	3.4*
Montana	5	3	5.9*	Indiana	12	10	3.1*
New Jersey	33	22	5.7	Delaware	1	1	3.0*
New York	85	56	5.4	Alabama	13	7	2.9*
Connecticut	16	9	5.4*	Tennessee	13	7	2.9*
Louisiana	18	14	5.3*	South Carolina	11	5	2.8*
Massachusetts	30	16	4.8*	Illinois	35	19	2.7*
Michigan	45	27	4.7	Kansas	13	4	2.7*
North Carolina	25	15	4.7*	New Mexico	2	2	2.3*
Alaska	2	1	4.7*	Washington	9	4	2.1*
Ohio	53	31	4.6	North Dakota	1	1	2.0*
Oregon	10	5	4.6*	Dist. of Col.	1	1	2.0*
Iowa	16	8	4.3*	Hawaii	1	1	2.0*
Arkansas	7	5	4.2*	Georgia	8	4	1.4*
Texas	46	30	4.2	Utah	4	1	1.3*
California	56	42	4.0	Mississippi	4	2	1.2*
Idaho	4	2	4.0*	Nebraska	2	1	1.0*
				New Hampshire	2	-	-

Table A.8.4 Composition of 24-center WHO cooperative study on congenital malformations among births, 1961-64

Country and city	Locus		Number of single births		Sets of multiple births	
	Lat.	Long.	Total	Stillborn	Twins	Triplets
Total			416,695	10,091	5,022	63[a]
Australia						
Melbourne (1)	37°S	145°E	7,844	169	98	2
Melbourne (2)	37°S	145°E	3,921	58	64	2
Brazil						
São Paulo	24°S	47°W	14,421	511	211	2
Chile						
Santiago	33°S	70°W	23,720	635	242	4
Colombia						
Bogotá	5°N	74°W	18,812	404	165	-
Medellín	6°N	75°W	20,459	268	193	3
Czechoslovakia[b]						
Prague et al.	50°W	13-18°E	20,074	196	170	3
United Arab Rep. (Egypt)						
Alexandria	31°N	30°E	9,598	788	391	7
Hong Kong						
Hong Kong[c]	22°N	114°E	9,872	137	126	3
India						
Bombay	19°N	73°E	39,498	1,729	490	5
Calcutta	22°N	88°E	19,191	887	269	5
Malaysia						
Kuala Lumpur	3°N	102°E	15,937	402	188	3
Singapore[d]	1°N	104°E	39,683	489	311	3
Mexico						
Mexico City (1)	19°N	99°W	24,700	386	291	1
Mexico City (2)	19°N	99°W	14,083	7	---	---
Northern Ireland						
Belfast	55°N	6°W	28,091	953	545	7
Panama						
Panama City	9°N	79°W	15,852	278	148	1
Philippines						
Manila	14°N	121°E	29,669	614	313	6[a]
Republic of So. Africa						
Cape Town[e]	34°S	18°E	3,051	113	40	1
Johannesburg[f]	26°S	28°E	11,176	205	124	1
Pretoria[g]	25°S	28°E	10,025	259	197	2
Spain						
Madrid	40°N	4°W	19,714	411	252	1
Yugoslavia						
Ljubljana	46°N	14°E	8,888	98	112	-
Zagreb	45°N	16°E	8,416	94	82	1

[a] Also one set of quadruplets.
[b] 5 centers.
[c] Chinese.
[d] More than one-half Chinese.
[e] Colored.
[f] White.
[g] Bantu.

Table A.9.1 Average annual age-adjusted[a] death rates per 100,000 population for monstrosity by sex: selected countries, various years, 1951-58
(ISC code 750)

Country	Years	Male	Female	M:F ratio[b]
Australia	1954-58	0.5	0.7	0.8
Belgium	1954-58	0.8	0.9	0.9
Canada[c]	1953-57	0.6	0.9	0.7
Denmark	1953-57	0.3	0.4	0.6
England and Wales	1953-57	0.3	0.5	0.6
Finland	1954-58	0.7	1.0	0.7
France	1953-57	0.1	0.1	0.8
Iceland	1951-55	0.2	0.7	0.3
Ireland	1954-58	0.7	1.8	0.4
Israel[d]	1956-58	0.3	0.9	0.4
Italy	1953-57	0.4	0.5	0.8
Japan	1953-57	0.03	0.02	1.5
Mexico	1956	0.1	0.1	0.8
Netherlands	1953-57	0.7	1.4	0.5
New Zealand[e]	1952-56	0.4	0.3	1.3
Norway	1953-57	0.3	0.3	1.1
Scotland	1951-55	0.3	0.5	0.5
Sweden	1953-57	0.4	0.5	0.9
Switzerland	1953-57	0.4	0.5	0.8
Union of So. Africa[f]	1953-57	0.1	0.3	0.2
United States (total)	1953-57	0.5	0.7	0.7
White	1953-57	0.5	0.8	0.7
Nonwhite	1953-57	0.2	0.4	0.7
Uruguay	1955-57	0.5	0.3	1.6

[a] Adjusted to the 1950 census population of the United States.

[b] Sex ratio computed from rates available to two decimal places.

[c] Yukon and Northwest Territories were included in 1956 and 1957 only.

[d] Jewish population only.

[e] Excludes Maori population.

[f] White population only.

Table A.9.2 Average annual age-adjusted[a] death rates per 100,000 population for spina bifida and meningocele by sex: selected countries, various years, 1951-58 (ISC code 751)

Country	Years	Male	Female	M:F ratio[b]
Australia	1954-58	0.9	1.2	0.7
Austria	1953-57	1.1	1.5	0.8
Belgium	1954-58	1.2	1.6	0.7
Canada[c]	1953-57	2.3	3.2	0.7
Colombia	1957	0.4	0.3	1.2
Denmark	1953-57	1.0	1.3	0.8
England and Wales	1953-57	2.6	3.8	0.7
Finland	1954-58	1.0	1.1	0.9
France	1953-57	0.5	0.6	0.8
Iceland	1951-55	1.5	0.9	1.6
Ireland	1954-58	2.8	4.0	0.7
Israel[d]	1956-58	1.5	1.9	0.8
Italy	1953-57	1.5	2.0	0.7
Japan	1953-57	0.2	0.2	1.0
Mexico	1956	0.5	0.6	0.9
Netherlands	1953-57	1.7	2.5	0.7
New Zealand				
European	1952-56	1.4	1.5	0.9
Maori	1952-56	0.3	0.4	0.9
Northern Ireland	1951-55	3.0	4.6	0.7
Norway	1953-57	0.8	1.0	0.8
Philippines	1956-57	0.04	0.03	1.3
Portugal	1955-58	0.9	0.9	1.0
Scotland	1951-55	2.5	4.3	0.6
Sweden	1953-57	0.8	1.1	0.7
Switzerland	1953-57	1.1	1.7	0.7
Union of So. Africa[e]	1953-57	0.6	0.7	0.8
United States (total)	1953-57	0.7	1.0	0.7
White	1953-57	0.8	1.1	0.7
Nonwhite	1953-57	0.4	0.4	1.0
Uruguay	1955-57	0.9	1.2	0.8
West Germany	1953-57	1.6	2.5	0.7

[a] Adjusted to the 1950 census population of the United States.
[b] Sex ratio computed from rates available to two decimal places.
[c] Yukon and Northwest Territories were included in 1956 and 1957 only.
[d] Jewish population only.
[e] White population only.

Table A.9.3 Average annual age-adjusted[a] death rates per 100,000 population for congenital hydrocephalus by sex: selected countries, various years, 1951-58
(ISC code 752)

Country	Years	Male	Female	M:F ratio[b]
Australia	1954-58	0.9	0.7	1.3
Belgium	1954-58	1.4	1.3	1.1
Canada[c]	1953-57	1.1	1.2	1.0
Denmark	1953-57	0.7	0.6	1.1
England and Wales	1953-57	0.6	0.6	1.0
Finland	1954-58	1.0	0.9	1.2
France	1953-57	0.5	0.5	1.2
Iceland	1951-55	0.2	0.7	0.3
Ireland	1954-58	1.8	1.9	1.0
Israel[d]	1956-58	1.5	1.1	1.3
Italy	1953-57	0.6	0.5	1.2
Japan	1953-57	0.3	0.2	1.4
Mexico	1956	0.4	0.4	1.0
Netherlands	1953-57	1.1	1.2	0.9
New Zealand[e]	1952-56	1.0	1.0	1.0
Norway	1953-57	0.8	0.6	1.3
Scotland	1951-55	1.5	1.5	1.0
Sweden	1953-57	0.8	0.6	1.4
Switzerland	1953-57	1.0	1.0	1.1
Union of So. Africa[f]	1953-57	1.0	1.1	0.9
United States (total)	1953-57	1.1	1.0	1.0
White	1953-57	1.1	1.0	1.0
Nonwhite	1953-57	1.0	0.8	1.2
Uruguay	1955-57	0.3	0.4	0.7

[a] Adjusted to the 1950 census population of the United States.
[b] Sex ratio computed from rates available to two decimal places.
[c] Yukon and Northwest Territories were included in 1956 and 1957 only.
[d] Jewish population only.
[e] Excludes Maori population.
[f] White population only.

Table A.9.4 Average annual age-adjusted[a] death rates per 100,000 population for other congenital malformations of the nervous system by sex: selected countries, various years, 1951-58

(ISC code 753)

Country	Years	Male	Female	M:F ratio[b]
Australia	1954-58	0.5	0.6	0.8
Belgium	1954-58	0.6	0.6	1.0
Canada[c]	1953-57	0.4	0.5	1.0
Denmark	1953-57	0.3	0.4	0.8
England and Wales	1953-57	0.3	0.4	0.9
Finland	1954-58	0.5	0.3	1.5
France	1953-57	0.2	0.2	1.1
Iceland	1951-55	0.2	0.5	0.5
Ireland	1954-58	0.3	0.3	1.2
Israel[d]	1956-58	1.3	0.9	1.4
Italy	1953-57	0.1	0.1	1.2
Japan	1953-57	0.05	0.04	1.3
Mexico	1956	0.1	0.1	0.9
Netherlands	1953-57	0.5	0.4	1.1
New Zealand[e]	1952-56	0.5	0.5	1.1
Norway	1953-57	0.3	0.2	1.4
Scotland	1951-55	0.4	0.5	0.9
Sweden	1953-57	0.3	0.3	1.0
Switzerland	1953-57	0.5	0.3	1.9
Union of So. Africa[f]	1953-57	0.8	1.0	0.8
United States (total)	1953-57	0.5	0.4	1.0
White	1953-57	0.5	0.5	1.0
Nonwhite	1953-57	0.4	0.3	1.2
Uruguay	1955-57	0.2	0.2	1.0

[a]Adjusted to the 1950 census population of the United States.
[b]Sex ratio computed from rates available to two decimal places.
[c]Yukon and Northwest Territories were included in 1956 and 1957 only.
[d]Jewish population only.
[e]Excludes Maori population.
[f]White population only.

Table A.9.5 Deaths and average annual death rates per 100,000 population for monstrosity by age, color and sex: United States, 1959-61
(ISC code 750)

Age	Total			White			Nonwhite		
	Total	Male	Female	Total	Male	Female	Total	Male	Female
	Number of deaths								
All ages	3,290	1,344	1,946	3,067	1,249	1,818	223	95	128
Under 1	3,263	1,331	1,932	3,042	1,237	1,805	221	94	127
1-4	11	5	6	10	4	6	1	1	-
5-14	4	2	2	4	2	2	-	-	-
15-24	2	1	1	2	1	1	-	-	-
25-34	1	1	-	1	1	-	-	-	-
35-44	1	-	1	1	-	1	-	-	-
45-54	1	-	1	-	-	-	1	-	1
55-64	3	1	2	3	1	2	-	-	-
65-74	1	1	-	1	1	-	-	-	-
75-84	2	1	1	2	1	1	-	-	-
85 & over	-	-	-	-	-	-	-	-	-
Unknown	1	1	-	1	1	-	-	-	-
	Death rate								
All ages crude	0.6	0.5	0.7	0.6	0.5	0.8	0.4	0.3	0.4
age adjusted	0.4*	0.3*	0.5*	0.4*	0.4*	0.5*	0.2*	0.2*	0.2*
Under 1	26.5	21.2	31.8	29.0	23.1	35.1	12.0	10.2	13.8
1 & over	0.0	0.0*	0.0*	0.0	0.0*	0.0*	0.0*	0.0*	0.0*

Table A.9.6 Deaths and average annual death rates per 100,000 population for spina bifida and meningocele by age, color and sex: United States, 1959-61

(ISC code 751)

Age	Total			White			Nonwhite		
	Total	Male	Female	Total	Male	Female	Total	Male	Female
	Number of deaths								
All ages	3,737	1,619	2,118	3,454	1,471	1,983	283	148	135
Under 1	3,339	1,455	1,884	3,081	1,321	1,760	258	134	124
1-4	254	100	154	236	89	147	18	11	7
5-14	82	30	52	79	29	50	3	1	2
15-24	41	24	17	40	24	16	1	-	1
25-34	5	2	3	5	2	3	-	-	-
35-44	8	3	5	8	3	5	-	-	-
45-54	3	2	1	3	2	1	-	-	-
55-64	2	2	-	1	1	-	1	1	-
65-74	1	-	1	-	-	-	1	-	1
75-84	2	1	1	1	-	1	1	1	-
85 & over	-	-	-	-	-	-	-	-	-
	Crude death rate								
All ages	0.7	0.6	0.8	0.7	0.6	0.8	0.5	0.5	0.4
Under 1	27.1	23.2	31.1	29.4	24.7	34.2	14.0	14.6	13.4
1-4	0.5	0.4	0.6	0.6	0.4	0.7	0.3*	0.3*	0.2*
Under 5	5.9	5.0	6.8	6.4	5.3	7.5	3.1	3.3	2.9
5-14	0.1	0.1	0.1	0.1	0.1	0.1	0.0*	0.0*	0.0*
Under 15	2.2	1.9	2.5	2.4	2.0	2.8	1.2	1.3	1.2
15-24	0.1	0.1	0.0*	0.1	0.1	0.1*	0.0*	-	0.0*
25 & over	0.0	0.0*	0.0*	0.0*	0.0*	0.0*	0.0*	0.0*	0.0*
	Age-adjusted death rate								
All ages	0.5*	0.4*	0.5*	0.5*	0.4*	0.6*	0.2*	0.2*	0.2*
Under 15	1.9	1.5	2.2	2.1	1.6	2.4	0.9*	0.9*	0.8*

APPENDIX / 367

Table A.9.7 Deaths and average annual death rates per 100,000 population for congenital hydrocephalus by age, color and sex: United States, 1959-61
(ISC code 752)

Age	Total			White			Nonwhite		
	Total	Male	Female	Total	Male	Female	Total	Male	Female
	\multicolumn{9}{c}{Number of deaths}								
All ages	4,790	2,471	2,319	4,118	2,112	2,006	672	359	313
Under 1	3,319	1,675	1,644	2,871	1,439	1,432	448	236	212
1-4	953	500	453	805	424	381	148	76	72
5-14	374	206	168	318	170	148	56	36	20
15-24	74	44	30	63	37	26	11	7	4
25-34	28	20	8	22	17	5	6	3	3
35-44	23	15	8	20	14	6	3	1	2
45-54	5	5	-	5	5	-	-	-	-
55-64	7	3	4	7	3	4	-	-	-
65-74	5	2	3	5	2	3	-	-	-
75-84	-	-	-	-	-	-	-	-	-
85 & over	-	-	-	-	-	-	-	-	-
Unknown	2	1	1	2	1	1	-	-	-
	\multicolumn{9}{c}{Crude death rate}								
All ages	0.9	0.9	0.8	0.9	0.9	0.8	1.1	1.2	1.0
Under 1	26.9	26.7	27.1	27.4	26.9	27.8	24.3	25.7	23.0
1-4	2.0	2.0	1.9	1.9	2.0	1.9	2.1	2.2	2.0
Under 5	7.0	7.0	7.0	7.1	7.0	7.1	6.7	7.0	6.4
5-14	0.4	0.4	0.3	0.3	0.4	0.3	0.4	0.5	0.3
Under 15	2.8	2.8	2.8	2.8	2.8	2.8	2.8	3.0	2.6
15-24	0.1	0.1	0.1	0.1	0.1	0.1	0.1*	0.2*	0.1*
25 & over	0.0	0.0	0.0	0.0	0.0	0.0	0.0*	0.0*	0.0*
	\multicolumn{9}{c}{Age-adjusted death rate}								
All ages	0.6	0.6*	0.6*	0.6	0.6*	0.6*	0.6*	0.7*	0.7*
Under 15	2.5	2.5	2.4	2.4	2.5	2.4	2.3	2.5	2.2

Table A.9.8 Deaths and average annual death rates per 100,000 population for other congenital malformations of the nervous system by age, color and sex: United States, 1959-61

(ISC code 753)

Age	Total			White			Nonwhite		
	Total	Male	Female	Total	Male	Female	Total	Male	Female
	Number of deaths								
All ages	2,631	1,383	1,248	2,312	1,214	1,098	319	169	150
Under 1	1,603	865	738	1,421	765	656	182	100	82
1-4	487	230	257	419	198	221	68	32	36
5-14	280	148	132	241	129	112	39	19	20
15-24	112	65	47	99	57	42	13	8	5
25-34	47	26	21	41	22	19	6	4	2
35-44	43	22	21	40	21	19	3	1	2
45-54	35	16	19	28	12	16	7	4	3
55-64	14	7	7	13	6	7	1	1	-
65-74	8	3	5	8	3	5	-	-	-
75-84	1	-	1	1	-	1	-	-	-
85 & over	1	1	-	1	1	-	-	-	-
	Crude death rate								
All ages	0.5	0.5	0.5	0.5	0.5	0.5	0.5	0.6	0.5
Under 1	13.0	13.8	12.2	13.5	14.3	12.8	9.9	10.9	8.9
1-4	1.0	0.9	1.1	1.0	0.9	1.1	1.0	0.9	1.0
Under 5	3.4	3.5	3.3	3.5	3.6	3.4	2.8	3.0	2.7
5-14	0.3	0.3	0.3	0.3	0.3	0.2	0.3	0.3*	0.3
Under 15	1.4	1.5	1.4	1.4	1.5	1.4	1.3	1.3	1.2
15-24	0.2	0.2	0.1	0.2	0.2	0.1	0.1*	0.2*	0.1*
25 & over	0.0	0.1	0.0	0.0	0.0	0.0	0.1*	0.1*	0.0*
	Age-adjusted death rate								
All ages	0.4	0.4	0.4	0.4	0.4	0.4*	0.3*	0.3*	0.3*
Under 15	1.2	1.2	1.2	1.3	1.3	1.2	1.0	1.1	1.0

Table A.9.9a Number of deaths under one year of age from congenital malformations of the nervous system by type of malformation: United States and each state, 1959-61

(ISC codes 750, 751, 752, 753)

State	ISC code[a]				State	ISC code[a]			
	750	751	752	753		750	751	752	753
United States	3,263	3,339	3,319	1,603					
Alabama	48	87	80	23	Missouri	78	63	80	28
Alaska	3	1	5	5	Montana	9	5	17	8
Arizona	19	27	33	15	Nebraska	28	24	41	19
Arkansas	23	25	26	21	Nevada	6	2	2	1
California	246	182	231	185	New Hampshire	13	17	9	6
Colorado	17	27	22	15	New Jersey	122	100	99	54
Connecticut	67	50	53	38	New Mexico	19	24	12	11
Delaware	16	15	3	3	New York	304	278	326	112
Dist. of Col.	7	8	22	7	North Carolina	71	88	109	47
Florida	71	115	90	46	North Dakota	10	15	8	10
Georgia	63	100	114	22	Ohio	200	192	214	85
Hawaii	21	6	8	6	Oklahoma	28	35	29	23
Idaho	6	7	8	4	Oregon	22	13	29	16
Illinois	186	188	174	82	Pennsylvania	199	221	170	90
Indiana	111	95	99	53	Rhode Island	25	29	13	4
Iowa	47	57	40	29	South Carolina	38	46	43	11
Kansas	35	27	35	21	South Dakota	12	12	12	10
Kentucky	43	78	57	30	Tennessee	56	90	77	18
Louisiana	61	73	53	27	Texas	192	186	162	88
Maine	29	26	18	13	Utah	10	8	17	6
Maryland	69	49	63	32	Vermont	8	8	9	3
Massachusetts	120	117	84	27	Virginia	70	98	105	32
Michigan	166	173	144	76	Washington	40	31	38	28
Minnesota	70	70	63	34	West Virginia	33	54	38	13
Mississippi	20	34	48	18	Wisconsin	103	60	82	45
					Wyoming	3	3	5	3

[a] 750-monstrosity; 751-spina bifida and meningocele; 752-congenital hydrocephalus; 753-other congenital malformations of the nervous system.

370 / APPENDIX

Table A.9.9b Average annual death rates per 100,000 population under one year of age for congenital malformations of the nervous system by type of malformation: United States and each state, 1959-61
(ISC codes 750, 751, 752, 753)

State	ISC code[a]				State	ISC code[a]			
	750	751	752	753		750	751	752	753
United States	26.5	27.1	26.9	13.0					
Alabama	20.2	36.6	33.7	9.7	Missouri	27.4	22.2	28.1	9.8
Alaska	14.1*	4.7*	23.5*	23.5*	Montana	17.7*	9.8*	33.5*	15.7*
Arizona	18.3*	26.0	31.8	14.5*	Nebraska	28.3	24.2	41.4	19.2*
Arkansas	19.5	21.1	22.0	17.8	Nevada	29.0*	9.7*	9.7*	4.8*
California	23.2	17.2	21.8	17.5	New Hampshire	32.1*	42.0*	22.3*	14.8*
Colorado	13.3*	21.1	17.2	11.7*	New Jersey	31.8	26.1	25.8	14.1
Connecticut	40.3	30.1	31.9	22.9	New Mexico	22.0*	27.8	13.9*	12.8*
Delaware	47.4*	44.5*	8.9*	8.9*	New York	29.3	26.8	31.4	10.8
Dist. of Col.	13.7*	15.7*	43.0	13.7*	North Carolina	22.2	27.5	34.1	14.7
Florida	21.4	34.6	27.1	13.9	North Dakota	20.3*	30.5*	16.2*	20.3*
Georgia	21.8	34.5	39.4	7.6	Ohio	29.6	28.4	31.6	12.6
Hawaii	41.5	11.9*	15.8*	11.9*	Oklahoma	19.0	23.8	19.7	15.6
Idaho	12.0*	14.0*	16.0*	8.0*	Oregon	20.3	12.0*	26.8	14.8*
Illinois	26.8	27.1	25.1	11.8	Pennsylvania	28.2	31.3	24.1	12.8
Indiana	34.0	29.1	30.3	16.2	Rhode Island	45.4	52.7	23.6*	7.3*
Iowa	25.1	30.4	21.3	15.5	South Carolina	21.2	25.7	24.0	6.1*
Kansas	23.5	18.1	23.5	14.1	South Dakota	23.4*	23.4*	23.4*	19.5*
Kentucky	20.5	37.3	27.2	14.3	Tennessee	23.5	37.8	32.3	7.6*
Louisiana	23.1	27.7	20.1	10.2	Texas	27.1	26.3	22.9	12.4
Maine	43.7	39.2	27.2*	19.6*	Utah	13.1*	10.5*	22.3*	7.9*
Maryland	31.2	22.2	28.5	14.5	Vermont	29.8*	29.8*	33.6*	11.2*
Massachusetts	36.0	35.1	25.2	8.1	Virginia	25.2	35.3	37.8	11.5
Michigan	28.9	30.1	25.1	13.2	Washington	21.1	16.3	20.0	14.8
Minnesota	27.2	27.2	24.5	13.2	West Virginia	28.6	46.9	33.0	11.3*
Mississippi	11.6	19.8	27.9	10.5*	Wisconsin	35.8	20.9	28.5	15.6
					Wyoming	12.1*	12.1*	20.2*	12.1*

[a] 750-monstrosity; 751-spina bifida and meningocele; 752-congenital hydrocephalus; 753-other congenital malformations of the nervous system.

Table A.9.10 Number of deaths under one year of age from congenital malformations of the nervous system by color, sex and type of malformation: United States and census regions, 1959-61
(ISC codes 750, 751, 752, 753)

Region, color and sex	ISC code[a]				Region, color and sex	ISC code[a]			
	750	751	752	753		750	751	752	753
United States	3,263	3,339	3,319	1,603					
New England	262	247	186	91	East South Central	167	289	262	89
White male	99	92	96	44	White male	62	110	106	29
White female	162	153	79	45	White female	85	153	96	41
Nonwhite male	-	-	5	1	Nonwhite male	9	12	31	11
Nonwhite female	1	2	6	1	Nonwhite female	11	14	29	8
Middle Atlantic	625	599	595	256	West South Central	304	319	270	159
White male	243	255	254	128	White male	105	113	103	75
White female	348	315	278	104	White female	164	160	110	58
Nonwhite male	16	21	31	8	Nonwhite male	15	27	31	16
Nonwhite female	18	8	32	16	Nonwhite female	20	19	26	10
East North Central	766	708	713	341	Mountain	89	103	116	63
White male	293	277	322	154	White male	37	47	52	29
White female	434	384	328	159	White female	48	43	56	26
Nonwhite male	15	19	32	14	Nonwhite male	2	5	5	3
Nonwhite female	24	28	31	14	Nonwhite female	2	8	3	5
West North Central	280	268	279	151	Pacific	332	233	311	240
White male	108	113	134	82	White male	127	101	156	124
White female	162	150	130	63	White female	171	115	127	94
Nonwhite male	2	1	10	3	Nonwhite male	16	8	15	15
Nonwhite female	8	4	5	3	Nonwhite female	18	9	13	7
South Atlantic	438	573	587	213					
White male	163	213	216	100					
White female	231	287	228	66					
Nonwhite male	19	41	76	29					
Nonwhite female	25	32	67	18					

[a] 750-monstrosity; 751-spina bifida and meningocele; 752-congenital hydrocephalus; 753-other congenital malformations of the nervous system.

Table A.9.11 Cases and incidence rates per 1,000 total (live plus stillborn) single births, standardized for maternal age, for major neural tube defects by type of defect: WHO study, by center, 1961-64

	Total[b] neural tube		Hydrocephalus				Spina bifida				Anencephaly alone	
			Alone		With spina bifida		Alone		With anencephaly			
Center[a]	Cases	Rate	Cases	Rate	Cases	Rate	Cases	Rate	Cases	Rate	Cases	Rate
Total	1,079	2.6	254	0.6	108	0.3	231	0.6	54	0.1	382	0.9
Melbourne (1)	28	3.8	12	1.6	2	0.3	3	0.4	4	0.5	4	0.6
Melbourne (2)	12	3.3	3	0.8	4	1.1	3	0.8	1	0.3	1	0.3
São Paulo	40	2.9	13	1.0	2	0.2	14	1.0	1	0.1	8	0.6
Santiago	29	1.2	8	0.3	1	0.0	10	0.4	1	0.0	6	0.3
Bogotá	22	1.2	16	0.9	1	0.0	1	0.1	-	-	2	0.1
Medellín	17	0.8	7	0.3	-	-	4	0.2	1	0.1	5	0.3
Czechoslovakia	38	2.1	7	0.6	5	0.3	12	0.6	1	0.0	10	0.4
Alexandria	76	7.9	20	2.0	6	0.6	8	0.8	6	0.6	30	3.2
Hong Kong	22	2.0	4	0.3	1	0.1	3	0.3	-	-	13	1.2
Bombay	142	3.8	30	0.7	12	0.3	30	0.8	6	0.2	60	1.7
Calcutta	11	0.6	1	0.1	-	-	2	0.1	1	0.1	6	0.3
Kuala Lumpur	37	2.3	16	1.0	-	-	3	0.2	1	0.1	17	1.0
Singapore	43	1.1[c]	9	0.2	-	-	5	0.1	2	0.1	26	0.7
Mexico City (1)	66	3.2	12	0.5	5	0.2	16	0.6	9	0.4	20	1.4
Mexico City (2)	15	1.1	3	0.2	3	0.2	4	0.3	-	-	2	0.1
Belfast	291	10.2	35	1.2	47	1.6	71	2.6	11	0.4	119	4.1
Panama City	37	2.5	15	0.9	2	0.1	10	0.7	2	0.1	7	0.5
Manila	30	1.0	8	0.3	1	0.0	1	0.0	-	-	15	0.5
Cape Town	7	2.7	2	0.8	-	-	2	0.8	-	-	2	0.8
Johannesburg	26	2.2	6	0.5	1	0.1	9	0.7	2	0.1	7	0.7
Pretoria	27	2.7	11	1.1	5	0.5	6	0.6	1	0.1	4	0.4
Madrid	35	1.4	7	0.3	4	0.2	8	0.4	-	-	16	0.6
Ljubljana	15	1.7	5	0.6	5	0.5	3	0.3	1	0.1	-	-
Zagreb	13	1.5	4	0.5	1	0.1	3	0.4	3	0.3	2	0.2

[a] See Table A.8.4 for composition of centers.

[b] Includes occipital meningocele and other neural tube defects but excludes microcephaly (27 cases) and the category of undefined "other nervous system" defects (3 cases) shown in Table 9.19.

[c] Rate shown is sum of standardized rates for specific neural malformations; standardized rate as published (2.09) seemed erroneous.

Table A.11.1 Average annual age-adjusted[a] death rates per 100,000 population for infantile cerebral palsy (cerebral spastic infantile paralysis) by sex: selected countries, various years, 1951-58
(ISC code 351)

Country	Years	Rate			M:F ratio[b]
		Total	Male	Female	
Australia	1954-58	0.3	0.4	0.3	1.4
Belgium	1954-58	0.2	0.3	0.2	2.1
Canada[c]	1953-57	0.3	0.4	0.3	1.4
Chile	1956,1958	0.2	---	---	---
Czechoslovakia	1953-57	0.5	---	---	---
Denmark	1953-57	0.7	0.7	0.7	1.0
England-Wales	1953-57	0.3	0.3	0.3	1.2
Finland	1954-58	0.7	0.9	0.6	1.5
France	1953-57	0.4	0.4	0.3	1.2
Ireland	1954-58	0.4	0.5	0.4	1.3
Israel[d]	1956-58	0.9	0.9	0.8	1.2
Italy	1953-57	0.2	0.3	0.2	1.3
Japan	1953-57	1.0	1.0	0.9	1.2
Mexico	1956	0.1	0.04	0.08	0.5
Netherlands	1953-57	0.5	0.5	0.4	1.4
New Zealand[e]	1952-56	0.4	0.5	0.3	1.4
Norway	1953-57	0.7	0.7	0.6	1.2
Scotland	1951-55	0.5	0.5	0.4	1.3
Sweden	1953-57	0.3	0.4	0.3	1.7
Switzerland	1953-57	0.4	0.4	0.3	1.3
Union of So. Africa[f]	1953-57	0.2	0.2	0.2	1.4
United States, white	1953-57	0.4	0.4	0.3	1.4
United States, nonwhite	1953-57	0.4	0.4	0.3	1.2
United States, total	1953-57	0.4	0.4	0.3	1.4
Uruguay	1955-57	0.3	0.3	0.4	0.7

[a] Adjusted to the 1950 United States census population.

[b] Sex ratio is computed from rates available to two decimal places.

[c] Yukon and Northwest Territories are included for 1956 and 1957 only.

[d] Jewish population only.

[e] Excludes Maori population.

[f] White population only.

Table A.11.2 Average annual death rates per 100,000 population under 5 years of age for neonatal cerebral palsy (intracranial and spinal injury at birth) by sex: selected countries, various years, 1951-58
(ISC code 760)

Country	Years	Rate Male	Rate Female	M:F ratio
Australia	1954-58	46.0	31.4	1.5
Belgium	1954-58	48.3	27.3	1.8
Canada[a]	1953-57	36.5	22.3	1.6
Denmark	1953-57	61.7	37.6	1.6
England-Wales	1953-57	54.7	33.7	1.6
Finland	1954-58	54.2	33.1	1.6
France	1953-57	43.7	28.3	1.5
Iceland	1951-55	29.8	23.3	1.3
Ireland	1954-58	60.4	31.9	1.9
Israel[b]	1956-58	49.7	28.4	1.8
Italy	1953-57	26.0	14.4	1.8
Japan	1953-57	9.8	5.9	1.7
Mexico	1956	10.2	6.1	1.7
Netherlands	1953-57	62.2	32.0	1.9
New Zealand[c]	1952-56	50.0	28.7	1.7
Norway	1953-57	45.4	27.5	1.7
Scotland	1951-55	57.6	35.2	1.6
Sweden	1953-57	58.2	38.9	1.5
Union of So. Africa[d]	1953-57	59.0	36.0	1.6
United States, white	1953-57	27.7	16.0	1.7
United States, nonwhite	1953-57	46.4	30.1	1.5
United States, total	1953-57	30.2	17.9	1.7
Uruguay	1955-57	53.7	32.9	1.6

[a] Yukon and Northwest Territories are included for 1956 and 1957 only.
[b] Jewish population only.
[c] Excludes Maori population.
[d] White population only.

Table A.11.3 Average annual crude death rates per 100,000 population, all ages, for neonatal cerebral palsy (intracranial and spinal injury at birth) by sex: selected countries, various years, 1951-58
(ISC code 760)

Country	Years	Rate			M:F ratio[a]
		Total	Male	Female	
Australia	1954-58	4.1	4.9	3.3	1.5
Belgium	1954-58	3.0	4.0	2.1	1.9
Canada[b]	1953-57	3.7	4.5	2.7	1.7
Chile	1956,1958	6.5	---	---	---
Czechoslovakia	1953-57	6.8	---	---	---
Denmark	1953-57	4.2	5.4	3.1	1.8
England-Wales	1953-57	3.3	4.3	2.4	1.8
Finland	1954-58	4.5	5.9	3.2	1.9
France	1953-57	3.3	4.2	2.4	1.7
Iceland	1951-55	3.4	3.9	2.9	1.3
Ireland	1954-58	4.8	6.3	3.3	1.9
Israel[c]	1956-58	5.1	6.5	3.6	1.8
Italy	1953-57	1.7	2.3	1.2	2.0
Japan	1953-57	0.8	1.1	0.6	1.8
Mexico	1956	1.3	1.6	0.9	1.7
Netherlands	1953-57	4.9	6.7	3.2	2.1
New Zealand[d]	1952-56	4.5	5.8	3.2	1.8
Norway	1953-57	3.3	4.2	2.4	1.8
Scotland	1951-55	4.0	5.4	2.8	1.9
Sweden	1953-57	3.6	4.5	2.8	1.6
Switzerland	1953-57	0.9	1.3	0.6	2.1
Union of South Africa[e]	1953-57	5.5	6.9	4.0	1.7
United States, white	1953-57	2.4	3.1	1.7	1.9
United States, nonwhite	1953-57	5.3	6.7	4.1	1.6
United States, total	1953-57	2.7	3.5	1.9	1.8
Uruguay	1955-57	4.6	5.8	3.4	1.7

[a] Sex ratio is computed from rates available to two decimal places.

[b] Yukon and Northwest Territories are included for 1956 and 1957 only.

[c] Jewish population only.

[d] Excludes Maori population.

[e] White population only.

Table A.11.4 Death certificates listing cerebral spastic infantile paralysis (ICP) and intracranial and spinal injury at birth (NCP) as primary or secondary causes of death, with percent listed as primary cause: selected countries, various years, 1953-61
(ISC codes 351 and 760)

Country and years	ICP (351)		NCP (760)	
	Total deaths	Percent primary	Total deaths	Percent primary
Norway (1956-60)[a]	196	58	---	---
United States (1955)[b]	1,294	49	4,742	92
Netherlands (1953-60)[c]	542	78	4,109	91
Netherlands (1961)[d]	99	81	503	95

[a] All secondary causes considered.

[b] Up to four secondary causes considered.

[c] Only one (most important) secondary cause considered; excludes deaths for 1958 (not available).

[d] Up to three secondary causes considered.

Table A.11.5 Deaths and average annual age-adjusted death rates per 100,000 population under 15 years of age for infantile cerebral palsy (cerebral spastic infantile paralysis): United States and each state, 1959-61
(ISC code 351)

State	Deaths	Rate	State	Deaths	Rate
United States	1,496	0.8	Louisiana	27	0.8*
			Michigan	67	0.8*
Hawaii	1	0.1*	North Carolina	40	0.8*
Montana	2	0.2*	Oklahoma	17	0.8*
Delaware	1	0.3*	South Carolina	21	0.8*
Connecticut	11	0.4*			
Rhode Island	3	0.4*	Illinois	92	0.9
			Texas	91	0.9
Nevada	1	0.4*	West Virginia	17	0.9*
Alaska	1	0.5*	Arkansas	18	1.0*
California	78	0.5	Maine	9	1.0*
Wyoming	2	0.5*			
Massachusetts	26	0.6*	Minnesota	36	1.0*
			Utah	10	1.0*
New Jersey	36	0.6*	Vermont	4	1.0*
New Mexico	8	0.6*	Virginia	41	1.0*
Nebraska	9	0.6*	Wisconsin	41	1.0*
North Dakota	4	0.6*			
Oregon	10	0.6*	Alabama	41	1.1*
			Arizona	16	1.1*
Colorado	13	0.7*	Idaho	8	1.1*
Kansas	15	0.7*	Kentucky	32	1.1*
Maryland	22	0.7*	Ohio	108	1.1
Mississippi	18	0.7*			
New York	101	0.7	Florida	60	1.2*
			Georgia	55	1.3
Pennsylvania	78	0.7	Missouri	50	1.3*
South Dakota	5	0.7*	Tennessee	48	1.3*
Washington	20	0.7*	Dist. of Col.	9	1.4*
Iowa	22	0.8*	New Hampshire	11	2.0*
Indiana	40	0.8*			

Table A.11.6 Average annual age-adjusted death rates per 100,000 population under 15 years of age for infantile cerebral palsy (cerebral spastic infantile paralysis) by color, sex and type of county: United States and census regions, 1959-61
(ISC code 351)

Region and color	Metropolitan counties			Nonmetropolitan counties		
	Total	Male	Female	Total	Male	Female
United States	0.8	0.8	0.7	0.9	1.1	0.8
Region						
New England	0.5*	0.6*	0.4*	1.1*	1.2*	0.9*
Middle Atlantic	0.6	0.6	0.7	0.8	1.0*	0.7*
East North Central	0.9	1.0	0.8	1.0	1.2*	0.8*
West North Central	1.0*	0.9*	1.0*	0.9	1.0*	0.7*
South Atlantic	0.9	0.9	1.0*	1.1	1.4	0.7*
East South Central	1.2*	1.1*	1.2*	1.0	1.0*	1.1*
West South Central	0.8	1.0*	0.6*	0.9	0.9*	0.9*
Mountain	0.8*	0.9*	0.7*	0.8*	0.8*	0.8*
Pacific	0.5	0.6*	0.4*	0.6*	0.5*	0.6*
Color						
White	0.8	0.8	0.7	0.9	1.1	0.8
Nonwhite	0.9	1.0	0.7	1.0	1.1*	0.8*

Table A.11.7 Average annual death rates per 100,000 population under 1 year of age for neonatal cerebral palsy (intracranial and spinal injury at birth) by color, sex and type of county: United States and census regions, 1959-61
(ISC code 760)

Region and color	Metropolitan counties			Nonmetropolitan counties		
	Total	Male	Female	Total	Male	Female
United States	80.4	100.9	59.2	74.0	91.8	55.5
Region						
New England	68.9	94.2	42.8	76.5	96.9	55.3
Middle Atlantic	85.6	105.4	65.1	76.6	95.2	57.3
East North Central	70.8	90.0	51.1	64.3	81.7	46.3
West North Central	67.6	83.4	51.1	56.2	73.5	38.2
South Atlantic	83.7	109.0	57.8	83.2	102.8	63.1
East South Central	73.8	96.7	50.3	79.2	93.4	64.7
West South Central	104.6	125.9	82.5	86.6	103.6	69.4
Mountain	73.2	90.8	55.1	70.5	93.4	46.9
Pacific	84.2	103.4	64.1	72.3	89.1	54.6
Color						
White	71.2	90.0	51.5	69.5	88.2	50.0
Nonwhite	132.7	164.0	101.6	99.8	113.1	86.6

Table A.12.1 Percentage distribution of first additions[a] to blindness register by major affection groups, by color and sex: MRA[b] total, 1966

Major affection group[c]	Total			White			Nonwhite		
	Total	Male	Female	Total	Male	Female	Total	Male	Female
All groups	100.0	100.0	100.0	100.0	100.0	100.0	100.0	100.0	100.0
Glaucoma (noncongenital)	10.9	12.0	10.0	8.6	9.1	8.2	21.2	25.4	17.7
Myopia	2.2	2.0	2.4	2.1	1.9	2.2	2.7	2.5	2.9
Keratitis	1.1	1.2	1.0	1.0	1.0	1.0	1.4	1.8	1.0
Other affect. of cornea, sclera	1.7	1.7	1.6	1.3	1.4	1.3	2.9	3.3	2.7
Cataract	18.9	17.4	20.2	19.1	17.6	20.3	19.6	17.4	21.4
Uveitis	3.2	3.7	2.8	3.1	3.7	2.6	3.6	3.0	4.1
Retrolental fibroplasia	1.0	1.0	1.0	1.1	1.2	1.0	0.2	0.3	0.2
Retinal degeneration	18.9	18.0	19.6	21.4	19.9	22.8	7.1	9.6	5.1
Other retinal affections	14.6	14.1	15.1	15.4	15.7	15.1	12.7	8.8	15.8
Optic nerve atrophy	5.2	6.9	3.7	5.1	6.9	3.6	5.0	6.8	3.5
Multiple affections[d]	9.2	6.7	11.4	9.3	7.0	11.3	8.8	4.8	12.1
Other	8.3	9.9	6.9	8.0	9.5	6.6	9.7	10.8	8.8
Unknown	4.8	5.3	4.3	4.5	5.0	4.1	5.1	5.5	4.7
(Number of first additions)	(4,965)[e]	(2,298)	(2,667)	(3,808)	(1,761)	(2,047)	(884)	(397)	(487)

[a] Data limited to first additions examined by ophthalmologists or eye-ear-nose-and-throat specialists.
[b] Model Reporting Area for Blindness Statistics, United States. Includes data on first additions for 14 states in 1966. (See Table 12.2)
[c] Standard Classification of Causes of Severe Vision Impairment and Blindness, 1966 Revision.
[d] There were 459 cases of multiple affections; i.e., two or more affections in the same eye of an individual.
[e] Includes 273 persons of unknown color.

Table A.12.2 Percentage distribution of first additions[a] to blindness register by major affection groups, by age[b]: MRA[c] total, 1966

Major affection group[d]	Total	Under 5	5-19	20-44	45-64	65-74	75-84	85 & over
Total	100.0	100.0	100.0	100.0	100.0	100.0	100.0	100.0
Glaucoma (noncongenital)	10.9	-	0.2	3.4	12.3	17.4	14.5	8.3
Myopia	2.2	2.2	6.9	4.0	2.8	1.0	0.5	0.8
Keratitis	1.1	0.7	0.9	2.3	1.9	0.7	0.4	0.2
Other affec. of cornea, sclera	1.7	1.4	0.7	4.6	1.7	1.6	1.2	0.6
Cataract	18.9	23.9	14.8	6.7	18.5	20.1	24.3	23.0
Uveitis	3.2	3.6	7.2	5.6	4.6	2.1	1.3	0.8
Retrolental fibroplasia	1.0	8.0	6.5	1.0	0.2	-	-	-
Retinal degeneration	18.9	1.4	8.5	17.6	9.9	18.0	28.3	34.0
Other retinal affections	14.6	9.4	3.9	20.3	24.0	17.7	9.3	4.2
Optic nerve atrophy	5.2	8.7	12.9	10.7	6.4	2.7	1.9	1.0
Multiple affections	9.2	-	-	1.5	6.0	12.3	13.2	22.0
Other	8.3	33.3	33.0	17.8	6.2	1.9	1.4	1.5
Unknown	4.8	7.2	4.4	4.4	5.6	4.5	3.6	3.7
(Number of first additions)	(4,965[e])	(138)	(433)	(522)	(1,241)	(821)	(1,124)	(518)

[a] Data limited to first additions examined by ophthalmologists or eye-ear-nose-and-throat specialists.
[b] Age at registration in MRA state.
[c] Model Reporting Area for Blindness Statistics, United States. Includes data on first additions for 14 states in 1966. (See Table 12.2)
[d] Standard Classification of Causes of Severe Vision Impairment and Blindness, 1966 Revision.
[e] Includes 168 persons of unknown age.

Table A.12.3 Percentage distribution of first additions[a] to blindness register by degree of vision in better eye, by major affection groups: MRA[b] total, 1966

Major affection group[c]	Total	Absolute blindness	Light perception	Light projection	Less than 5/200	5/200 to less than 10/200	10/200 to less than 20/200	20/200	Restricted field	Unknown	Number of first additions
Total	100.0	4.8	8.8	1.2	16.5	10.2	18.7	28.2	6.2	5.5	(4,965)
Glaucoma (noncongenital)	100.0	7.4	9.4	1.7	17.5	5.7	9.0	15.8	27.4	6.1	(543)
Myopia	100.0	-	-	0.9	15.5	10.9	23.6	41.8	-	7.3	(110)
Keratitis	100.0	7.5	9.4	1.9	13.2	11.3	18.9	34.0	1.9	1.9	(53)
Other affec. of cornea, sclera	100.0	2.4	10.8	-	22.9	10.8	14.5	27.7	3.6	7.2	(83)
Cataract	100.0	1.4	11.0	2.1	19.2	9.2	18.7	31.9	1.1	5.5	(938)
Uveitis	100.0	3.7	8.1	0.6	14.4	8.1	21.9	31.9	1.9	9.4	(160)
Retrolental fibroplasia	100.0	26.0	26.0	-	2.0	6.0	8.0	24.0	-	8.0	(50)
Retinal degeneration	100.0	1.1	2.8	0.6	14.5	13.1	25.3	32.7	6.5	3.3	(936)
Other retinal affections	100.0	4.5	12.5	1.8	21.2	11.3	18.7	26.1	1.9	1.9	(727)
Optic nerve atrophy	100.0	12.4	13.1	0.4	13.1	13.5	15.8	13.9	10.8	6.9	(259)
Multiple affections	100.0	3.1	8.3	1.1	17.2	13.3	21.8	30.7	2.0	2.6	(459)
Other	100.0	10.0	9.8	0.5	10.0	5.6	16.8	33.4	3.2	9.8	(410)
Unknown	100.0	10.1	6.8	0.4	14.3	8.9	14.3	23.2	6.3	15.6	(237)

[a] Data limited to first additions examined by ophthalmologists or eye-ear-nose-and-throat specialists.
[b] Model Reporting Area for Blindness Statistics, United States. Includes data on first additions for 14 states in 1966. (See Table 12.2)
[c] Standard Classification of Causes of Severe Vision Impairment and Blindness, 1966 Revision.

Table A.12.4 Percentage distribution of first additions[a] to blindness register by major cause groups, by color and sex: MRA[b] total, 1966

Major cause group[c]	Total			White			Nonwhite		
	Total	Male	Female	Total	Male	Female	Total	Male	Female
Total	100.0	100.0	100.0	100.0	100.0	100.0	100.0	100.0	100.0
Infectious diseases	2.5	2.8	2.2	2.3	2.6	2.1	2.4	2.8	2.1
Injuries, poisonings	2.8	4.3	1.5	2.4	3.7	1.2	4.8	7.6	2.5
Neoplasms	1.1	1.5	0.9	1.3	1.5	1.0	0.5	0.8	0.2
Diabetes	11.6	9.6	13.3	11.8	10.3	13.0	11.8	7.1	15.6
Senile degeneration	33.0	28.8	36.7	36.0	31.3	39.9	22.5	19.6	24.8
Vascular diseases	3.0	3.6	2.5	3.1	3.8	2.4	2.5	2.0	2.9
Other general diseases[d]	1.4	1.7	1.2	1.3	1.8	1.0	1.5	1.5	1.4
Prenatal influenced	13.7	16.0	11.7	13.6	15.7	11.7	13.2	15.4	11.5
Multiple causes	4.9	3.9	5.8	5.0	4.1	5.7	4.9	3.0	6.4
Unknown to science	11.8	12.6	11.1	9.4	9.8	9.1	22.1	25.9	18.9
Not reported or determined	14.1	15.2	13.1	14.0	15.4	12.8	14.0	14.4	13.8
(Number of first additions)	(4,965)[e]	(2,298)	(2,667)	(3,808)	(1,761)	(2,047)	(884)	(397)	(487)

[a] Data limited to first additions examined by ophthalmologists or eye-ear-nose-and-throat specialists.
[b] Model Reporting Area for Blindness Statistics, United States. Includes data on first additions for 14 states in 1966. (See Table 12.2)
[c] Standard Classification of Causes of Severe Vision Impairment and Blindness, 1966 Revision.
[d] See Table 12.1 for description.
[e] Includes 273 persons of unknown color.

Table A.12.5 Percentage distribution of first additions[a] to blindness register by major cause groups, by age[b]: MRA[c] total, 1966

Major cause group[d]	Total	Under 5	5-19	20-44	45-64	65-74	75-84	85 & over
All causes	100.0	100.0	100.0	100.0	100.0	100.0	100.0	100.0
Infectious diseases	2.5	23.2	5.5	3.3	2.3	1.6	0.5	-
Injuries, poisonings	2.8	8.0	5.5	11.1	2.7	0.9	-	0.2
Neoplasms	1.1	7.2	4.2	1.3	1.3	0.2	0.3	0.2
Diabetes	11.6	-	-	17.8	21.0	17.1	5.0	2.3
Senile degeneration	33.0	-	0.2	1.3	21.3	38.4	56.5	70.1
Vascular diseases	3.0	0.7	0.2	0.4	3.6	3.5	4.7	2.3
Other general diseases	1.4	0.7	2.3	5.4	1.7	0.2	0.3	0.2
Prenatal influence[e]	13.7	47.8	64.4	33.7	8.8	2.4	1.0	0.8
Multiple causes	4.9	-	-	3.4	3.4	6.3	8.1	8.9
Unknown to science	11.8	-	1.4	7.1	13.1	17.7	14.9	8.3
Not reported or determined	14.1	12.3	16.2	17.4	20.8	11.7	8.7	6.8
(Number of first additions)	(4,965[f])	(138)	(433)	(522)	(1,241)	(821)	(1,124)	(518)

[a] Data limited to first additions examined by ophthalmologists or eye-ear-nose-and-throat specialists.
[b] Age at registration in MRA state.
[c] Model Reporting Area for Blindness Statistics, United States. Includes data on first additions for 14 states in 1966. (See Table 12.2)
[d] Standard Classification of Causes of Severe Vision Impairment and Blindness, 1966 Revision.
[e] See Table 12.1 for description.
[f] Includes 168 persons of unknown age.

Table A.12.6 Percentage distribution of first additions[a] to blindness register by degree of vision in better eye, by major cause groups: MRA[b] total, 1966

Major cause group[c]	Total	Absolute blindness	Light perception	Light projection	Less than 5/200	5/200 to less than 10/200	10/200 to less than 20/200	20/200	Restricted field	Unknown	Number of first additions
Total	100.0	4.8	8.8	1.2	16.5	10.2	18.7	28.2	6.2	5.5	(4,965)
Infectious diseases	100.0	6.6	15.6	0.8	14.8	4.9	17.2	20.5	2.5	17.2	(122)
Injuries, poisonings	100.0	24.3	20.0	0.7	12.9	6.4	11.4	16.4	3.6	4.3	(140)
Neoplasms	100.0	28.1	15.8	—	8.8	14.0	7.0	12.3	8.8	5.3	(57)
Diabetes	100.0	3.3	12.7	1.2	22.4	12.5	20.6	24.1	1.7	1.6	(577)
Senile degeneration	100.0	0.9	5.9	1.5	17.6	12.3	22.7	35.2	0.7	3.3	(1,640)
Vascular diseases	100.0	4.1	14.9	2.0	20.3	10.8	21.6	16.9	7.4	2.0	(148)
Other general diseases[d]	100.0	10.0	11.4	—	14.3	11.4	22.9	21.4	4.3	4.3	(70)
Prenatal influence	100.0	4.1	5.7	0.6	9.7	7.6	19.0	32.8	9.0	11.5	(680)
Multiple causes	100.0	4.9	9.4	1.2	18.8	12.2	20.0	29.4	2.0	2.0	(245)
Unknown to science	100.0	6.8	8.9	1.5	17.4	6.0	9.9	17.7	25.8	6.0	(586)
Not reported or determined	100.0	7.3	9.9	1.1	15.4	9.7	15.9	27.1	5.9	7.7	(700)

[a] Data limited to first additions examined by ophthalmologists or eye-ear-nose-and-throat specialists.
[b] Model Reporting Area for Blindness Statistics, United States. Includes data on first additions for 14 states in 1966. (See Table 12.2)
[c] Standard Classification of Causes of Severe Vision Impairment and Blindness, 1966 Revision.
[d] See Table 12.1 for description.

Table A.12.7 Percentage distribution of total on blindness register as of end of year by degree of vision in better eye, by age: MRA[a] total, 1966

Degree of vision	Total	Under 5	5-19	20-44	45-64	65-74	75-84	85 & over
Total	100.0	100.0	100.0	100.0	100.0	100.0	100.0	100.0
Absolute blindness	11.7	22.8	15.9	13.4	12.7	11.6	9.4	7.7
Light perception	11.9	19.9	13.4	11.8	12.1	13.0	11.1	10.8
Light projection	1.1	2.8	0.7	1.0	1.2	1.2	1.0	1.2
Less than 5/200	15.7	3.8	8.6	13.8	17.6	18.7	17.2	16.8
5/200 to less than 10/200	9.5	1.5	6.3	8.6	9.8	9.8	11.1	12.2
10/200 to less than 20/200	14.5	3.6	12.7	14.5	14.3	13.8	15.9	16.4
20/200	20.8	4.1	26.5	23.7	18.5	18.8	21.8	20.7
Restricted field	5.5	–	1.3	6.3	7.9	6.7	4.3	2.5
Unknown	9.3	41.4	14.7	7.0	6.0	6.5	8.2	11.7
(Number on register)	(61,037)[b]	(391)	(6,072)	(9,969)	(16,704)	(10,128)	(9,728)	(6,135)

[a]Model Reporting Area for Blindness Statistics, United States. Includes data on persons on register for 15 states in 1966. (See Table 12.2)

[b]Includes 1,910 persons of unknown age.

APPENDIX / 387

Table A.12.8 Prevalence rates per 100,000 population for blindness by definition of blindness: selected countries,[a] various years, 1940-65

Definition, continent and country	Year and method[b]	Rate	Source
20/200 (6/60)			
America			
Canada	1965 R	128	MacDonald 1965
United States	1960 E	214	Hurlin 1962
Europe			
Bulgaria	1945 C	57	AFB[d]
Finland	1961-62 S	79	Vannas and Raivio 1964
U.S.S.R. (exclusive of Moldavia)	1962 R	117	Tatimov 1966
13/200 (4/60)			
Europe			
Denmark	1949 E	100	AFB[d]
10/200 (3/60)			
Africa			
Algeria	1946 E	304	AFB[d]
Kenya	1955 E	1050-1150	BESB[e]
Tunisia	1960 S	450	WHO[f]
United Arab Republic	1960 C	463	WHO[f]
Asia			
Iran	1960 E	750	WHO[f]
Israel	1961 S	250	WHO[f]
Europe			
France	1946 C	107	AFB[d]
Gibraltar	1961 C	647	WHO[g]
Iceland	1950 S	272	Björnsson 1955
Malta and Gozo	1958 S	194	Damato 1960
Netherlands	1959 E	50-60	Schappert-Kimmijser[h]
Poland	1959 E	65	Rostkowski and Korczak[i]
United Kingdom			
England and Wales	1963 R	205	GB[j]
Northern Ireland	1963 R	161	NI[k]
Scotland	1964 R	194	S[l]
U.S.S.R. (exclusive of Moldavia)	1962 R	69	Tatimov 1966

(continued)

Table A.12.8 Prevalence rates per 100,000 population for blindness by definition of blindness: selected countries,[a] various years, 1940-65 (continued)

Definition, continent and country	Year and method[b]	Rate	Source
7/200 (2/60)			
Asia			
Kuwait	1965 E	436	Hamdan 1968
Europe			
Austria	1949 E	66	AFB[d]
3/200 (1/60)			
Africa			
Cameroons			
North	1952 S	1800	Rodger 1959
South	1952 S	400	Rodger 1959
Ghana (North)	1952 S	3000	Rodger 1959
United Arab Republic	1960 C	355	UAR[m]
Europe			
Norway	1948 S	100	Holst 1952
Spain	1947-52 E	56	Alcalá-Lopez 1953
Switzerland	1950 C	60	Sorsby et al. 1955
Absolute blindness			
Africa			
Malawi	1945 C	225	GBC[t]
Southern Rhodesia	1962 C	332	WHO[g]
United Arab Republic	1960 C	296	WHO[f]
Asia			
Iraq	1961 E	500-1000	WHO[f]
Syria	1958-60 S	91	WHO[f]
Yemen	1960 E	4000	WHO[f]
Europe			
Portugal	1960 C	93	WHO[g]
Qualitative def.			
Africa			
Zambia	1961 E	500-750	Phillips 1961
Asia			
Kuwait	1957 C	230	WHO[f]

(continued)

Table A.12.8 Prevalence rates per 100,000 population for blindness by definition of blindness: selected countries,[a] various years, 1940-65 (continued)

Definition, continent and country	Year and method[b]	Rate	Source
No definition given			
Africa			
Ethiopia	1962 E	380-450	WHO[f]
Gambia	1955 E	983	BESB[e]
Mauritius	1960 C	39	RCSB[n]
Sierra Leone	1955 E	952	BESB[e]
South Africa	1960 R	216	SANCB[o]
European pop.		86	
Colored pop.		155	
Asiatic pop.		65	
Bantu pop.		272	
Tanganyika	1955 E	569	BESB[e]
Uganda	1955 E	636	BESB[e]
America			
Argentina	1947 C	90	WHO[g]
Bermuda	1957 E	139	RCSB[n]
Brazil	1940 C	147	WHO[g]
Cuba	1943 C	97	WHO[g]
Dominican Republic	1950 C	134	WHO[g]
Guatemala	1940 C	72	Soper 1951
Honduras	1940 C	108	Soper 1951
Jamaica	1955 S	304	RCSB[n]
Mexico[c]	1940 C	101	WHO[g]
Nicaragua	1950 E	100	Lacayo 1950
Peru	1940 C	145	WHO[g]
Trinidad and Tobago	1947 C	125	WHO[g]
Venezuela	1941 C	124	WHO[g]
Asia			
Aden	1957 E	1403	RCSB[n]
Ceylon	1963 E	470	Around the World 1964
China	1947 E	450	Mackenzie and Flowers[p]
Cyprus	1962 E	224	RCSB[n]
Hong Kong	1963 E	1392	Around the World 1964
India	1962 E	460	WHO[q]
Japan	1958 E	210	Nakajima 1961
Malaysia	1963 E	470	Around the World 1964
Pakistan	1963 E	400	Around the World 1964
Saudi Arabia	1961 E	3000	WHO[f]
Singapore	1957 E	189	RCSB[n]
Turkey	1955 C	132	WHO[g]

(continued)

Table A.12.8 Prevalence rates per 100,000 population for blindness by definition of blindness: selected countries,[a] various years, 1940-65 (continued)

Definition, continent and country	Year and method[b]	Rate	Source
No definition given (continued)			
Europe			
Belgium	1963 R	51	BINS[r]
W. Germany	1961 E	74	Rohrschneider 1962
Greece	1951 C	170	WHO[g]
Sweden	1965 E	130	von Bahr 1965
Yugoslavia	1959 E	100	Hudolin and Laktic[s]
Oceania			
Fiji Islands	1955 E	1190	BESB[e]
New Zealand	1962 R	112	Tennent 1962

[a] Excluding United States MRA data.
[b] C=census; E=estimate; R=register; S=survey.
[c] Based on census of the blind 5 years old or older.
[d] American Foundation for the Blind, Inc. 1949.
[e] British Empire Society for the Blind 1954-56.
[f] World Health Organization, Regional Office for the Eastern Mediterranean 1963.
[g] World Health Organization 1966.
[h] Schappert-Kimmijser 1959.
[i] Rostkowski and Korczak 1962.
[j] Great Britain, Ministry of Health 1964.
[k] Northern Ireland, Ministry of Health and Local Government 1964.
[l] Scotland, Scottish Home and Health Department 1965.
[m] United Arab Republic, Department of Statistics and Census 1963.
[n] Royal Commonwealth Society for the Blind 1957-64.
[o] South African National Council for the Blind 1958-60.
[p] Mackenzie and Flowers 1949.
[q] World Health Organization, Regional Office for South-East Asia 1962.
[r] Belgique Institut National de Statistique 1963.
[s] Hudolin and Laktic 1959.
[t] Great Britain, Colonial Office 1948.

APPENDIX / 391

Table A.12.9 Prevalence rates per 100,000 population for blindness by definition of blindness, age and sex: selected countries[a], various years, 1941-65

| Definition, continent and country | Year and method[b] | Sex | All ages | \multicolumn{6}{c}{Various age groups} | Source |

Definition, continent and country	Year and method[b]	Sex	All ages							Source
20/200 (6/60)				0-39	40-64	65-69	70+			
America										
Canada	1965 R	T	128	40	173	461	940			MacDonald 1965
		M	131	---	---	---	---			
		F	126	---	---	---	---			
Europe				0-14	15-64	65+				
Finland	1961-62 S	T	79	12	69	384				Vannas and Raivio 1964
				0-6	7-15	16-59	65+			
U.S.S.R. (exclusive of Moldavia)	1962 R	T	139	1	29	160	505			Tatimov 1966
10/200 (3/60)				0-14	15-19	20-29	30-39	40-49	50-59	60-69	70+	
Asia												
Israel Jewish	1956 S	T	88	9	75	69	98	102	163	285	517	Israeli Ministry of Social Welfare, Division of Research and Planning 1957
		M	108	7	92	89	136	147	203	324	613	
		F	67	12	58	49	61	57	119	245	436	
Non-Jewish	1956 S	T	117	9	38	98	105	263	353	496	949	
		M	123	16	52	112	86	383	348	431	902	
		F	111	—	21	83	119	156	358	563	993	
Europe				0-4	5-9	10-14	15-19	20-29	30-39	40-59	60+	
France	1946 C	T	107	7	11	17	21	28	37	88	434	American Foundation for the Blind, Inc. 1949
		M	111	7	12	20	25	38	48	113	458	
		F	104	7	10	14	18	19	26	67	418	
				0-4	5-14	15-24	25-34	35-44	45-54	55-64	65+	
Gibraltar	1961 C	T	647	—	28	69	159	244	441	818	5,095	World Health Organization 1966
		M	307	—	55	69	188	135	281	490	2,432	
		F	960	—	—	69	129	335	592	1,101	6,571	

Table A.12.9 Prevalence rates per 100,000 population for blindness by definition of blindness, age and sex: selected countries[a], various years, 1941-65 (continued)

Definition, continent and country	Year and method[b]	Sex	All ages	Various age groups								Source
Iceland	1950 S	T	272	0-4: 5	5-14: 19	15-19: 25	20-39: 27	40-59: 86	60-69: 349	70+: 4,446		Björnsson 1955
		M	303	9	24	17	22	101	324	6,019		
		F	241	–	6	35	32	71	373	3,296		
Malta and Gozo	1958 S	T	194	0-4: 23	5-14: 19	15-19: 31	20-39: 34	40-59: 249	60-69: 761	70+: 1,902		Damato 1960
		M	193	15	24	49	44	259	720	1,804		
		F	196	31	13	14	26	239	794	1,986		
United Kingdom												
England and Wales	1963 R	T	205	0-4: 8	5-10: 22	11-20: 28	21-29: 36	30-49: 75	50-64: 192	65-79: 741	80+: 3,256	Great Britain, Ministry of Health 1964
3/200 (1/60)												
Africa												
U.A.R.	1960 C	T	355	0-4: 12	5-9: 29	10-19: 95	20-29: 177	30-39: 288	40-49: 447	50-59: 903	60+: 2,912	United Arab Republic, Department of Statistics and Census 1963
		M	338	13	31	97	200	243	440	860	2,785	
		F	373	10	26	89	157	214	455	946	3,024	
Absolute blindness												
Africa												
Malawi	1945 C	T	225	0-18: 53	18+: 421							Great Britain, Colonial Office 1948
		M	237	60	493							
		F	214	46	371							
Asia												
Syria	1958-60 S	T	91	0-6: 6	7-11: 23	12-17: 40	18-29: 54	30-39: 70	40-59: 199	60+: 586		World Health Organization, Regional Office for the Eastern Mediterranean 1963
		M	104	---	---	---	---	---	---	---		
		F	77	---	---	---	---	---	---	---		
Europe												
Portugal	1960 C	T	93	0-9: 23	10-19: 31	20-29: 43	30-39: 50	40-49: 67	50-59: 111	60-69: 223	70+: 704	World Health Organization 1966
		M	94	---	---	---	---	---	---	---	---	
		F	91	---	---	---	---	---	---	---	---	
No definition given												
America												
Cuba	1943 C	T	97	1-9: 17	10-19: 35	20-29: 67	30-39: 95	40-49: 119	50-59: 175	60+: 671		World Health Organization 1966
		M	110	21	43	80	112	137	202	669		

APPENDIX / 393

Country	Year	T/M/F									Source
Jamaica	1943 C		0-9	10-19	20-39	40+					World Health Organization 1966
		T	277	38	70	1,104					
		M	256	36	77	1,029					
		F	297	41	63	1,171					
Trinidad and Tobago	1947 C		0-4	5-14	15-24	25-44	45-64	65+			World Health Organization 1966
		T	125	9	12	118	269	1,576			
		M	104	13	13	120	218	1,346			
		F	147	5	12	115	325	1,763			
Venezuela	1941 C		0-9	10-19	20-29	30-39	40-49	50-59	60-69	70+	World Health Organization 1966
		T	124	34	46	80	166	345	807	2,386	
		M	121	40	55	99	185	341	795	2,487	
		F	126	28	38	61	146	349	816	2,325	
Asia											
Ceylon	1946 C		0-14	15-24	25-39	40-59	60+				World Health Organization 1966
		T	69	44	58	111	400				
		M	69	43	58	104	387				
		F	69	45	57	120	416				
Hong Kong	1961 C		0-4	5-14	15-24	25-44	45-64	65+			World Health Organization 1966
		T	27	16	31	23	53	168			
		M	25	14	29	23	60	189			
		F	29	19	34	24	46	158			
Turkey	1955 C		0-9	10-14	15-24	25-44	45-64	65+			World Health Organization 1966
		T	132	54	67	111	301	1,149			
		M	128	61	77	128	298	1,083			
		F	137	47	49	94	305	1,192			
Greece	1951 C		0-4	5-14	15-24	25-44	45-64	65+			World Health Organization 1966
		T	170	22	36	70	211	1,525			
		M	182	27	49	90	228	1,698			
		F	159	17	23	51	196	1,388			
Netherlands	1948 S		0-13	14-21	22-35	36-45	46-64	65+			Netherlands, Centraal Bureau voor de Statistiek 1954
		T	51	14	31	49	81	244			
		M	60	16	38	58	102	277			
		F	42	12	24	32	60	217			

[a] Excluding United States.
[b] C = census; E = estimate; R = register; S = survey.

394 / APPENDIX

Table A.12.10 Number of blind persons and percentage distribution by site and by type of affection[a], by definition of blindness: selected countries[b], various years, 1944-68

Definition, continent and country	Year	No. of blind	Total	Glaucoma (exclusive of congenital)	Structural anomalies	Refractory errors, degenerative changes	Conjunctiva	Cornea	Lens	Uveal tract	Retina	Optic nerve, optic pathway and cortical visual centers	Vitreous	Site and type unspecified or not reported	Source
20/200 (6/60)															
Africa															
U.A.R.[c] (urban)	1965-66	74	19	5	1	12	–	31	36	1	5	4	–	3	Said et al. 1967
(rural)		274	9	7	1	1	–	54	33	1	2	1	–	–	
America															
Argentina	1955	14,309	21	–	–	–	–	21	23	22	–	13	–	–	Diez et al. 1955
Canada	1965	24,605	37	10	18	9	–	6	16	7	23	10	1	–	MacDonald 1965
Venezuela	1949-54	216	53	47	1	4	–	11	2	8	6	19	–	1	Espino 1954
Europe															
Denmark	1952	145	18	6	8	3	–	18	4	–	17	21	–	23	Denmark, Labor and Social Ministries 1955
Finland	1961-62	1,991	9	6	–	3	–	–	6	14	22	8	–	41	Vannas and Raivio 1964
France[d]	1955	1,630	25	9	–	16	–	13	8	19	14	16	1	3	Desvignes et al. 1955
Italy[e]	1958	500[f]	37	11	2	24	–	7	30	7	10	6	–	2	Pascucci 1958
Oceania															
New Zealand	1968	3,687	16	10	–	2	–	4	12	5	34	8	–	21	Sturman 1969
13/200 (4/60)															
Europe															
Denmark[g]	1958-60	1,000	23	15	–	8	–	3	6	9	48	8	–	3	Vedel-Jensen 1962
10/200 (3/60)															
America															
Bolivia	1956	229	27	11	1	12	–	25	–	25	1	22	–	–	Solares 1956
Asia															
Iran	1955	145	9	9	–	–	40	14	6	2	2	3	–	24	Mohsénine and Darougar 1955

Location	Year	Total												Reference
Europe														
Czechoslovakia	1962	74	30	12	4	14	1	5	8	7	16	15	–	18	Štefek and Štruplová 1963
Iceland	1950	143	57	52	1	4	–	8	8	7	13	4	–	2	Björnsson 1955
Malta and Gozo	1958	638	38	17	2	19	–	12	21	2	1	7	–	18	Damato 1960
Netherlands	1959	4,180	28	9	12	7	1	4	6	13	31	13	–	4	Schappert-Kimmijser 1959
United Kingdom															
England and Wales	1960	10,050	24	13	–	9	–	2	22	3	44	4	–	1	Great Britain, Ministry of Health 1961
7/200 (2/60)															
Asia															
Kuwait	1965	400	31	26	3	2	36	25	4	–	–	1	–	3	Holmes 1966
Europe															
Sweden	1967	3,557[h]	19	15	–	–	1	6	5	15	33	14	–	7	Lindstedt 1967
3/200 (1/60)															
Africa															
Cameroons	1952	332	12	7	–	5	–	36	17	12	10	4	–	8	Rodger 1959
Ghana (North)	1952	1,230	5	1	–	4	–	49	7	33	3	2	–	–	Rodger 1959
Nigeria (North)	1952	2,330	8	2	–	5	–	52	18	12	4	5	–	1	Rodger 1959
U.A.R.	1952	44,082	58	23	–	35	–	28	7	1	1	–	–	4	United Arab Republic, Ministry of Public Health, Ophthalmic Section 1953
U.A.R.[c] (urban)	1965-66	25	16	8	–	8	–	16	52	4	8	4	–	–	Said et al. 1967
(rural)		107	12	11	–	1	–	51	30	3	3	1	–	–	
Europe															
Norway	1948	3,146	14	5	6	3	2	11	12	14	17	14	–	16	Holst 1952
Spain[i]	1947-52	900	19	16	–	–	2	37	8	12	7	14	–	–	Alcalá-Lopez 1953
Absolute blindness															
Africa															
Kenya	1953-55	1,093	22	5	–	1	–	20	46	2	1	6	–	3	Calcott 1956
Oceania															
New Zealand	1962	304	28	16	–	3	–	4	7	3	33	5	–	19	Tennent 1962
No definition given															
Africa															
Burundi	1951-53	153	12	10	2	–	–	–	40	–	–	34	–	–	Kivits 1955
Nigeria	1944	254	5	4	–	–	41	–	10	–	–	–	–	44	Stock 1946
South Africa	1945	32,873	6	3	–	–	7	4	39	–	–	–	–	44	South African National Council for the Blind 1944-45
European pop.		2,218	37	7	–	–	4	14	11	–	–	–	–	36	
Colored pop.		2,080	19	13	–	–	6	9	16	–	–	–	–	41	
Asiatic pop.		133	8	4	–	–	11	18	44	–	–	–	–	23	
Bantu pop.		28,442	3	2	–	–	8	3	42	–	–	–	–	45	

(continued)

Table A.12.10 Number of blind persons and percentage distribution by site and by type of affection[a], by definition of blindness; selected countries[b], various years, 1944-68 (continued)

Definition, continent and country	Year	No. of blind	Eyeball in general										Site and type unspecified or not reported	Source
			Total	Glaucoma (exclusive of congenital)	Structural anomalies	Refractory errors, degenerative changes	Conjunctiva	Cornea	Lens	Uveal tract	Retina	Optic nerve, optic pathway and cortical visual centers	Vitreous	
No definition given (continued)															
Africa (continued)															
Southern Rhodesia	1960	1,032	4	4	-	-	-	31	46	-	-	6	-	13	Executive Sub-Committee, Coordinating Committee for Blind Welfare 1960
Tunisia	1954	243	52	51	1	-	25	17	-	1	2	1	-	2	Malnou 1954
America															
Nicaragua	1950	100	35	27	2	-	9	5	-	10	10	10	-	21	Lacayo 1950
Europe															
Netherlands	1954	306	26	12	7	7	-	2	6	10	23	3	-	30	Schappert-Kimmijser 1956
Oceania															
Australia	1953-58	2,806	25	16	-	9	1	7	20	4	22	9	-	12	Yates 1963
Tasmania	1953-58	157	20	15	-	-	-	4	24	10	22	18	1	1	Phillips 1959
Kimberly District	1953	149	3	2	1	-	3	75	14	-	-	-	-	5	Mann 1954
New Guinea and Papua	1954-55	96	13	1	1	11	1	33	40	7	-	5	-	-	Mann and Loschdorfer 1956

[a]These data are based on surveys of specific towns, villages, or regions, or on examinations of blind persons seen at certain institutions for the blind, or registered as blind in order to secure certain benefits or services. The data refer only to those blind for whom site or type of affection data were available and not to total prevalence.
[b]Excluding United States.
[c]Alexandria area only.
[d]Paris area only.
[e]Umbrian region only.
[f]Approximately.
[g]Newly registered.
[h]All above age 16 as of January 1, 1964, who had lost their locomotor vision before age 60.
[i]Malaga province only.

APPENDIX / 397

Table A.12.11 Number of blind persons and percentage distribution by cause of blindness[a], by definition of blindness[b]: selected countries[b], various years, 1944-68

Definition, continent and country	Year	No. of blind	Infectious diseases Total	Gonorrhoea	Smallpox	Syphilis	Trachoma	Onchocerciasis	Leprosy	Accidents and poisonings	Neoplasm not elsewhere classified (NEC)	General diseases NEC	Prenatal influence NEC	Cause undetermined or not specified	Source
20/200 (6/60)															
Africa															
U.A.R.[c] (urban)	1965-66	74	31	-	-	-	-	-	-	1	-	41	1	26	Said et al. 1967
(rural)		274	54	-	-	-	1	-	-	1	-	32	4	9	
America															
Argentine	1955	14,309	38	-	-	-	-	-	-	9	-	2	25	26	Diez et al. 1955
Canada	1965	24,605	12	3	-	3	1	-	-	7	1	16	32	31	MacDonald 1965
Venezuela	1949-54	216	15	2	-	12	1	-	-	-	1	-	-	84	Espino 1954
Europe															
Denmark	1952	145	-	-	-	-	-	-	-	7	-	-	12	81	Denmark, Labor and Social Ministries 1955
Finland	1961-62	1,991	-	-	-	-	-	-	-	26	-	2	23	49	Vannas and Raivio 1964
France[e]	1955	1,630[f]	-	-	-	-	-	-	-	1	-	3	1	94	Desvignes et al. 1955
Italy[e]	1958	500[f]	-	-	-	-	-	-	-	8	-	1	26	65	Pascucci 1958
Oceania															
New Zealand	1968	3,687	3	-	-	-	-	-	-	5	1	34	18	38	Sturman 1969
13/200 (4/60)															
Europe															
Denmark[g]	1958-60	1,000	-	-	-	-	-	-	-	-	-	24	4	72	Vedel-Jensen 1962
10/200 (3/60)															
America															
Bolivia	1956	229	43	1	10	13	1	-	-	13	-	6	1	37	Solares 1956
Asia															
Iran	1955	145	70	-	16	-	14	-	-	7	-	1	2	20	Mohsenine and Darougar 1955

(continued)

Table A.12.11 Number of blind persons and percentage distribution by cause of blindness[a], by definition of blindness: selected countries[b], various years, 1944-68 (continued)

Location	Year	Number										Reference
Europe												
7/200 (2/60)												
Czechoslovakia	1962	74	3	–	1	1	–	13	–	3	19	62	Štefek and Štruplová 1963
Iceland	1950	143	–	–	–	–	–	2	1	–	4	94	Björnsson 1955
Malta and Gozo	1958	638	13	–	–	12	–	2	1	15	9	59	Damato 1960
Netherlands	1959	4,180	7	–	1	–	–	7	4	8	41	33	Schappert-Kimmijser 1959
United Kingdom													
England and Wales	1960	10,050	1	–	–	–	–	1	1	13	5	80	Great Britain, Ministry of Health 1961
Asia												
Kuwait	1965	400	62	–	–	7	–	3	–	5	29	1	Holmes 1966
Europe												
Sweden	1967	3,557[h]	9	1	2	–	–	11	–	20	34	26	Lindstedt 1967
3/200 (1/60)												
Africa												
Cameroons	1952	332	64	–	5	6	27	23	2	1	–	33	Rodger 1959
Ghana (North)	1952	1,230	80	–	2	3	20	45	1	2	–	18	Rodger 1959
Nigeria (North)	1952	2,330	65	–	7	7	31	2	1	1	–	31	Rodger 1959
U.A.R.	1952	44,082	28	–	–	–	–	–	–	–	–	71	U.A.R., Ministry of Public Health, Opthalmic Section 1953
U.A.R.[c] (urban)	1965-66	25	16	–	–	–	–	–	–	60	4	20	Said et al. 1967
(rural)		107	51	–	–	–	–	3	–	29	3	14	
Europe												
Norway	1948	3,146	9	2	4	–	–	–	2	2	50	23	Holst 1952
Spain[i]	1947-52	900	38	1	4	–	23	–	13	1	16	7	31	Alcalá-Lopez 1953
Absolute blindness												
Africa												
Kenya	1953-55	1,093	5	–	–	4	–	–	2	–	–	93	Calcott 1956
Oceania												
New Zealand	1962	304	2	–	1	1	–	–	4	10	–	83	Tennent 1962
No definition given												
Africa												
Burundi	1951-53	153	10	–	–	–	5	–	2	–	–	88	Kivits 1955
Nigeria	1944	254	42	–	41	–	16	–	1	–	–	3	57	Stock 1946
South Africa	1945	32,873	20	1	6	–	1	–	2	6	3	69	So. African Natl. Council for the Blind 1944-45
European pop.		2,218	31	2	11	–	–	–	8	8	34	19	
Colored pop.		2,080	50	3	20	–	16	–	6	8	7	29	
Asiatic pop.		133	35	2	9	–	1	–	3	1	6	56	

APPENDIX / 399

Definition, continent and country	Year	No. of blind	Infectious diseases							Accidents and poisonings	Neoplasm NEC	General diseases NEC	Prenatal influence NEC	Cause undetermined or not specified	Source
			Total	Gonorrhoea	Smallpox	Syphilis	Trachoma	Onchocerciasis	Leprosy						
No definition given (continued)															
Africa (continued)															
Southern Rhodesia	1960	1,032	17	-	-	-	17	-	-	-	-	-	-	83	Exec. Sub-Comm., Coordinating Comm. for Blind Welfare 1960
Tunisia	1954	243	42	-	-	-	2	-	-	2	-	-	-	56	Malnou 1954
America															
Nicaragua	1950	100	27	9	-	7	-	-	-	22	1	1	5	44	Lacayo 1950
Europe															
Netherlands	1954	306	9	-	-	3	-	-	-	9	-	9	53	19	Schappert-Kimmijser 1956
Oceania															
Australia	1953-58	2,806	6	1	-	-	2	-	-	6	1	16	15	56	Yates 1963
Tasmania	1953-58	157	9	-	-	-	-	-	-	8	1	30	14	38	Phillips 1959
Kimberly Distr.	1953	149	76	3	-	-	72	-	1	9	-	-	1	13	Mann 1954
New Guinea and Papua	1954-55	96	21	1	-	-	20	-	-	6	-	-	-	73	Mann and Loschdorfer 1956

[a] These data are based on surveys of specific towns, villages, or regions, or on examinations of blind persons seen at certain institutions for the blind, or registered as blind in order to secure certain benefits or services. The data refer only to those blind for whom site or type of affection data were available and not to total prevalence.
[b] Excluding United States.
[c] Alexandria area only.
[d] Paris area only.
[e] Umbrian region only.
[f] Approximately.
[g] Newly registered.
[h] All above age 16 as of January 1, 1964, who had lost their locomotor vision before age 60.
[i] Malaga province only.

REFERENCES

Acheson, E.D., "Multiple sclerosis in British Commonwealth countries in the Southern Hemisphere," *Brit J Prev Soc Med*, 15:118-125 (1961).

───── "The epidemiology of multiple sclerosis," in D. McAlpine, C.E. Lumsden, and E.D. Acheson, eds., *Multiple sclerosis: a reappraisal* (Edinburgh: Livingstone, 1965), pp. 3-58.

───── C.A. Bachrach, and F.M. Wright, "Some comments on the relationship of the distribution of multiple sclerosis to latitude, solar radiation, and other variables," *Acta Psychiat Neurol Scand*, 35 suppl 147:132-147 (1960).

Ackermann, A., "Die multiple Sklerose in der Schweiz: Enquete von 1918-22," *Schweiz Med Wschr*, 61:1245-1250 (1931).

Adams, J.M., and D.T. Imagawa, "Measles antibodies in multiple sclerosis," *Proc Soc Exp Biol Med*, 111:562-566 (1962).

Adams, R.D., D. Denny-Brown, and C.M. Pearson, *Diseases of muscle: a study in pathology*, ed. 2 (New York: Hoeber Medical Division, Harper, 1962), 735 pp.

───── L.M. Eaton, and G.M. Shy, eds., "Neuromuscular disorders (the motor unit and its disorders)," *Proc Assn Res Nerv Ment Dis*, 38:1-813 (1960).

Adler, F.H., *Gifford's textbook of ophthalmology*, ed. 6 (Philadelphia: Saunders, 1957), p. 358.

Alcalá-Lopez, A., "A description of classification of the causes of blindness and statistics on the blind of Malaga," *Arch Soc Oftal Hisp-Amer*, 13:642-658 (1953).

Allan, W., "Inheritance of shaking palsy," *Arch Intern Med* (Chicago), 60:424-436 (1937).

Allen, J.H., *May's manual of the diseases of the eye for students and general practitioners*, ed. 23 (Baltimore: Williams & Wilkins, 1963), p. 94.

Allison, R.S., "Disseminated sclerosis in North Wales: an inquiry into its incidence, frequency, distribution and other aetiological factors," *Brain*, 53:391-430 (1931).

───── "Some neurological aspects of medical geography," *Proc Roy Soc Med*, 56:71-76 (1963).

───── "Multiple sclerosis in Northern Ireland," read at the Symposium on Multiple Sclerosis sponsored by the National Multiple Sclerosis Society, New York, 24 September 1969.

───── and J.H.D. Millar, "Prevalence of disseminated sclerosis in Northern Ireland," *Ulster Med J*, 23 suppl 2:5-22 (1954).

Alter, M., "Anencephalic births in a northern and a southern community: a comparison," *Amer J Dis Child*, 106:536-544 (1963a).

───── "Familial aggregation of Bell's palsy," *Arch Neurol* (Chicago), 8:557-564 (1963b).

───── Personal communication, September 1969.

───── and J.F. Kurtzke, *The epidemiology of multiple sclerosis* (Springfield, Ill.: Charles C Thomas, 1968), 204 pp.

―― and J. Speer, "Clinical evaluation of possible etiology factors in multiple sclerosis," *Neurology (Minneap)*, 18:109-116 (1968).

―― and O.R. Talbert, unpublished data.

―― R.S. Allison, O.R. Talbert, and L.T. Kurland, "Geographic distribution of multiple sclerosis: a comparison of prevalence in Charleston County, South Carolina, U.S.A., and Halifax County, Nova Scotia, Canada," *World Neurol*, 1:55-68 (1960).

―― L. Halpern, L.T. Kurland, B. Bornstein, U. Leibowitz, and J. Silberstein, "Multiple sclerosis in Israel: prevalence among immigrants and native inhabitants," *Arch Neurol (Chicago)*, 7:253-263 (1962).

―― U. Leibowitz, and J. Speer, "Risk of multiple sclerosis related to age at immigration to Israel," *Arch Neurol (Chicago)*, 15:234-237 (1966).

―― A. Antonovsky, and U. Leibowitz, "Epidemiology of multiple sclerosis in Israel," in M. Alter and J.F. Kurtzke, eds., *The epidemiology of multiple sclerosis* (Springfield, Ill.: Charles C Thomas, 1968), pp. 83-109.

Altmann, F., "Histopathology and etiology of otosclerosis: a critical review," in H.F. Schuknecht, ed., *Otosclerosis* (Boston: Little, Brown, 1962), pp. 15-42.

American Foundation for the Blind, Inc., *Proceedings of the International Conference of Workers for the Blind*, Merton College. Oxford (American Foundation for the Blind, New York, and National Institute for the Blind, London, with the participation of the United Nations Organization and UNESCO, 4-12 August 1949).

Ancona, F., and A. Tomaino, "Risultati delle campagne di audiometria scolastica relative agli anni 1959-1963," *Arcisped S Anna Ferrara*, 17:489-501 (1964).

Andersen, B., "Cerebral palsy," *J Oslo City Hosp*, 4:65-87 (1954).

Andrade, C., "A peculiar form of peripheral neuropathy: familiar atypical generalized amyloidosis with special involvement of the peripheral nerves," *Brain*, 75:408-427 (1952).

Annotation, "Rubella and congenital defects," *Brit Med J*, 2:1005 (1960).

―― "Viral infections during pregnancy and their effects on the offspring," *Quart Rev Pediat*, 16:57-59 (1961).

Antonovsky, A., U. Leibowitz, J.M. Medalie, H.A. Smith, L. Halpern, and M. Alter, "Epidemiological study of multiple sclerosis in Israel. Part III. Multiple sclerosis and socio-economic status," *J Neurol Neurosurg Psychiat*, n.s. 30:1-6 (1967).

Around the World, "Northern Rhodesia: Study of blindness in children," *Sightsav Rev*, 33:48 (1963).

―― *Sightsav Rev*, 34:40-44 (1964).

Babbott, J.G., and T.H. Ingalls, "Field studies of selected congenital malformations occurring in Pennsylvania," *Amer J Public Health*, 52:2009-2017 (1962).

Bamford, J.A.C., and C.A.P. Boundy, "The natural history of herpes zoster (shingles)," *Med J Aust*, 1:524-528 (1968).

Barlow, J.S., "Correlation of the geographic distribution of multiple sclerosis with cosmic-ray intensities," *Acta Psychiat Neurol Scand*, 35 suppl 147:108-130 (1960).

——— "Solar-flare induced increases in sea-level cosmic ray intensities and other geophysical phenomena in relation to multiple sclerosis," *Acta Neurol Scand*, 42 suppl 19:118-136 (1966).

——— "Multiple sclerosis in North Korea and China: translations of original papers from the Bulgarian and the Chinese," *Neurology (Minneap)*, 17:802-812 (1967).

"Current brain research in China" (abstr.), *Excerpta Medica International Congress Series* No. 193, 1969a, pp. 306-307.

——— "The geography of multiple sclerosis—some contributions from the recent non-English literature" (abstr.), *Excerpta Medica International Congress Series* No. 193, 1969b, p. 307.

Barr, B., and R. Lundström, "Deafness following maternal rubella: retrospective and prospective studies," *Acta Otolaryng (Stockholm)*, 53:413-423 (1961).

Barton, M.E., S.D. Court, and W. Walker, "Causes of severe deafness in schoolchildren in Northumberland and Durham," *Brit Med J*, 1:351-355 (1962).

Barwick, D.D., and J.N. Walton, "Polymyositis," *Amer J Med*, 35:646-660 (1963).

Batsakis, J.G., and R.H. Nishiyama, "Deafness with sporadic goiter: Pendred's syndrome," *Arch Otolaryng (Chicago)*, 76:401-406 (1962).

Beasley, W.C., "Characteristics and distribution of impaired hearing in the population of the United States," *J Acoust Soc Amer*, 12:114-121 (1940).

Becker, P.E., "Two new families of benign sex-linked recessive muscular dystrophy," *Rev Canad Biol*, 21:551-566 (1962).

Beebe, G.W., J.F. Kurtzke, L.T. Kurland, T.L. Auth, and B. Nagler, "Studies on the natural history of multiple sclerosis. 3. Epidemiologic analysis of the Army experience in World War II," *Neurology (Minneap)*, 17:1-17 (1967).

Behrend, R.C., "Prevalence of multiple sclerosis in Hamburg and Marseille," *Acta Neurol Scand*, 42 suppl 19:27-41 (1966).

——— "A basis for discussion of an MS epidemiological research programme in Europe" (abstr.), *Excerpta Medica International Congress Series* No. 193, 1969, p. 188.

Belgique Institut national de Statistique, *Annuaire statistique de la Belgique*, 1963.

Bell, E.A., personal communication, 1966.

Belloc, N.B., D.H. Fowler, and W.D. Simmons, "Causes of blindness in California," *Sightsav Rev*, 27:98-111 (1957).

Berens, C., F.M. Foote, and C.E. Kerby, "Prevention of blindness in children: statistical and sociologic aspects," in *XVII Concilium Ophthalmologicum, 1954, Canada, United States of America, Acta*, vol. 3 (Toronto: University of Toronto Press, 1955), pp. 2052-2058.

Berry, R.J., "Genetic factors in the aetiology of multiple sclerosis," *Acta Neurol Scand*, 45:459-483 (1969).

Bickford, J.A.R., and R.M. Ellison, "The high incidence of Huntington's chorea in the Duchy of Cornwall," *J Ment Sci*, 99:291-294 (1953).

Bing, R., and H. Reese, "Die multiple Sklerose in der Nordwestschweiz (Kantone Basel, Solothurn, Aargau, Luzern)," *Schweiz Med Wschr*, 56:30-34 (1926).

Bird, A.V., H.J. Heinz, and G. Klintworth, "Convulsive disorders in Bantu mine-workers," *Epilepsia (Amst)*, s.4. 3:175-187 (1962).

Björnsson, G., "Prevalence and causes of blindness in Iceland: with special reference to glaucoma simplex," *Amer J Ophthal*, 39:202-208 (1955).
——— "The primary glaucoma in Iceland: epidemiological studies," *Acta Ophthal (Kobenhavn)*, suppl 91:3-99 (1967).
Bonduelle, M.M., P. Bouygues, J. Delahousse, and C. Faveret, "Evolution simultanée chez un même malade d'une maladie de Parkinson et d'une sclérose latérale amyotrophique: discussion," *Rev Neurol (Paris)*, 101:63-66 (1959).
Bornstein, M.B., and S.M. Crain, "Functional studies of cultured brain tissues as related to 'demyelinative disorders'," *Science*, 148:1242-1244 (1965).
Boughton, C.R., "Varicella-zoster in Sydney. 3. Herpes zoster and complications," *Med J Aust*, 2:502-504 (1966).
Brandt, S., *Werdnig-Hoffmann's infantile progressive muscular atrophy: clinical aspects, pathology, heredity and relation to Oppenheim's amyotonia congenita and other morbid conditions with laxity of joints or muscles in infants* (Copenhagen: Ejnar Munksgaard, 1950), 344 pp.
Brendle, P., E. Elsässer, A. Löwe, and O. Martin, "Hörschäden bei Volks- und Hilfsschülern," *Neue Blätter für Taubstummenbildung*, 15:200-211 (1961).
Brewis, M., D.C. Poskanzer, C. Rolland, and H. Miller, "Neurological disease in an English city," *Acta Neurol Scand*, 42 suppl 24:9-89 (1966).
British Empire Society for the Blind, *Annual report and accounts* (London, 1954-56).
Broman, T., "Parkinson's syndrome, prevalence and incidence in Göteborg," *Acta Neurol Scand*, 39 suppl 4:95-101 (1963).
Brothers, C.R.D., "Huntington's chorea in Victoria and Tasmania," *J Neurol Sci*, 1:405-420 (1964).
——— and A.W. Meadows, "An investigation of Huntington's chorea in Victoria," *J Ment Sci*, 101:548-563 (1955).
Brown, K.S., "The genetics of childhood deafness," in F. McConnell and P.H. Ward, eds., *National symposium on deafness in childhood* (Nashville, Tenn.: Vanderbilt University Press, 1967), pp. 177-202.
Brown, W.J., J.F. Donohue, N.W. Axnick, J.H. Blount, N.H. Ewen, and O.G. Jones, *Syphilis and other venereal diseases* (APHA monograph; Cambridge, Mass.: Harvard University Press, 1970), 241 pp.
Bunina, T.L., "On intracellular inclusions in familial amyotrophic lateral sclerosis," *Zh Nevropat Psikhiat Korsakov*, 62:1293-1299 (1962).
Burch, T.A., W.M. O'Brien, R. Need, and L.T. Kurland, "Hyperuricaemia and gout in the Mariana Islands," *Ann Rheum Dis*, 25:114-116 (1966).

Calcott, R.D., *Blindness in Kenya* (London: British Empire Society for the Blind, 1956), 28 pp.
Campanelli, P.A., and J.D. Schein, "Inter-observer agreement in judging auditory responses in neonates," *Eye Ear Nose Throat Monthly*, 48:697-702 (1969).
Campbell, A.M.G., G. Herdan, W.F.T. Tatlow, and E.G. Whittle, "Lead in relation to disseminated sclerosis," *Brain*, 73:52-70 (1950).
——— R.M. Norman, and R.J. Sandry, "Subacute encephalitis in an adult associated with necrotising myelitis and results of animal inoculation experiments," *J Neurol Neurosurg Psychiat*, 26:439-446 (1963).
Canadian Sickness Survey, 1950-51, special compilation no. 5: *Volume of*

sickness (Ottawa: Dominion Bureau of Statistics and Department of National Health and Welfare, April 1954).

Carter, S., "Diagnosis and treatment: management of the child who has had one convulsion," *Pediatrics*, 33:431-434 (1964).

Caruso, G., A. Uras, and A. Coni, "La sclerosi a placche in Sardegna: sua prevalenza e distribuzione in rapporto alle variazioni altimetriche del suolo," *Acta Neurol (Napoli)*, 23:382-392 (1968).

Cassady, G., K. Brown, M. Cohen, and W. DeMaria, "Hereditary renal dysfunction and deafness," *Pediatrics*, 35:967-979 (1965).

Cendrowski, W., "Niektóre dane o geografii plasawicy dziedzicznej" [Some data on the geography of hereditary chorea], *Neurol Neurochir Psychiat Pol*, 14:63-66 (1964).

Central Bureau of Statistics, The Hague, Netherlands, personal communication, 1961.

Chalfant, J.C., *Factors related to special education services in Illinois*, unpublished doctoral dissertation, University of Illinois, 1965.

Charcot, J.M., *Lectures on the diseases of the nervous system*, translated from the second edition by G. Sigerson (Philadelphia: Henry C. Lea, 1879), 271 pp.

Chen, K., J.A. Brody, and L.T. Kurland, "Patterns of neurologic diseases on Guam. I. Epidemiologic aspects," *Arch Neurol (Chicago)*, 19:573-578 (1968).

Chipman, M., "Multiple sclerosis in Houston, Texas, 1954-1959: a study of the methodology used in determining a prevalence rate in a large southern city," *Acta Neurol Scand*, 42 suppl 19:77-82 (1966).

Cockburn, W.C., "World aspects of the epidemiology of rubella," *Amer J Dis Child*, 118:112-122 (1969).

Coffey, V.P., and W.J.E. Jessop, "A study of 137 cases of anencephaly," *Brit J Prev Soc Med*, 11:174-180 (1957).

Collmann, R.D., and A. Stoller, "A survey of mongolism and congenital anomalies of the central nervous system in Victoria," *New Zealand Med J*, 61:24-32 (1962*a*).

────── "A survey of mongoloid births in Victoria, Australia, 1942-1957," *Amer J Public Health*, 52:813-829 (1962*b*).

Comision Nacional del Censo, Argentine Republic, *Tercer Censo Nacional: Levantado el 1 de Junio de 1914*, vol. 1 (Buenos Aires: Comision, 1916), 656 pp.

Commission on Terminology (International League against Epilepsy), "A proposed international classification of epileptic seizures," *Epilepsia (Amst)*, s.4. 5:297-306 (1964).

Conway, H., and K.J. Wagner, "Congenital anomalies of the head and neck as reported on birth certificates in New York City, 1952 to 1962, inclusive," *Plast Reconstr Surg*, 36:71-79 (1965).

Cooper, J.E., "Epilepsy in a longitudinal survey of 5,000 children," *Brit Med J*, 1:1020-1022 (1965).

Cotzias, G.C., P.S. Papavasiliou, and R. Gellene, "Modification of parkinsonism: chronic treatment with L-dopa," *New Eng J Med*, 280:337-345 (1969).

Crombie, D.L., K.W. Cross, J. Fry, R.J.F.H. Pinsent, and C.A.H. Watts, "A survey of the epilepsies in general practice: a report by the Research Committee of the College of General Practitioners," *Brit Med J*, 2:416-422 (1960).

Cruickshank, E.K., "Neuromuscular disease in relation to nutrition," *Fed Proc*, 20 suppl 7:345-352 (1961).

Dada, T.O., *Epilepsy in Nigeria: a study of the incidence, pathogenesis, clinical patterns and socio-psychological problems of epilepsy*, M.D. thesis, Bristol, England, September 1968.

Dalby, M.A., "Epilepsy and 3 per second spike and wave rhythms: a clinical, electroencephalographic and prognostic analysis of 346 patients," *Acta Neurol Scand*, 45 suppl 40:1-183 (1969).

Damato, F.J., "Incidence and causes of blindness in the Maltese Islands: a survey based on the examination of 638 blind persons," *Brit J. Ophthal*, 44:164-171 (1960).

Dauer, C.C., R.F. Korns, and L.M. Schuman, *Infectious diseases* (APHA monograph; Cambridge, Mass.: Harvard University Press, 1968), 262 pp.

Davis, H., ed., "The young deaf child: identification and management," *Acta Otolaryng (Stockholm)*, suppl 206:1-258 (1965).

―――― and F.W. Kranz, "The international standard reference zero for pure-tone audiometers and its relation to the evaluation of impairment of hearing," *J Speech Hearing Res*, 7:7-16 (1964).

―――― and S.R. Silverman, *Hearing and deafness*, ed. 3 (New York: Holt, Rinehart & Winston, 1970), 522 pp.

Dean, G., "Disseminated sclerosis in South Africa: its relationship to swayback disease and suggested treatment," *Brit Med J*, 1:842-845 (1949).

―――― "Annual incidence, prevalence, and mortality of multiple sclerosis in white South-African-born and in white immigrants to South Africa," *Brit Med J*, 2:724-730 (1967).

―――― and J.F. Kurtzke, "A critical age for the acquisition of multiple sclerosis" (abstr.), *Trans Amer Neurol Assn*, 95:232-233 (1970).

―――― ―――― "On the risk of multiple sclerosis according to age at immigration to South Africa," *Brit Med J*, 3:725-729 (1971).

DeJong, D., "Parkinson's disease—V.A.-D.V.A. Study Group. Part 1. Biostatistics and case reporting," *Med Serv J Canada*, 16:3-12 (1960).

―――― "Parkinson's disease: statistics," *J Neurosurg*, 24:149-158 (1966).

Denmark, Labor and Social Ministries, *Follow-up study of students suffering from blindness*, a report by the scientific advisor to the ministries, Economic and statistical studies no. 21 (Copenhagen, 1955).

De Reynier, J.P., "La surdi-mutité en Suisse en 1953," *Bibl Otorhinolaryng*, 5:1-73 (1959).

DeSanto, L.W., and H.A. Schubert, Bell's palsy: ten cases in a family," *Arch Otolaryng (Chicago)*, 89:700-702 (1969).

Desvignes, P., Michaut, and Gouray, "The causes of invalidism from blindness in the Paris region," *Bull Soc Ophtal Franc*, 7:466-467 (1955).

Diez, M.A., E. Adroqué, and E.C. Adroqué, "Causes of blindness in the Argentine Republic," *Oftal (B Air)*, 30:350-356 (1955).
Dimsdale, H., "Changes in the parkinsonian syndrome in the twentieth century," *Quart J Med*, n.s. 15:155-170 (1946).
Dirrecion Nacional de Estadistica, *Censo Nacional de Poblacion de 1940*, vol. 1 (Lima, Peru: Ministerio de Hacienda y Comercio, 1943), 673 pp.
Dixon, W.J., and F.J. Massey, Jr., *Introduction to statistical analysis*, ed. 3 (New York: McGraw-Hill, 1969), 638 pp.
Doctor, P.V., "A proposed study of the incidence of deafness structured geographically by school enrollment in states, 1848-1964," in *Proceedings of the conference on the collection of statistics of severe hearing impairments and deafness in the United States, 1964* Public Health Service Publication No. 1227 (Washington, D.C.: Government Printing Office, 1964), pp. 24-27.
Dorn, H.F., "Some applications of biometry in the collection and evaluation of medical data," *J Chronic Dis*, 1:638-664 (1955).
Doxiadis, S., S. Pantelakis, and T. Valaes, "Down's syndrome and infectious hepatitis" (letter to the editor), *Lancet*, 1:897 (1970a).
────── ────── ────── "Infectious hepatitis and Down's syndrome" (letter to the editor), *Lancet*, 2:826 (1970b).
Duff, F.L., *Effects of geography, season and length of military service upon common respiratory diseases in United States Army*, graduate school thesis, Johns Hopkins University, Baltimore, 1953.
Dunn, O.J., *Basic statistics: a primer for the biomedical sciences* (New York: John Wiley, 1964), 184 pp.
Duvoisin, R.C., and M.D. Schweitzer, "Paralysis agitans mortality in England and Wales, 1855-1962," *Brit J Prev Soc Med*, 20:27-33 (1966).
────── and M.D. Yahr. "Encephalitis and parkinsonism," *Arch Neurol (Chicago)*, 12:227-239 (1965).
────── ────── M.D. Schweitzer, and H.H. Merritt, "Parkinsonism before and since the epidemic of encephalitis lethargica," *Arch Neurol (Chicago)*, 9:232-236 (1963).
Dyck, P.J., and E.H. Lambert, "Lower motor and primary sensory neuron diseases with peroneal muscular atrophy. II. Neurologic, genetic, and electrophysiologic findings in various neuronal degenerations," *Arch Neurol (Chicago)*, 18:619-625 (1968).

Eadie, M.J., J. M. Sutherland, and R.L. Doherty, "Encephalitis in etiology of parkinsonism in Australia," *Arch Neurol (Chicago)*, 12:240-245 (1965).
Eagles, E.L., "Methodological problems in collecting data on the deaf: the survey," in *Proceedings of the conference on the collection of statistics of severe hearing impairments and deafness in the United States, 1964*, Public Health Service Publication No. 1227 (Washington, D.C.: Government Printing Office, 1964), pp. 41-44.
────── S.M. Wishik, L.G. Doerfler, W. Melnick, and H.S. Levine, *Hearing sensitivity and related factors in children* (Pittsburgh: University of Pittsburgh Graduate School of Public Health, 1963), 220 pp.
Educational Research and Development Council of the Twin Cities Metropolitan Area, Inc., *Children with hearing handicaps* (Minneapolis: privately published, 1964), 82 pp.

Eldridge, R., "The torsion dystonias: literature review and genetic and clinical studies," *Neurology (Minneap)*, 20(pt 2):1-78 (1970).
───── E. Ryan, J. Brody, and I. Cooper, "Dystonia musculorum deformans: evidence for two hereditary forms," *Excerpta Medica International Congress Series* No. 175, 1967, pp. 772-788.
Elizan, T.S., K.-M. Chen, K.V. Mathai, D. Dunn, and L.T. Kurland, "Amyotrophic lateral sclerosis and parkinsonism-dementia complex: a study in non-Chamorros of the Mariana and Caroline Islands," *Arch Neurol (Chicago)* 14:347-355 (1966a).
───── A. Hirano, B.M. Abrams, R.L. Need, C. Van Nuis, and L.T. Kurland, "Amyotrophic lateral sclerosis and parkinsonism-dementia complex of Guam: neurological reevaluation," *Arch Neurol (Chicago)*, 14:356-368 (1966b).
Espino, J.M., "Causes of blindness in Venezuela," *Gac Med Caracas*, 62:625-628 (1954).
Espinosa, R.E., M.M. Okihoro, D.W. Mulder, and G.P. Sayre, "Hereditary amyotrophic lateral sclerosis: a clinical and pathologic report with comments on classification," *Neurology (Minneap)*, 12:1-7 (1962).
Evans, J.H., "Post-traumatic epilepsy," *Neurology (Minneap)*, 12:665-674 (1962).
Everberg, G., "Unilateral anacusis: clinical, radiological, and genetic investigations," *Acta Otolaryng (Stockholm)*, suppl 158-366-374 (1960a).
───── "Unilateral total deafness in children: clinical problems with a special view to vestibular function," *Acta Otolaryng (Stockholm)*, 52:253-269 (1960b).
Executive Sub-Committee, Co-ordinating Committee for Blind Welfare, "Some facts and figures on the survey of African blindness," *Cent Afr J Med*, 6:267-270 (1960).

Fahey, D.J., "Otologic care of cleft palate cases," *Laryngoscope*, 75:570-587 (1965).
Farrant, R.H., *The audiometric testing of children in schools and kindergartens*, Report C.A.L. No. 14 (Sydney, Australia: Commonwealth Acoustic Laboratories, March 1958), 57 pp.
Feinmesser, M., L. Bauberger-Tell, and R. Bilski-Hirsch, "A hearing survey in the public schools of Jerusalem," *Israel Med J*, 18:59-63 (1959).
Field, E.J., H. Miller, and D.S. Russell, "Observations on glial inclusion bodies in a case of acute disseminated sclerosis," *J Clin Path*, 15:278-284 (1962).
Forssman, H., and H.O. Åkesson, "Mortality in patients with Down's syndrome," *J Ment Defic Res*, 9:146-149 (1965).
Fox, J.P., C.E. Hall, and L.R. Elveback, *Epidemiology: man and disease* (London: Macmillan, 1970), 339 pp.
Frantzen, E., M. Lennox-Buchthal, and A. Nygaard, "Longitudinal EEG and clinical study of children with febrile convulsions," *Electroenceph Clin Neurophysiol*, 24:197-212 (1968).
Fraser, G.R., "Profound childhood deafness," *J Med Genet*, 1:118-151 (1964).
Freeman, M.S., and R.J. Freeman, "Serous otitis media," *Amer J Dis Child*, 99:683-687 (1960).
Friedman, A.P., and D. Freedman, "Amyotrophic lateral sclerosis," *J Nerv Ment Dis*, 111:1-18 (1950).

Fullmer, H.M., H.D. Siedler, R.S. Krooth, and L.T. Kurland, "A cutaneous disorder of connective tissue of amyotrophic lateral sclerosis: a histochemical study," *Neurology (Minneap)*, 10:717-724 (1960).

Gajdusek, D.C., "Motor-neuron disease in natives of New Guinea," *New Eng J Med*, 268:474-476 (1963).

———"Kuru in New Guinea and the origin of the NINDB study of slow, latent, and temperate virus infections of the nervous system of man," in D.C. Gajdusek, C.J. Gibbs, Jr., and M. Alpers, eds., *Slow, latent, and temperate virus infections*, NINDB Monograph No. 2, Public Health Service Publication No. 1378 (Washington, D.C.: Government Printing Office, 1965), pp. 3-12.

———C.J. Gibbs, Jr., and M. Alpers, "Transmission and passage of experimental 'kuru' to chimpanzees," *Science*, 155:212-214 (1967).

Gardner-Medwin, D., "Mutation rate in Duchenne type of muscular dystrophy," *J Med Genet*, 7:334-337 (1970).

Garland, H., and A.N.G. Clark, "Myasthenia gravis: a personal study of 60 cases," *Brit Med J*, 1:1259-1262 (1956).

Gastaut, H., "Clinical and electroencephalographical classification of epileptic seizures," *Epilepsia (Amst)*, s.4. 10 suppl:S2-S13 (1969).

——— and M. Fischer-Williams, "The physiopathology of epileptic seizures," in J. Field, H.W. Magoun, and V.E. Hall, eds., *Handbook of physiology, section 1: neurophysiology*, vol. 1 (Washington, D.C.: American Physiological Society, 1959), pp. 329-363.

Gentile, A., and S. DiFrancesca, *Academic achievements test performance of hearing impaired students, United States: spring 1969* (Washington, D.C.: Gallaudet College Press, 1969), 45 pp.

———J.D. Schein, and K. Haase, "Characteristics of persons with impaired hearing," *Vital Health Statist*, Series 10, No. 35, 1967, pp. 1-64.

Georgi, F., and P. Hall, "Studies on multiple sclerosis frequency in Switzerland and East Africa," *Acta Psychiat Neurol Scand*, 35 suppl 147:75-84 (1960).

Georgia's Deaf, Official Project No. 665-34-3-90 (Atlanta: Works Project Administration of Georgia, 1942), 19 pp.

Giaquinto, M., and F.M. Lyons, "International activities in the field of trachoma and other communicable eye diseases," in *XVII Concilium Ophthalmologicum, 1954, Canada, United States of America, Acta*, vol. 3 (Toronto: University of Toronto Press, 1955), pp. 2044-2051.

Gibbs, C.J., [Jr.], "Discussion," in F.H. Norris, Jr., and L.T. Kurland, eds., *Motor neuron diseases: research on amyotrophic lateral sclerosis and related disorders* (New York: Grune & Stratton, 1969), pp. 282-283.

——— and D.C. Gajdusek, "Infection as the etiology of spongiform encephalopathy (Creutzfeldt-Jakob disease)," *Science*, 165:1023-1025 (1969).

Gibson, J.B., and L.T. Kurland, unpublished data.

Glorig, A., and R. Gallo, "Comments on sensorineural hearing loss in otosclerosis," in H.F. Schuknecht, ed., *Otosclerosis* (Boston: Little, Brown, 1962), pp. 63-78.

——— and J. Roberts, "Hearing levels of adults by age and sex," *Vital Health Statist*, Series 11, No. 11, 1965, pp. 1-34.

Goldberg, I.D., and L.T. Kurland, "Mortality in 33 countries from diseases of the nervous system," *World Neurol*, 3:444-465 (1962).
───── ─────unpublished data.
Goldberger, J., G.A. Wheeler, and E. Sydenstricker, "A study of the relation of family income and other economic factors to pellagra incidence in seven cotton-mill villages of South Carolina in 1916," *Public Health Rep*, 35:2673-2714 (1920).
Goldstein, G., "Thymitis and myasthenia gravis," *Lancet*, 2:1164-1167 (1966).
───── and W.H. Hofmann, "Experimental myasthenia gravis," read at the meeting of the Association for Research in Nervous and Mental Disease, New York, 6 December 1969.
Goldstein, H., "The role of blindness statistics in prevention and control," *Sightsav Rev*, 36:133-140 (1966).
Grant, H.C., A.V. Hoffbrand, and D.G. Wells, "Folate deficiency and neurological disease," *Lancet*, 2:763-767 (1965).
Grashchenkov, N.I., B.M. Hekht, A.B. Rogover, and A.M. Vein, "Characteristics of the geographical distribution of disseminated sclerosis in the Soviet Union," *Acta Psychiat Neurol Scand*, 35 suppl 147:148-158 (1960).
Great Britain, Colonial Office, *Blindness in British African and Middle East territories* (London: Her Majesty's Stationery Office, 1948).
Great Britain, Ministry of Health, *Report of the ministry of health for the year 1960. Part II. On the state of the public health, being the annual report of the chief medical officer* (London, 1961).
─────*Report of the ministry of health for the year ended December 31, 1963* (London, 1964).
Greenfield, J.G., *The spino-cerebellar degenerations* (Oxford: Blackwell, 1954), 112 pp.
Greenslade, C., *The incidence and causes of blindness* (London: British Empire Society for the Blind, 1956).
Greenwald, I., "The history of goiter in the Inca empire: Peru, Chile and the Argentine Republic; its significance for the etiology of the disease," *Texas Rep Biol Med*, 15:874-889 (1957).
Gregory, P., *Deafness and public responsibility: the provision of hearing aids*, occasional papers on social administration, No. 7 (London: G. Bell, 1964), 56 pp.
Grove, R.D. and A.M. Hetzel, *Vital statistics rates in the United States, 1940-1960*, Public Health Service Publication No. 1677 (Washington, D.C.: Government Printing Office, 1968), 881 pp.
Gudmundsson, G., "Epilepsy in Iceland: a clinical and epidemiological investigation," *Acta Neurol Scand*, 43 suppl 25:1-124 (1966).
Gudmundsson, K.R., "Cerebral palsy in Iceland," *Acta Neurol Scand*, 43 suppl 34:1-32 (1967*a*).
───── "A clinical survey of parkinsonism in Iceland," *Acta Neurol Scand*, 43 suppl 33:1-61 (1967*b*).
───── personal communication, 4 July 1968*a*.
───── "The prevalence of some neurological diseases in Iceland," *Acta Neurol Scand*, 44:57-69 (1968*b*).

_____ "The prevalence and occurrence of some rare neurological diseases in Iceland," *Acta Neurol Scand*, 45:114-118 (1969).
_____ personal communication, 20 February 1970.
_____ and G. Gudmundsson, "Studies in multiple sclerosis. V. Multiple sclerosis in Iceland," *Acta Neurol Scand*, 38 suppl 2:1-63 (1962).
Gusic, D.-B., "Le goitre endémique et les troubles cochléo-vestibulaires," *Rev Laryng (Bordeaux)*, 85:189-194 (1964).
Guyot, R., "Quelques réflexions au suject des résultats de six années de dépistage de la surdité," *J Franc Otorhinolaryng*, 12:619-621 (1963).

Hamdan, Y., "Survey on blindness in Kuwait," *J Kuwait Med Assn*, 2:35-38 (1968).
Hamtoft, H., and J. Mosbech, "Om primaere og sekundaere dødsårsager," *Ugeskr Laeg*, 123:1363-1364 (1961).
Hansen, E., "Cerebral palsy in Denmark: a discussion of its occurrence, disease types, etiology and social aspects, based on a material of 2621 patients born in the period 1925-1953," *Acta Psychiat Neurol Scand*, 35 suppl 146:1-148 (1960).
Harvald, B., and M. Hauge, "Hereditary factors elucidated by twin studies," in J.V. Neel, M.W. Shaw, and W.J. Schull, eds., *Genetics and the epidemiology of chronic diseases*, Public Health Service Publication No. 1163 (Washington, D.C.: Government Printing Office, 1965), pp. 61-76.
Hatchuel, W., "The importance of performing adequate hearing tests in children with cerebral palsy," *S Afr Med J*, 36:237-238 (1962).
Hatfield, E.M., "Causes of blindness in school children," *Sightsav Rev*, 33:218-233 (1963).
Hauser, W.A., L.T. Kurland, M.R. Gomez, and L.R. Elveback, "Prognosis of patients with febrile convulsions in Rochester, Minnesota, 1945-1967" (abstr.), *Trans Amer Neurol Assn*, 95:257-259 (1970).
_____ W.E. Karnes, J. Annis, and L.T. Kurland, "Incidence and prognosis of Bell's palsy in the population of Rochester, Minnesota," *Mayo Clin Proc*, 46:258-264 (1971).
_____ _____ and L.T. Kurland, "Convulsive disorders in Rochester, Minnesota: a 30-year study," unpublished data.
Health Statistics, National Health Survey, *Impairments by type, sex and age, United States, July 1957-June 1958*, Public Health Service Publication No. 584-B9 (Washington, D.C.: Government Printing Office, 1959), 28 pp.
_____ *Selected impairments by etiology and activity limitation, United States, July 1959-June 1961*, Public Health Service Publication No. 584-B35 (Washington, D.C.: Government Printing Office, 1962), 50 pp.
Heasman, M.A., "Accuracy of death certification," *Proc Roy Soc Med*, 55:733-736 (1962).
_____ and L. Lipworth, *Accuracy of certification of cause of death: a report on a survey conducted in 1959 in 75 hospitals of the National Health Service to obtain information on the extent of agreement between clinical and post-mortem diagnoses* (London: Her Majesty's Stationery Office, 1966), 133 pp.
Heathfield, K.W.G., "Huntington's chorea: investigation into the prevalence of

this disease in the area covered by the North East Metropolitan Regional Hospital Board," *Brain*, 90:203-232 (1967).

Henriksen, G.F., personal communication, 23 September 1969.

──── and W.H. Krohn, "The organization of a national system for the medical care of epileptics" (abstr.), *Excerpta Medica International Congress Series* No. 193, 1969, p. 5.

Herlitz, G., and B. Redin, "The prevalence of cerebral palsy," *Acta Paediat*, 44:146-154 (1955).

Herndon, C.N., "Three North Carolina surveys," *Amer J Hum Genet*, 6:65-74 (1954).

Herrmann, C., Jr., "Myasthenia gravis occurring in families," *Neurology (Minneap)*, 16:75-85 (1966).

Hewitt, D., "Geographical variations in the mortality attributed to spina bifida and other congenital malformations," *Brit J Prev Soc Med*, 17:13-22 (1963).

Hill, A.B., *Statistical methods in clinical and preventive medicine* (London: Livingstone, 1962), 610 pp.

Hinchcliffe, R., "Hearing levels of elderly in Jamaica: a pilot survey," *Ann Otol*, 73:1012-1019 (1964).

Hirano, A., N. Malamud, and L.T. Kurland, "Parkinsonism–dementia complex, an endemic disease on the island of Guam. II. Pathological features," *Brain*, 84:662-679 (1961).

──── L.T. Kurland, and G.P. Sayre, "Familial amyotrophic lateral sclerosis: a subgroup characterized by posterior and spinocerebellar tract involvement and hyaline inclusions in the anterior horn cells," *Arch Neurol (Chicago)*, 16:232-243 (1967).

──── N. Malamud, L.T. Kurland, and H.M. Zimmerman, "A review of the pathologic findings in amyotrophic lateral sclerosis," in F.H. Norris, Jr., and L.T. Kurland, eds., *Motor neuron diseases: research on amyotrophic lateral sclerosis and related disorders* (New York: Grune & Stratton, 1969), pp. 51-60.

Hirsch, A., *Handbook of geographical and historical pathology*, vol. 1, *Acute infective diseases*, translated from the second German edition by C. Creighton (London: New Sydenham Society, 1883), pp. 1, 2.

──── *Handbook of geographical and historical pathology*, vol. 3, *Diseases of organs and parts*, translated from the second German edition by C. Creighton (London: New Sydenham Society, 1886), p. 510.

Hokkanen, E., "Epidemiology of myasthenia gravis in Finland," *J Neurol Sci*, 9:463-478 (1969).

Holmes, W.J., "Report on a survey on ocular leprosy and general ophthalmology," *J Soc Ophthal*, 23:21-23 (1958*a*).

──── "Blindness and the prevention of blindness in Asia," *J Soc Ophthal*, 24-25:8-13 (1958*b*).

──── "Preventable eye diseases and blindness: in the newly developing countries," *Amer J Ophthal*, 62:983-985 (1966).

Holst, J.C., "The occurrence of blindness in Norway," *Amer J Ophthal*, 35:1153-1166 (1952).

Hope-Simpson, R.E., "The nature of herpes zoster: a long-term study and a new hypothesis," *Proc Roy Soc Med*, 58:9-20 (1965).

Hudolin, V., and N. Laktic, "Centre for the study and prevention of blindness," *J Soc Ophthal*, 26:10-12 (1959).

Huntington, G., "On chorea," *Med Surg Reporter*, 26:317-321 (1872).

―― "Recollections of Huntington's chorea as I saw it at East Hampton, Long Island, during my boyhood," *J Nerv Ment Dis*, 37:255-257 (1910).

Hurlin, R.G., *Estimated prevalence of blindness in the United States* (New York: American Foundation for the Blind, 1953).

―― "Estimated prevalence of blindness in the United States and in individual states, 1960," *Sightsav Rev*, 32:4-12 (1962).

Hyllested, K., *Disseminated sclerosis in Denmark: prevalence and geographical distribution*, thesis (Copenhagen: J. Jørgensen, 1956), 147 pp.

―― and L.T. Kurland, "Studies in multiple sclerosis. VI. Further explorations on the geographic distribution of multiple sclerosis," *Acta Neurol Scand*, 42 suppl 19:1-176 (1966).

Illinois Census of Exceptional Children, *The prevalence of exceptional children in Illinois in 1958*, circular―Census 1A (Springfield, Ill.: Superintendent of Public Instruction, 1959), 17 pp.

Ingram, T.T.S., "A study of cerebral palsy in the childhood population of Edinburgh," *Arch Dis Child*, 30:85-98 (1955).

Innes, J.R.M., personal communication, 1966.

Inoue, Y.K., Y. Nishibe, and Y. Nakamura, "Virus associated with S.M.O.N. in Japan" (letter to the editor), *Lancet*, 1:853-854 (1971).

Israeli Ministry of Social Welfare, Division of Research and Planning, *The blind in Israel: a survey* (Jerusalem, 1957).

Jablon, S., D.M. Angevine, Y.S. Matsumoto, and M. Ishida, "On the significance of cause of death as recorded on death certificates in Hiroshima and Nagasaki, Japan," *Nat Cancer Inst Monogr*, 19:445-465 (1966).

Jackson, A.D.M., "Infection and congenital abnormalities," *Practitioner*, 191:152-158 (1963).

James, G., R.E. Patton, and A.S. Heslin, "Accuracy of cause-of-death statements on death certificates," *Public Health Rep*, 70:39-51 (1955).

Jenkins, A.C., "Epidemiology of parkinsonism in Victoria," *Med J Aust*, 2:496-502 (1966).

Jepsen, O., "Topognosis (topographic diagnosis) of facial nerve lesions," *Arch Otolaryng (Chicago)*, 81:446-456 (1965).

Johnson, R.T., "Virologic studies and summary of Soviet experiments on the transmission of amyotrophic lateral sclerosis (ALS) to monkeys," in F.H. Norris, Jr., and L.T. Kurland, eds., *Motor neuron diseases: research on amyotrophic lateral sclerosis and related disorders* (New York: Grune & Stratton, 1969), pp. 280-282.

Joseph, R.B., and J.P. Frazer, "Otosclerosis incidence in Caucasians and Japanese," *Arch Otolaryng (Chicago)*, 80:256-257 (1964).

Juul-Jensen, P., "Epilepsy: a clinical and social analysis of 1,020 adult patients with epileptic seizures," *Acta Neurol Scand*, 40 suppl 5:1-148 (1964).

Kakar, P.K., K.L. Sawhney, and P.S. Saharia, "Familial Bell's palsy (case report)," *J Laryng*, 80:628-630 (1966).

REFERENCES / 413

Kelly, D.R., E.R. Nilo, and R.B. Berggren, "Deafness after topical neomycin wound irrigation," *New Eng J Med*, 280:1338-1339 (1969).
Kennedy, W.P., "Epidemiologic aspects of the problem of congenital malformations," in D. Bergsma, ed., *Birth defects original article series*, vol. 3, no. 2 (New York: National Foundation, December 1967), 18 pp.
Kerby, C.E., "Causes and prevention of blindness in children," *Sightsav Rev*, 20:67-80 (1950).
―――― "Causes and prevention of blindness in children of school age," *Sightsav Rev*, 22:22-31 (1952).
―――― "Causes of blindness in children of school age," *Sightsav Rev*, 28:10-21 (1958).
Kessler, I.I., "Epidemiologic studies of Parkinson's disease. II. A hospital-based survey," *Amer J. Epidem*, 95:308-318 (1972).
―――― "Epidemiologic studies of Parkinson's disease. III. A community-based survey" (unpublished data).
―――― and E.L. Diamond, "Epidemiologic studies of Parkinson's disease. I. Smoking and Parkinson's disease: a survey and explanatory hypothesis," *Amer J Epidem*, 94:16-25 (1971).
Khodos, K.G., "K geographii rasseiannogo sklerosa" [On the geography of multiple sclerosis], translated by J.S. Barlow, *Zh Nevropat Psikhiat Korsakov*, 60:1435-1443 (1960).
Kimura, K., Y. Yase, Y. Higashi, S. Uno, K. Yamamoto, M. Iwasaki, I. Tsumoto, M. Sugiura, S. Yoshimura, K. Namikawa, J. Kumura, S. Iwamoto, I. Yamamoto, Y. Handa, M. Yata, and Y. Yata, "Epidemiological and geomedical studies on amyotrophic lateral sclerosis," *Dis Nerv Syst*, 24:155-159 (1963).
Kivits, M., "La cécité au Congo Belge et au Ruanda-Urundi," *Ann Soc Belge Med Trop*, 35:39-45 (1955).
Krohn, W., "A study of epilepsy in Northern Norway, its frequency and character," *Acta Psychiat Neurol Scand*, 36 suppl 150:215-225 (1961).
Krooth, R.S., M.T. Macklin, and T.F. Hilbish, "Diaphysial aclasis (multiple exostoses) on Guam," *Amer J Hum Genet*, 13:340-347 (1961).
Kryter, K.D., C. Williams, and D.M. Green, "Auditory acuity and the perception of speech," *J Acoust Soc Amer*, 34:1217-1223 (1962).
Kučera, J., "Down's syndrome and infectious hepatitis" (letter to the editor), *Lancet*, 1:569-570 (1970).
Kurland, L.T., "The frequency and geographic distribution of multiple sclerosis as indicated by mortality statistics and morbidity surveys in the United States and Canada," *Amer J Hyg*, 55:457-476 (1952).
―――― "Definitions of cerebral palsy and their role in epidemiologic research," *Neurology (Minneap)*, 7:641-654 (1957a).
―――― "Epidemiologic investigations of amyotrophic lateral sclerosis. III. A genetic interpretation of incidence and geographic distribution," *Proc Staff Meet Mayo Clin*, 32:449-462 (1957b).
―――― "Descriptive epidemiology of selected neurologic and myopathic disorders with particular reference to a survey in Rochester, Minnesota," *J Chronic Dis*, 8:378-418 (1958a).
―――― "Epidemiology: incidence, geographic distribution and genetic consider-

_____ations," in W.S. Fields, ed., *Pathogenesis and treatment of parkinsonism* (Springfield, Ill.: Charles C Thomas, 1958*b*), pp. 5-43.

_____"The incidence and prevalence of convulsive disorders in a small urban community," *Epilepsia (Amst)*, s.4. 1:143-161 (1959).

_____"The geographic and genetic characteristics of amyotrophic lateral sclerosis and other selected chronic neurological diseases," in J.V. Neel, M.W. Shaw, and W.J. Schull, eds., *Genetics and the epidemiology of chronic diseases*, Public Health Service Publication No. 1163 (Washington, D.C.: Government Printing Office, 1965), pp. 145-162.

_____"The epidemiologic characteristics of multiple sclerosis," in P.J. Vinken and G.W. Bruyn, eds., *Handbook of clinical neurology*, vol. 9, *Multiple sclerosis and other demyelinating diseases* (Amsterdam: North-Holland Publishing Co., 1970), pp. 63-84.

_____"Geography of neural tumors," in J. Minckler, ed., *Pathology of the nervous system*, vol. 3 (New York: McGraw-Hill, 1972), pp. 2803-2808.

_____and M. Alter, "Current status of the epidemiology and genetics of myasthenia gravis," in H.R. Viets, ed., *Myasthenia gravis*, second international symposium, Los Angeles, 1959 (Springfield, Ill.: Charles C Thomas, 1961), pp. 307-336.

_____and N.W. Choi, unpublished data.

_____and J.F. Kurtzke, "Geographic neuropathology," in J. Minckler, ed., *Pathology of the nervous system*, vol. 3 (New York: McGraw-Hill, 1972), pp. 2771-2803.

_____and D.W. Mulder, "Epidemiologic investigations of amyotrophic lateral sclerosis: preliminary report on geographic distribution, with special reference to the Mariana Islands, including clinical and pathologic observations," *Neurology (Minneap)*, 4:355-378; 438-448 (1954).

_____ _____"Epidemiologic investigations of amyotrophic lateral sclerosis. 2. Familial aggregations indicative of dominant inheritance," *Neurology (Minneap)*, 5:182-196; 249-268 (1955).

_____and K.B. Westlund, "Epidemiologic factors in the etiology and prognosis of multiple sclerosis," *Ann NY Acad Sci*, 58:682-701 (1954).

_____S.N. Faro, and H. Siedler, "Minamata disease: the outbreak of a neurologic disorder in Minamata, Japan, and its relationship to the ingestion of seafood contaminated by mercuric compounds," *World Neurol*, 1:370-391 (1960).

_____A. Hirano, N. Malamud, and S. Lessell, "Parkinsonism-dementia complex, an endemic disease on the island of Guam: clinical, pathological, genetic and epidemiological features," *Trans Amer Neurol Assn*, 86:115-120 (1961).

_____A. Stazio, and D. Reed, "An appraisal of population studies of multiple sclerosis," *Ann NY Acad Sci*, 122:520-541 (1965).

_____G.W. Beebe, J.F. Kurtzke, B. Nagler, T.L. Auth, S. Lessell, and M.D. Nefzger, "Studies on the natural history of multiple sclerosis. 2. The progression of optic neuritis to multiple sclerosis," *Acta Neurol Scand*, 42 suppl 19:157-176 (1966).

_____N.W. Choi, and G.P. Sayre, "Implications of incidence and geographic patterns on the classification of amyotrophic lateral sclerosis," in F.H. Norris, Jr., and L.T. Kurland, eds., *Motor neuron diseases: research on amyotrophic lateral sclerosis and related disorders* (New York: Grune & Stratton, 1969a), pp. 28-50.

―――― W.A. Hauser, R.H. Ferguson, and K.E. Holley, "Epidemiologic features of diffuse connective tissue disorders in Rochester, Minnesota, 1951 through 1967, with special reference to systemic lupus erythematosus," *Mayo Clin Proc*, 44:649-663 (1969b).

―――― ――――H. Okazaki, and F.T. Nobrega, "Epidemiologic studies of parkinsonism with special reference to the cohort hypothesis," in *Third symposium on Parkinson's disease* (Edinburgh: Livingstone, 1969c), pp. 12-16.

Kuroiwa, Y., "Multiple sclerosis and allied demyelinating encephalomyelitis in Japan," in *Zukunft der Neurologie* (Stuttgart: Thieme, 1967), pp. 70-84.

Kurtzke, J.F., "Normal ceruloplasmin in Wilson's disease," *Arch Neurol (Chicago)*, 7:371-376 (1962).

―――― "General features of the prevalence of multiple sclerosis," *J Indian Med Prof*, 11:4896-4901, 4895 (1964).

―――― "Familial incidence and geography in multiple sclerosis," *Acta Neurol Scand*, 41:127-139 (1965a).

―――― "Medical facilities and the prevalence of multiple sclerosis," *Acta Neurol Scand*, 41:561-579 (1965b).

―――― "On the time of onset in multiple sclerosis," *Acta Neurol Scand*, 41:140-158 (1965c).

―――― "The distribution of multiple sclerosis and other diseases," *Acta Neurol Scand*, 42:221-243 (1966a).

―――― "An epidemiologic approach to multiple sclerosis," *Arch Neurol (Chicago)*, 14:213-222 (1966b).

―――― "An evaluation of the geographic distribution of multiple sclerosis," *Acta Neurol Scand*, 42 suppl 19:91-110 (1966c).

―――― "Further considerations on the geographic distribution of multiple sclerosis," *Acta Neurol Scand*, 43:283-298 (1967a).

―――― "On the fine structure of the distribution of multiple sclerosis," *Acta Neurol Scand*, 43:257-279 (1967b).

―――― "A Fennoscandian focus of multiple sclerosis," *Neurology, (Minneap)*, 18:16-20 (1968a).

―――― "Multiple sclerosis and infection from an epidemiologic aspect," *Neurology (Minneap)*, 18 (pt 2):170-175 (1968b).

―――― "Some epidemiologic and clinical features of adult seizure disorders," *J Chronic Dis*, 21:143-156 (1968c).

―――― "Comments on the epidemiology of amyotrophic lateral sclerosis (ALS)," in F.H. Norris, Jr., and L.T. Kurland, eds., *Motor neuron diseases: research on amyotrophic lateral sclerosis and related disorders* (New York: Grune & Stratton, 1969a), pp. 85-89.

―――― *Epidemiology of cerebrovascular disease* (Berlin: Springer-Verlag, 1969b), 197 pp.

―――― "Clinical manifestations of multiple sclerosis," in P.J. Vinken and G.W. Bruyn, eds., *Handbook of clinical neurology*, vol. 9, *Multiple sclerosis and other demyelinating diseases* (Amsterdam: North-Holland Publishing Co., 1970), pp. 161-216.

416 / REFERENCES

───── unpublished data.
───── and L.T. Kurland, "Epidemiology of cerebrovascular disease," in R.G. Siekert, ed., *Cerebrovascular survey report, for Joint Council Subcommittee on Cerebrovascular Disease*, revised (Rochester, Minn.: Whiting, July 1970), pp. 163-175.
───── G.W. Beebe, B. Nagler, T.L. Auth, L.T. Kurland, and M.D. Nefzger, "Studies on the natural history of multiple sclerosis. 4. Clinical features of the onset bout," *Acta Neurol Scand*, 44:467-494 (1968a).
───── C.S. Park, and S.J. Oh, "Multiple sclerosis in Korea: clinical features and prevalence," *J Neurol Sci*, 6:463-475 (1968b).
───── G.W. Beebe, B. Nagler, M.D. Nefzger, T.L. Auth, and L.T. Kurland, "Studies on the natural history of multiple sclerosis. V. Long-term survival in young men," *Arch Neurol (Chicago)*, 22:215-225 (1970a).
───── G. Dean, and D.P.J. Botha, "A method for estimating the age at immigration of white immigrants to South Africa, with an example of its importance," *S Afr Med J*, 44:663-669 (1970b).
───── L.T. Kurland, and I.D. Goldberg, "Mortality and migration in multiple sclerosis," *Neurology (Minneap)*, 21:1186-1197 (1971).

Lacayo, C.R., "La oftalmologia y la ceguera en Nicaragua," *Arch Soc Oftal Litoral*, 3:234-238 (1950).
Lancaster, H.O., "Deafness as an epidemic disease in Australia: a note on census and institutional data," *Brit Med J*, 2:1429-1432 (1951).
Larsson, A., "Genetic problems in otosclerosis," in H.F. Schuknecht, ed., *Otosclerosis* (Boston: Little, Brown 1962), pp. 109-117.
Larsson, T., and T. Sjögren, "Dystonia musculorum deformans: a genetic and clinical population study of 121 cases," *Acta Neurol Scand*, 42 suppl 17:3-232 (1966).
Laurence, K.M., "The survival of untreated spina bifida cystica," *Develop Med Child Neurol*, suppl 11:10-19 (1966).
Leck, I., "Incidence of malformations following influenza epidemics," *Brit J. Prev Soc Med*, 17:70-80 (1963).
───── "Changes in the incidence of neural-tube defects," *Lancet*, 2:791-793 (1966).
───── and E.L.M. Millar, "Short-term changes in the incidence of malformations," *Brit J Prev Soc Med*, 17:1-12 (1963).
Leibowitz, U., and M. Alter, "Epilepsy in Jerusalem, Israel," *Epilepsia (Amst)*, s.4. 9:87-105 (1968).
───── E. Kahana, and M. Alter, "Population studies of multiple sclerosis in Israel," in E.J. Field, T.M. Bell, and P.R. Carnegie, eds., *Multiple sclerosis: progress in research* (Amsterdam: North-Holland Publishing Co., 1972), pp. 179-196.
Leneman, F., "The Guillain-Barré syndrome: definition, etiology, and review of 1,100 cases," *Arch Intern Med (Chicago)*, 118:139-144 (1966).
Lenz, W., "Epidemiology of congenital malformations," *Ann NY Acad Sci*, 123:228-236 (1965).
Lessell, S., A. Hirano, J. Torres, and L.T. Kurland, "Parkinsonism-dementia complex: epidemiological considerations in the Chamorros of the Mariana Islands and California," *Arch Neurol (Chicago)*, 7:377-385 (1962a).

———— J.M. Torres, and L.T. Kurland, "Seizure disorders in a Guamanian village," *Arch Neurol (Chicago)*, 7:37-44 (1962b).
Lesser, R.P., W.A. Hauser, and L.T. Kurland, unpublished data.
Levy, L.F., J.I. Forbes, and T.S. Parirenyatwa, "Epilepsy in Africans," *Cent Afr J Med*, 10:241-249 (1964).
Lilienfeld, A.M., and C.H. Benesch, *Epidemiology of mongolism* (Baltimore: Johns Hopkins Press, 1969), 145 pp.
———— M.L. Levin, and I.I. Kessler, *Cancer in the United States* (APHA monograph; Cambridge, Mass.: Harvard University Press, 1972), 546 pp.
Limburg, C.C., "The geographic distribution of multiple sclerosis and its estimated prevalence in the United States," *Proc Assn Res Nerv Ment Dis*, 28:15-24 (1950).
Lindenov, H., *The etiology of deaf-mutism with special reference to heredity* (Copenhagen: Ejnar Munksgaard, 1945), 268 pp.
Lindstedt, E., "Blindhetsorsaker i Sverige," *Lakartidningen*, 64:1620-1628 (1967).
Logan, R.G., J.M. Bandera, W.M. Mikkelsen, and I.F. Duff, "Polymyositis: a clinical study," *Ann Intern Med*, 65:996-1007 (1966).
Logan, W.P.D., and A.A. Cushion, *Studies on medical and population subjects*, No. 14, *Morbidity statistics from general practice*, vol. 1, *General* (London: Her Majesty's Stationery Office, 1958), 174 pp.
Lumio. J.S., and P. Paljakka, "Tutkimuksia suomen Kuurojenkeskisistä Avioliitoista," *Duodecim*, suppl 43:1-15 (1964).
Lunde, A.S., and S.K. Bigman, *Occupational conditions among the deaf* (Washington, D.C.: Gallaudet College Press, 1959), 66 pp.
Lundström, R., "Rubella during pregnancy: a follow-up study of children born after an epidemic of rubella in Sweden, 1951, with additional investigations on prophylaxis and treatment of maternal rubella," *Acta Paediat Scand*, suppl 133:1-110 (1962).

Macchi, G., M. Saginario, and S. Valla, "La Sclérose en Plaques dans la Province de Parma (Italie)," *World Neurol*, 3:731-738 (1962).
MacDonald, A.E., "Causes of blindness in Canada: an analysis of 24,605 cases registered with the Canadian National Institute for the Blind," *Canad Med Assn J*, 92:264-279 (1965).
Mackay, R.P., and N.C. Myrianthopoulos, "Multiple sclerosis in twins and their relatives: final report," *Arch Neurol (Chicago)*, 15:449-462 (1966).
Mackenzie, C.N., and W.S. Flowers, *Blindness in China. Report to the Government of China*, 1949.
MacLean, A.R., J. Berkson, H.W. Woltman, and L. Schionneman, "Multiple sclerosis in a rural community," *Proc Assn Res Nerv Ment Dis*, 28:25-27 (1950).
MacMahon, B., and T.F. Pugh, *Epidemiology: principles and methods* (Boston: Little, Brown 1970), 376 pp.
———— and S. Yen, "Unrecognised epidemic of anencephaly and spina bifida," *Lancet*, 1:31-33 (1971).
———— T.F. Pugh, and J. Ipsen, *Epidemiologic methods* (Boston: Little, Brown, 1960), 302 pp.

Macrae, J.H., "Deterioration of the residual hearing of children with sensorineural deafness," *Acta Otolaryng (Stockholm)*, 66:33-39 (1968).
Maggiore, L., "Causes of juvenile blindness in Italy: statistics and general discussion," *J Soc Ophthal*, 12:29-35 (1951).
Malnou, F., "Blindness in South Tunis," *Tunisie Med*, 42:1009-1029 (1954).
Mann, I., *Ophthalmic survey of the Kimberley division of Western Australia* (Perth, Western Australia, 1954).
———"Trachoma in Australia," *Oriental Arch Ophthal*, 1:8-18 (1963).
———and J. Loschdorfer, *Ophthalmic survey of the territories of Papua and New Guinea* (Port Moresby, 1956).
Manson, M.M., W.P.D. Logan, and R.M. Loy, "Rubella and other virus infections during pregnancy," in "Clinics: viral infections during pregnancy and their effects on the offspring," *Quart Rev Pediat*, 16:57-59 (1961).
Mapelli, G., and E. Ramelli, "Ricerche epidemiologiche sulla sclerosi a placche nella Provincia di Ferrara," *Arcisped S Anna Ferrara*, 20 suppl 6:1071-1088 (1967).
Marsden, P.D., and R. Knight, "Halogenated oxyquinoline derivatives" (letter to the editor), *Lancet*, 1:854 (1971).
Mathai, K.V., D.P. Dunn, L.T. Kurland, and F.A. Reeder, "Convulsive disorders in the Mariana Islands," *Epilepsia (Amst)*, s.4. 9:77-85 (1968).
Matzker, J., "Schizophrenie und Taubheit," *Z Laryng Rhinol Otol*, 39:85-91 (1960).
McArdle, B., "Metabolic myopathies: the glycogenoses affecting muscle, and hypo- and hyperkalemic periodic paralysis," *Amer J Med*, 35:661-672 (1963).
McCall, M.G., personal communication, 12 July 1968.
——— T. Le G. Brereton, A. Dawson, K. Millingen, J. M. Sutherland, and E.D. Acheson, "Frequency of multiple sclerosis in three Australian cities—Perth, Newcastle, and Hobart," *J Neurol Neurosurg Psychiat*, 31:1-9 (1968).
McFarland, H.R., and G.L. Heller, "Guillain-Barré disease complex: a statement of diagnostic criteria and analysis of 100 cases," *Arch Neurol (Chicago)*, 14:196-201 (1966).
McGregor, R.M., "Herpes zoster, chicken-pox, and cancer in general practice," *Brit Med J*, 1:84-87 (1957).
McIlroy, W.J., and J. C. Richardson, "Syringomyelia: a clinical review of 75 cases," *Canad Med Assn J*, 93:731-734 (1965).
McKeown, T., and R.G. Record, "Seasonal incidence of congenital malformations of the central nervous system," *Lancet*, 1:192-196 (1951).
Melnick, S.C., and T.H. Flewett, "Role of infection in the Guillain-Barré syndrome," *J Neurol Neurosurg Psychiat*, 27:395-407 (1964).
Mélotte, G., "Idiopathic paralysis of the facial nerve," *Practitioner*, 187:349-353 (1961).
Mena, I., J. Court, S. Fuenzalida, P.S. Papavasiliou, and G.C. Cotzias, "Modification of chronic manganese poisoning: treatment with L-dopa or 5-OH tryptophane," *New Eng J Med*, 282:5-10 (1970).
Merritt, H.H., *A textbook of neurology*, ed. 4 (Philadelphia: Lea & Febiger, 1967), 844 pp. (For Chapter 6 see pp. 535-548; for Chapter 7 see pp. 548-556.)
Merselis, J.G., Jr., D. Kaye, and E.W. Hook, "Disseminated herpes zoster: a report of 17 cases," *Arch Intern Med (Chicago)*, 113:679-686 (1964).

Mesolella, C., and F. Laurini, "Contributo allo studio della funzione uditiva nei portatori di palatoschisi," *Arch Ital Laring*, 69:417-428 (1961).

Metrakos, K., and J.D. Metrakos, "Genetics of convulsive disorders. II. Genetic and electroencephalographic studies in centrencephalic epilepsy," *Neurology (Minneap)*, 11:474-483 (1961).

Metropolitan Life Insurance Company, "Blindness: prevalence and longevity," *Statist Bull Metrop Life Insur Co*, 47:6-9 (August 1966).

Mikelson, O., personal communication, 15 February 1970.

Millichap, J.G., *Febrile convulsions* (New York: Macmillan, 1968), 222 pp.

Mjönes, H., "Paralysis agitans: a clinical and genetic study," *Acta Psychiat Neurol Scand*, suppl 54:1-195 (1949).

Moffie, D., "De geografische verbreiding van multipele sclerose," *Nederl T. Geneesk*, 110:1454-1457 (1966).

Mohsénine, H., and S. Darougar, "Preliminary report on the study and causes of blindness in Iran," *Rep Univ Sch Med Iran*, pp. 1-9 (1955).

Monif, G.R.G., J.B. Hardy, and J.L. Sever, "Studies in congenital rubella, Baltimore 1964-65. I. Epidemiologic and virologic," *Bull Hopkins Hosp*, 118:85-96 (1966).

Montgomery, R.D., E.K. Cruickshank, W.B. Robertson, and W.H. McMenemey, "Clinical and pathological observations on Jamaican neuropathy: a report on 206 cases," *Brain*, 87:425-462 (1964).

Moriyama, I.M., W.S. Baum, W.M. Haenszel, and B.F. Mattison, "Inquiry into diagnostic evidence supporting medical certifications of death," *Amer J Public Health*, 48:1376-1387 (1958).

―――― T.R. Dawber, and W.B. Kannel, "Evaluation of diagnostic information supporting medical certifications of deaths from cardiovascular disease," *Nat Cancer Inst Monogr*, 19:405-419 (1966).

―――― D.E. Krueger, and J. Stamler, *Cardiovascular diseases in the United States* (APHA monograph; Cambridge, Mass.: Harvard University Press, 1971), 496 pp.

Morton, N.E., and C.S. Chung, "Formal genetics of muscular dystrophy," *Amer J Hum Genet*, 11:360-379 (1959).

Mosbech, J., *Heredity in pernicious anaemia: a proband study of the heredity and the relationship to cancer of the stomach* (Copenhagen: Ejnar Munksgaard, 1953), 107 pp.

Mulder, D.W., "The clinical syndrome of amyotrophic lateral sclerosis," *Proc Staff Meet Mayo Clin*, 32:427-436 (1957).

―――― and L.T. Kurland, "Amyotrophic lateral sclerosis in Micronesia," *Proc Staff Meet Mayo Clin*, 29:666-670 (1954).

―――― ―――― and L.L.G. Iriarte, "Neurologic diseases on the island of Guam," *US Armed Forces Med J*, 5:1724-1739 (1954).

Müller, R., "Genetic aspects of multiple sclerosis," *Arch Neurol Psychiat (Chicago)*, 70:733-740 (1953).

Munck, W., "Autopsy finding and clinical diagnosis: Comparative study of 1000 cases," *Acta Med Scand*, 142 Suppl 266:775-781 (1952).

Murray, N.E., "Deafness following maternal rubella," *Med J Aust*, 1:126-130 (1949).

Myrianthopoulos, N.C., "Genetics and public health," *Public Health Rep*, 74:1098-1106 (1959).

———and P.T. Rowley, "Monozygotic twins concordant for Huntington's chorea," *Neurology (Minneap)*, 10:506-511 (1960).

———A.A. Kurland, and L.T. Kurland, "Hereditary predisposition in drug induced parkinsonism," *Arch Neurol (Chicago)*, 6:5-9 (1962).

Naggan, L., "The recent decline in prevalence of anencephaly and spina bifida," *Amer J Epidem*, 89:154-160 (1969).

———and B. MacMahon, "Ethnic differences in the prevalence of anencephaly and spina bifida in Boston, Massachusetts," *New Eng J Med*, 277:1119-1123 (1967).

Nakajima, A., "Congenital and hereditary blindness in Japan," *J Soc Ophthal*, 30:9-22 (1961).

National Center for Health Statistics, *International classification of diseases, adapted for indexing hospital records by diseases and operations*, rev. ed., vol. 1, *Tabular list*; vol. 2, *Alphabetic index*; Public Health Service Publication No. 719 (Washington, D.C.: Government Printing Office, 1962), vol. 1, 375 pp.; vol. 2, 417 pp.

———"Binocular visual acuity of adults: United States, 1960-62; vision testing methods and binocular visual acuity findings, by age, sex, and race among adults aged 18-79 years," *Vital Health Statist*, Series 11, No. 3, 1964, pp. 1-27.

———*Vital Statistics of the United States. 1955 supplement: Mortality data, multiple causes of death, estimated number of conditions coded on death certificates* (Washington, D.C.: Government Printing Office, 1965), 51 and 149 pp.

———*Eighth revision international classification of diseases, adapted for use in the United States*, vol. 1, *Tabular list*; vol. 2, *Alphabetical index*; Public Health Service Publication No. 1693 (Washington, D.C.: Department of Health, Education, and Welfare, 1968a), vol. 1, 671 pp.; vol. 2, 685 pp.

———"Prevalence of selected impairments: United States, July 1963-June 1965," *Vital Health Statist*, Series 10, No. 48, 1968b, pp. 1-78.

———*Vital Statistics of the United States, 1967*, vol. 1, *Natality* (Washington, D.C.: Government Printing Office, 1969).

National Institute of Neurological Diseases and Blindness, *The Model Reporting Area for blindness statistics: purpose, development, standards, program*, Public Health Service Publication No. 1003 (Washington, D.C.: Government Printing Office, 1963), 14 pp.

———*The Model Reporting Area for blindness statistics: annual statistical report, 1965*, Public Health Service Publication No. 1601 (Washington, D.C.: Government Printing Office, 1966), 34 pp.

———*Statistics for 1966 on blindness in Model Reporting Area [MRA]*, Public Health Service Publication (Washington, D.C.: Government Printing Office, 1969), 63 pp.

National Office of Vital Statistics, *Nosology guidelines*, supplement to *Cause of death coding manual* (Washington, D.C.: Department of Health, Education, and Welfare, August 1958), pp. 1-4.

National Society for the Prevention of Blindness, *NSPB fact book: estimated statistics on blindness and vision problems* (New York, 1966), 109 pp.

Netherlands, Centraal Bureau voor de Statistiek, *Jaarcijfers voor Nederland, 1951-52* (Utrecht, 1954).

Nilsson, L.R., N. Borgfors, I. Gamstorp, H.-E. Holst, and G. Lidén, "Non-endemic goitre and deafness," *Acta Paediat (Stockholm)*, 53:117-131 (1964).

Nobrega, F.T., E. Glattre, L.T. Kurland, and H. Okazaki, "Comments on the epidemiology of parkinsonism including prevalence and incidence statistics for Rochester, Minnesota, 1935-1966," *Excerpta Medica International Congress Series* No. 175, 1967, pp. 474-485.

Norris, F.H., Jr., and W.K. Engel, "Carcinomatous amyotrophic lateral sclerosis," in W.R. Brain, and F.H. Norris, Jr., eds., *The remote effects of cancer on the nervous system* (New York: Grune & Stratton, 1965), pp. 24-34.

Northern Ireland, Ministry of Health and Local Government, *Report on health and local government administration in Northern Ireland during the two years ended December 31, 1963* (Belfast, 1964).

Oey-Khoenlian, "Efforts toward preventing blindness in Indonesia," *Oriental Arch Ophthal*, 1:159-166 (1963).

Oftedal, S.-I., "Multiple sclerosis in Vestfold, Norway," *Acta Neurol Scand*, 42 suppl 19:19-25 (1966).

Okinaka, S., D. McAlpine, K. Miyagawa, N. Suwa, Y. Kuroiwa, H. Shiraki, S. Araki, and L.T. Kurland, "Multiple sclerosis in northern and southern Japan," *World Neurol*, 1:22-38 (1960).

Osler, W., "On heredity in progressive muscular atrophy as illustrated in the Farr family of Vermont," *Arch Med NY*, 4:316-320 (1880).

Øster, J., *Mongolism: a clinicogenealogical investigation comprising 526 mongols living on Seeland and neighbouring islands in Denmark* (Copenhagen: Ejnar Munksgaard, 1953), 206 pp.

Pantelakos, C.G., "Audiometric and otolaryngolic survey of retarded students," *N Carolina Med J*, 24:238-242 (1963).

Parker, G.F., "The incidence of mongoloid imbecility in the newborn infant: a 10-year study covering 27,931 live births," *J Pediat*, 36:493-494 (1950).

Pascucci, I., "Some considerations concerning the Italian law on the care of the non-military blind: the main causes of blindness in the Umbrian region as recorded during visits to those assisted," *Arch Ottal*, 62:269-286 (1958).

Paul, J.R., *Clinical epidemiology*, rev. ed. (Chicago: University of Chicago Press, 1966), 305 pp.

Pearson, C.M., "Polymyositis," *Ann Rev Med*, 17:63-82 (1966).

Pearson, E.S., and H.O. Hartley, eds., *Biometrika tables for statisticians*, vol. 1 (London. Cambridge University Press, 1954), 238 pp.

Pearson, J.S., M.C. Petersen, J.A. Lazarte, H.E. Blodgett, and I.B. Kley, "An educational approach to the social problem of Huntington's chorea," *Proc Staff Meet Mayo Clin*, 30:349-357 (1955).

Pendred, V., cited by W.R. Trotter (1960).

Pennington, G.W., and A. Wilson, "Incidence of myasthenia gravis in the Merseyside conurbation," in H.R. Viets, ed., *Myasthenia gravis*, second international symposium, Los Angeles, 1959 (Springfield, Ill.: Charles C Thomas, 1961), pp. 337-345.

Penrose, L.S., "Genetics of anencephaly," *J Ment Defic Res*, 1:4-15 (1957).
―― and G.F. Smith, *Down's anomaly* (Boston: Little, Brown, 1966), 218 pp.
Penry, J.K., "NIH collaborative study of *absence* seizures," unpublished data.
Percy, A.K., L.T. Kurland, F.T. Nobrega, E. Glattre, and H. Okazaki, "Multiple sclerosis in Rochester, Minnesota—a 60-year appraisal" (abstr.), *Trans Amer Neurol Assn*, 93:264-265 (1968).
Phillips, C.M., "Blindness in Africans in Northern Rhodesia," *Cent Afr J Med*, 7:153-158 (1961).
Phillips, F., "Causes of blindness among blind pension applicants in Tasmania, five-year period beginning July 1, 1953," *J Soc Ophthal*, 27-28:15 (1959).
Phillips, J.W., and H. Lehman, "Mastoid disease in Alaska," *Amer J. Nurs*, 61:58-60 (1961).
Pleydell, M.J., "Huntington's chorea in Northamptonshire," *Brit Med J*, 2:1121-1128 (1954).
―― "Mongolism and other congenital abnormalities: an epidemiological study in Northamptonshire," *Lancet*, 1:1314-1319 (1957).
Pollock, M., and R.W. Hornabrook, "The prevalence, natural history and dementia of Parkinson's disease," *Brain*, 89:429-448 (1966).
Pond, D.A., B.H. Bidwell, and L. Stein, "A survey of epilepsy in fourteen general practices. I. Demographic and medical data," *Psychiat Neurol Neurochir*, 63:217-236 (1960).
Poser, C.M., personal communication.
―― *The relationship between syringomyelia and neoplasm* (Springfield, Ill.: Charles C Thomas, 1956), 98 pp.
Poskanzer, D.C., "Tonsillectomy and multiple sclerosis," *Lancet*, 2:1264-1266 (1965).
―― "Neurological disorders," in D.W. Clark and B. MacMahon, eds., *Preventive medicine* (Boston: Little, Brown, 1967), pp. 373-402.
―― "Etiology of multiple sclerosis: analogy suggesting infection in early life," in M. Alter and J.F. Kurtzke, eds., *The epidemiology of multiple sclerosis* (Springfield, Ill.: Charles C Thomas, 1968), pp. 62-82.
―― and R.W. Schwab, "Cohort analysis of Parkinson's syndrome: evidence for a single etiology related to subclinical infection about 1920," *J Chronic Dis*, 16:961-973 (1963).
―― K. Schapira, and H. Miller, "Epidemiology of multiple sclerosis in the counties of Northumberland and Durham," *J Neurol Neurosurg Psychiat*, n.s. 26:368-376 (1963a).
―― ―― ―― "Multiple sclerosis and poliomyelitis," *Lancet*, 2:917-921 (1963b).
Post, R.H., "Hearing acuity variation among Negroes and whites," *Eugen Quart*, 11:65-81 (1964).
Powers, M.H., "The prevalence of deafness in school age children," *Amer Ann Deaf*, 109:410-417 (1964).
Pratt, R.T.C., *The genetics of neurological disorders* (London: Oxford University Press, 1967), 310 pp.
―― N.D. Compston, and D. McAlpine, "The familial incidence of disseminated sclerosis and its significance," *Brain*, 74:191-214 (1951).
Presthus, J., "Multiple sclerosis in Møre og Romsdal County, Norway," *Acta Neurol Scand*, 42 suppl 19:12-18 (1966).

"Proceedings of the third conference on the toxicity of cycads," *Fed Proc*, 23:1333-1388 (1964).

Rainer, J.D., K.Z. Altshuler, and F.J. Kallmann, *Family and mental health problems in a deaf population* (New York: New York State Psychiatric Institute, Columbia University, 1963), 260 pp.

Ravn, H., "The Landry-Guillain-Barré syndrome: a survey and a clinical report of 127 cases," *Acta Neurol Scand*, 43 suppl 30:9-64 (1967).

Record, R.G., and A. Smith, "Incidence, mortality, and sex distribution of mongoloid defectives," *Brit J Prev Soc Med*, 9:10-15 (1955).

Reed, D., J. Sever, J. Kurtzke, and L.T. Kurland, "Measles antibody in patients with multiple sclerosis," *Arch Neurol (Chicago)*, 10:402-409 (1964).

──── C. Plato, T. Elizan, and L.T. Kurland, "The amyotrophic lateral sclerosis/parkinsonism-dementia complex: a ten-year follow-up on Guam. Part I. Epidemiologic studies, *Amer J Epidem*, 83:54-73 (1966).

Renwick, D.H.G., "Estimating prevalance of certain chronic childhood conditions by use of a central registry," *Public Health Rep*, 82:261-269 (1967).

Research Committee of the Council of the College of General Practitioners, *Studies on medical and population subjects*, No. 14. *Morbidity statistics from general practice*, vol. 3, *Disease in general practice* (London: Her Majesty's Stationery Office, 1962).

Rigrodsky, S., F. Prunty, and L. Glovsky, "A study of the incidence, types and associated etiologies of hearing loss in an institutionalized mentally retarded population," *Train Sch Bull (Vineland)*, 58:30-44 (1961).

Rischbieth, R.H., "The prevalence of disseminated sclerosis in South Australia," *Med J Aust*, 1:774-776 (1966).

Robb, P., *Epilepsy: a review of basic and clinical research*, Public Health Service Publication No. 1357 (Washington, D.C.: Department of Health, Education, and Welfare, 1965), 69 pp.

Roberts, J., and D. Bayliss, "Hearing levels of adults by race, region, and area of residence," *Vital Health Statist*, Series 11, No. 26, 1967, pp. 1-33.

──── and J. Cohrssen, "Hearing levels of adults by education, income, and occupation," *Vital Health Statist*, Series 11, No. 31, 1968, pp. 1-41.

Robertson, E.E., "Progressive bulbar paralysis showing heredofamilial incidence and intellectual impairment," *Arch Neurol Psychiat (Chicago)*, 69:197-207 (1953).

Rodger, F.C., "Eye diseases in the African continent," *Amer J Ophthal*, 45:343-358 (1958).

──── *Blindness in West Africa* (London: H.K. Lewis, 1959), 262 pp.

Rodin, E., and S. Gonzalez, "Hereditary components in epileptic patients: electroencephalogram family studies," *JAMA*, 198:221-225 (1966).

Rogot, E., I.D. Goldberg, and H. Goldstein, "Survivorship and causes of death among the blind," *J Chronic Dis*, 19:179-197 (1966).

Rohrschneider, W., "Preservation of eyesight—prevention of blindness," *Munchen Med Wschr*, 104:1407-1414 (1962).

Rose, A.L., and J.N. Walton, "Polymyositis: a survey of 89 cases with particular reference to treatment and prognosis," *Brain*, 89:747-768 (1966).

Rosen, S., D. Plester, A. El-Mofty, and H.V. Rosen, "Relation of hearing loss to

cardiovascular disease," *Trans Amer Acad Ophthal Otolaryng*, 68:433-444 (1964).
Rostkowski, L., and C.W. Korczak, "Blindness prevention in Poland," *Zdrow Publiczne*, 77:367-374 (1962).
Royal Commonwealth Society for the Blind, *Annual reports and accounts*, 1957-64.
Rozanski, J., "Contribution to the incidence of multiple sclerosis among Jews in Israel," *Monatsschr Psychiat Neurol*, 123:65-72 (1952).

Said, M.E., A. Korra, and K. El-Kashlan, "The blindness register survey in Egypt," in *Proceedings of the fifth annual conference of the Model Reporting Area for blindness statistics, 1966*, Public Health Service Publication No. 1593 (Washington, D.C.: Government Printing Office, 1967).
Saint, E.G., and M. Sadka, "The incidence of multiple sclerosis in Western Australia," *Med J Aust*, 2:249-250 (1962).
Sato, S., "The epidemiological and clinico-statistical study of epilepsy in Niigata City. Part 2. The epidemiological study of epilepsy in Niigata City," *Clin Neurol (Japan)*, 4:413-424 (1964).
Schapira, K., D.C. Poskanzer, and H. Miller, "Familial and conjugal multiple sclerosis," *Brain*, 86:315-332 (1963).
Schappert-Kimmijser, J., "A statistical study on the causes of blindness in blind persons living in the Hague and surrounding districts," *Ophthalmologica (Basel)*, 132:176-180 (1956).
_____ *The causes of blindness in the Netherlands* (Assen, Netherlands: Van Gorcum, 1959).
Schein, J.D., "Factors in the definition of deafness as they relate to incidence and prevalence," in *Proceedings of the conference on the collection of statistics of severe hearing impairments and deafness in the United States, 1964*, Public Health Service Publication No. 1227 (Washington, D.C.: Government Printing Office, 1964), pp. 28-37.
_____ *The deaf community: studies in the social psychology of deafness* (Washington, D.C.: Gallaudet College Press, 1968), 101 pp.
_____ "Report of the first annual meeting on the national census of the deaf," *The Deaf American*, 22:36-45 (1969).
_____ "The national census of deaf persons," *J Rehabil Deaf*, 4:144-150 (1971).
_____ and S.M. Bushnaq, "Higher education for the deaf in the United States: a retrospective investigation," *Amer Ann Deaf*, 107:416-420 (1962).
_____ A. Gentile, and K. Haase, "Methodological aspects of a hearing ability interview survey," *Vital Health Statist*, Series 2, No. 12, 1965, pp. 1-19.
_____ _____ _____ "Development and evaluation of an expanded hearing loss scale questionnaire," *Vital Health Statist*, Series 2, No. 37, 1970, pp. 1-42.
Schumacher, G.A., G. Beebe, R.F. Kibler, L.T. Kurland, J.F. Kurtzke, F. McDowell, B. Nagler, W.A. Sibley, W.W. Tourtellotte, and T.L. Willmon, "Problems of experimental trials of therapy in multiple sclerosis: report by the panel on the evaluation of experimental trials of therapy in multiple sclerosis," *Ann NY Acad Sci*, 122:552-568 (1965).
Schwab, R.S., L.J. Doshay, H. Garland, P. Bradshaw, E. Garvey, and B. Crawford, "Shift to older age distribution in parkinsonism: a report on

1,000 patients covering the past decade from three centers," *Neurology (Minneap)*, 6:783-790 (1956).
Scotland, Scottish Home and Health Department, *Health and welfare services in Scotland: report* (Edinburgh: Her Majesty's Stationery Office, 1965).
Seiler, H.E., "A study of herpes zoster particularly in its relationship to chickenpox," *J Hyg (Camb)*, 47:253-262 (1949).
Sever, J.L., and W. Zeman, eds., "Conference on measles virus and subacute sclerosing panencephalitis," *Neurology (Minneap)*, 18(pt 2):1-192 (1968).
Shapiro, S., E.R. Schlesinger, and R.E.L. Nesbitt, Jr., *Infant, perinatal, maternal, and childhood mortality in the United States* (APHA monograph; Cambridge, Mass.: Harvard University Press, 1968), 388 pp.
Shiraki, H., "The neuropathology of amyotrophic lateral sclerosis (ALS) in the Kii Peninsula and other areas of Japan," in F.H. Norris, Jr. and L.T. Kurland, eds., *Motor neuron diseases: research on amyotrophic lateral sclerosis and related disorders* (New York: Grune & Stratton, 1969), pp. 80-84.
Sibley, W.A., and J.M. Foley, "Infection and immunization in multiple sclerosis," *Ann NY Acad Sci*, 122:457-468 (1965).
Siedler, H.D., W. Nicholl, and L.T. Kurland, "The prevalence and incidence of multiple sclerosis in Missoula County, Montana," *J Lancet*, 78:358-360 (1958).
Sirken, M.G., "The potential impact (of the decennial undercount) on vital statistics," read at the meeting of the Washington Statistical Society, Washington, D.C., 25 October 1967.
Smithells, R.W., "The Liverpool Congenital Abnormalities Registry," *Develop Med Child Neurol*, 4:320-324 (1962).
―――― and E.R. Chinn, "Spina bifida in Liverpool," *Develop Med Child Neurol*, 7:258-268 (1965).
―――― ―――― and D. Franklin, "Anencephaly in Liverpool," *Develop Med Child Neurol*, 6:231-240 (1964).
Sobue, I., K. Ando, M. Iida, T. Takayanagi, Y. Yamamura, and Y. Matsuoka, "Neuromyelopathy with gastro-intestinal disorders: its clinico-pathology and epidemiology" (abstr.), *Excerpta Medica International Congress Series* No. 193, 1969, p. 283.
―――― ―――― ―――― ―――― ―――― ―――― "Myeloneuropathy with abdominal disorders in Japan: a clinical study of 752 cases," *Neurology (Minneap)*, 21:168-173 (1971).
Solares, A., "Causes of blindness in Bolivia," *J Soc Ophthal*, 17:27-31 (1956).
Soll, R.W., "Delayed hypersensitivity: a possible mechanism in the etiology of multiple sclerosis," in M. Alter, and J.F. Kurtzke, eds., *The epidemiology of multiple sclerosis* (Springfield, Ill.: Charles C Thomas, 1968), pp. 110-128.
Soper, F.L., "Hemispheric control of eye infection," *J Soc Ophthal*, 12:6-7 (1951).
Sorsby, A., *The incidence and causes of blindness: an international survey*, Brit J Ophthal Monograph Suppl XIV, 1950.
―――― "The incidence and causes of blindness in England and Wales, 1948-1962," in *Ministry of health reports on public health and medical subjects*, No. 114 (London: Her Majesty's Stationery Office, 1966), 94 pp.
―――― A. Franceschetti, and H. Koenig, "The decline of blindness in children

from infectious disease," in *XVII Concilium Ophthalmologicum, 1954, Canada, United States of America, Acta*, vol. 3 (Toronto: University of Toronto Press, 1955), pp. 2082-2089.

South African National Council for the Blind, *8th Biennial report, 1944-45*, Pretoria.

――― *15th Biennial report, 1958-60*, Pretoria.

Spiegelman, M., "The organization of the Vital and Health Statistics Monograph Program," in *Emerging techniques in population research*, proc. 39th annual conference Milbank Memorial Fund, 18-19 September 1962 (New York: Milbank Memorial Fund, 1963), pp. 230-249.

Statistisk Sentralbyrå, Oslo, Norway, personal communication, 1961.

Stazio, A., L.T. Kurland, L.G. Bell, M.G. Saunders, and E. Rogot, "Multiple sclerosis in Winnipeg, Manitoba: methodological considerations of epidemiologic survey; ten year follow-up on a communitywide study, and population re-survey," *J Chronic Dis*, 17:415-438 (1964).

――― R.M. Paddison, and L.T. Kurland, "Multiple sclerosis in New Orleans, Louisiana, and Winnipeg, Manitoba, Canada: follow-up of a previous survey in New Orleans, and comparison between the patient populations in the two communities," *J Chronic Dis*, 20:311-331 (1967).

Štefek, J., and V. Štruplová, "[Statistical analysis of blindness in the Opava district obtained by screening]," *CS Oftal*, 19:338-342 (1963).

Stevenson, A.C., and E.A. Cheeseman, "Hereditary deaf mutism, with particular reference to Northern Ireland," *Ann Hum Genet*, 20:177-231 (1956).

――― H.A. Johnston, D.R. Golding, and M.I.P. Stewart, *Comparative study of congenital malformations: basic tabulations in respect of consecutive post 28-week births recorded in the co-operating centres* (Oxford: Medical Research Council Population Genetics Research Unit, 1966a).

――― ――― M.I.P. Stewart, and D.R. Golding, "Congenital malformations: a report of a study of series of consecutive births in 24 centres," *Bull WHO*, 34 suppl:9-127 (1966b).

Stock, F.E., "Blindness in an urban centre in Nigeria," *Brit Med J*, 1:525-526 (1946).

Stoller, A., and R.D. Collmann, "Incidence of infective hepatitis followed by Down's syndrome nine months later," *Lancet*, 2:1221-1223 (1965).

Storm-Mathisen, A., *Myasthenia gravis: a clinical study with special reference to prevalence and prognosis* (Stockholm: Almqvist & Wiksell, 1961), 132 pp.

――― "Epidemiological and prognostical aspects of myasthenia gravis in Norway," *Ann NY Acad Sci*, 135:431-435 (1966).

Sturman, D., "A statistical approach to the eye problems in New Zealand," *Trans Ophthal Soc New Zeal*, 21:74-84 (1969).

Sutherland, J.M., "Observations on the prevalence of multiple sclerosis in northern Scotland," *Brain*, 79:635-654 (1956).

――― J.H. Tyrer, M.J. Eadie, J.H. Casey, and L.T. Kurland, "The prevalence of multiple sclerosis in Queensland, Australia: a field survey," *Acta Neurol Scand*, 42 suppl 19:57-67 (1966).

Sveinsson, K., "Glaucoma and heredity in Iceland," *Acta Ophthal (Kobenhavn)*, 37:191-198 (1959).

Swank, R.L., O. Lerstad, A. Strøm, and J. Backer, "Multiple sclerosis in rural

Norway: its geographic and occupational incidence in relation to nutrition," *New Eng J Med*, 246:721-728 (1952).

Swartout, H.O., and R.G. Webster, "To what degree are mortality statistics dependable?" *Amer J Public Health*, 30:811-815 (1940).

Szanton, V.L., and W.C. Szanton, "Hearing disturbances in allergic children," *Ann Allerg*, 19:1177-1187 (1961).

Tatimov, M., "Some statistical data on blindness," *Vestn Statistiki*, 11:29-36 (1966).

Tato, J.M., A. Arabel, J.M. Tato, Jr., L. Anderedson, M. Lauberer, and E. Tato, "Estudios oto-audiologicos en indigenas Argentinos," *Otolaringológica (Argentine)*, 6:372-377 (1961).

Taverner, D., "Bell's palsy: a clinical and electromyographic study," *Brain*, 78:209-228 (1955).

———"Electrodiagnosis in facial palsy," *Arch Otolaryng (Chicago)*, 81:470-477 (1965).

Taylor, W.W., and I.W. Taylor, *Special education of physically handicapped children in western Europe* (New York: International Society for the Welfare of Cripples, 1960), 497 pp.

Tennent, A.A., "Blindness in New Zealand," *New Zeal Med J*, 61:463-465 (1962).

Thomasen, E., *Myotonia: Thomsen's disease (myotonia congenita), paramyotonia, and dystrophia myotonica: a clinical and heredobiologic investigation*, translated from the Danish by F.B. Carlsen (Aarhus, Denmark: Universitetsforlaget, 1948), 251 pp.

Thomsen, J., "Nachträgliche Bemerkungen über Myotonia congenita (Strümpell), Thomsen'sche Krankheit (Westphal)," *Arch Psychiat Nervenkr*, 24:918-923 (1892).

Thong, N.N., *Contribution à l'étude de la sclerose en plaques au Viet-Nam (à propos de deux cas observés à la clinique médicale de Cho-Ray Départment de Neurologie du Professeur Agrégé Bui Quoc Huong)*, Medical school thesis, University of Saigon, No. 563/42, 1965, 129+ pp.

Thould, A.K., and E.F. Scowen, "The syndrome of congenital deafness and simple goitre," *J Endocr*, 30:69-77 (1964).

Torgersruud, T., "Ocular findings by blindness in Ethiopia," *J Soc Ophthal*, 20:12-18 (1957).

Toyokura, Y., H. Tsukagoshi, and A. Igata, "An obscure neuromyelopathy occurring in Japan: a clinical and neuropathological study" (abstr.), *Excerpta Medica International Congress Series* No. 193, 1969, p. 290.

Trotter, W.R., "The association of deafness with thyroid dysfunction," *Brit Med Bull*, 16.92-98 (1960).

Tsubaki, T., Y. Honma, and M. Hoshi, "Neurological syndrome associated with clioquinol" (letter to the editor), *Lancet*, 1:696-697 (1971).

Tsuiki, T., "Clinical studies on streptomycin deafness," *Tohoku Igaku Z*, 67:155-179 (1963).

Tyler, F.H., and F.E. Stephens, "Studies in disorders of muscle. II. Clinical manifestations and inheritance of facioscapulohumeral dystrophy in a large family," *Ann Intern Med*, 32:640-660 (1950).

_____"Studies in disorders of muscle. IV. Clinical manifestations and inheritance of childhood progressive muscular dystrophy," *Ann Intern Med*, 35:169-185 (1951).

United Arab Republic, Department of Statistics and Census, *1960 Census of population*, vol. 2, *General tables* (Cairo, 1963).

United Arab Republic, Ministry of Public Health, Ophthalmic Section, *Report for the year 1952*, 1953.

United States Bureau of the Census, *The blind and deaf-mutes in the United States: 1930* (Washington, D.C.: Government Printing Office, 1931), 23 pp.

Van Bogaert, L., and M.A. Radermecker, "XXII. Scléroses latérales amyotrophiques typiques et paralysies agitantes héréditaires, dans une même famille, avec une forme de passage possible entre les deux affections," *Monatsschr Psychiat Neurol*, 127:185-203 (1954).

Vannas, S., and T. Raivio, "Occurrence and causes of blindness in Finland," *Acta Ophthal (Kobenhavn)*, 42 pt. 1:307-318 (1964).

Van Wart, R.M., "A note on the frequency of multiple sclerosis in Louisiana," *New Orleans Med Surg J*, 57:549-551 (1905).

Vedel-Jensen, N., "The causes of blindness in 1000 consecutive new members of the Danish Society for the Blind," *Danish Med Bull*, 9:185-188 (1962).

Venkataswamy, G., "Malnutrition blindness in India," *J Indian Med Assn*, 47:67-74 (1966).

Vercelletto, P., and J. Courjon, "Heredity and generalized epilepsy," *Epilepsia (Amst)*, s.4. 10:7-21 (1969).

Vogel, F., "Some remarks on the theoretical basis of the investigation of isolates," *J Genet Hum*, 13:3-9 (1964).

von Bahr, G., "Blindher, dess orsaker och bekämpande," *Nord Med*, 73:121-125 (1965).

Waaler, E., and M. Grimstvedt, "The clinical diagnoses of the causes of death and their reliability," *Acta Path Microbiol Scand*, 43:330-338 (1958).

Waggoner, L.G., "Secretory otitis media," *Harper Hosp Bull*, 22:50-58 (1964).

Walton, J.N., "Clinical aspects of human muscular dystrophy," in G.H. Bourne and M.N. Golarz, eds., *Muscular dystrophy in man and animals* (New York: Hafner, 1963), pp. 263-321.

_____ "Muscular dystrophy: some recent advances in knowledge," *Brit Med J*, 1:1344-1348 (1964).

_____ (ed.) *Disorders of voluntary muscle*, ed. 2 (London: Churchill, 1969), 941 pp.

_____ and F.J. Nattrass, "On the classification, natural history and treatment of the myopathies," *Brain*, 77:169-231 (1954).

Warren, H.V., R.E. Delavault, and C.H. Cross, "Possible correlations between geology and some disease patterns," *Ann NY Acad Sci*, 136:657-710 (1967).

Webb, C., S. Kinde, B. Weber, and R. Beedle, "Incidence of hearing loss in institutionalized mental retardates," *Amer J Ment Defic*, 70:563-568 (1966).

Westlund, K.B., and L.T. Kurland, "Studies on multiple sclerosis in Winnipeg, Manitoba, and New Orleans, Louisiana. I. Prevalence. Comparison between the patient groups in Winnipeg and New Orleans," *Amer J Hyg*, 57:380-396 (1953).

Whisnant, J.P., J.P. Fitzgibbons, L.T. Kurland, and G.P. Sayre, "Natural history of stroke in Rochester, Minnesota, 1945 through 1954," *Stroke*, 2:11-22 (1971).

White, D.N., and L. Wheelan, "Disseminated sclerosis: a survey of patients in the Kingston, Ontario, area," *Neurology (Minneap)*, 9:256-272 (1959).

White, L.R., J.L. Sever, and F.P. Alepa, "Maternal and congenital rubella before 1964: frequency, clinical features, and search for isoimmune phenomena," *J Pediat*, 74:198-207 (1969).

Wiederholt, W.C., D.W. Mulder, and E.H. Lambert, "The Landry-Guillain-Barré-Strohl syndrome or polyradiculoneuropathy: historical review, report on 97 patients, and present concepts," *Mayo Clin Proc*, 39:427-451 (1964).

Williams, G.R., L.T. Kurland, and I.D. Goldberg, "Morbidity and mortality with parkinsonism," *J Neurosurg*, 24:138-143, 158 (1966).

Williamson, E.M., "Incidence and family aggregation of major congenital malformations of central nervous system," *J Med Genet*, 2:161-170 (1965).

Wilson, J.F., "The blind in a changing world: the extent, causes, and distribution of blindness; a statistical survey," *J Soc Ophthal*, 36:27-33 (1965).

Wishik, S.M., and E.R. Kramm, "Audiometric testing of hearing of school children," *J Speech Hearing Dis*, 18:360-365 (1953).

World Health Organization, "The prevalence of blindness and deaf-mutism in various countries," *WHO Epidem Vital Statist Rep*, 6:1-31 (1953).

——— *Manual of the international statistical classification of diseases, injuries, and causes of death*, 1955 rev. (Geneva: World Health Organization, 1957), vol. 1, 393 pp.; vol. 2, 540 pp.

——— "Blindness: information collected from various sources," *WHO Epidem Vital Statist Rep*, 19:437-511 (1966).

——— *Manual of the international statistical classification of diseases, injuries, and causes of death*, 1965 rev. (Geneva: World Health Organization), vol. 1, 1967, 478 pp.; vol. 2, 1969, 616 pp.

——— Regional Office for the Eastern Mediterranean, *Prevalence of blindness and care of blind persons in the countries of the eastern Mediterranean region: results of an enquiry by the regional office, 1962*, 1963.

——— Regional Office for South-East Asia, *World Health Day, April 7, 1962: "preserve sight—prevent blindness"* (New Delhi, 1962).

Yassin, A., and M. Taha, "Sensory neural deafness in pellagra," *J Laryng*, 77:992-1000 (1963).

Yates, P.C., "Blindness in Australia, 1953 to 1958," *Med J Aust*, 50:828-830 (1963).

Zeman, W., and P. Dyken, "Dystonia musculorum deformans: clinical, genetic and pathoanatomical studies," *Psychiat Neurol Neurochir*, 70:77-121 (1967).

Ziegler, D.K., "Multiple sclerosis and rheumatic fever: related diseases," *Dis Nerv Syst*, 20:221-224 (1959).

Zil'ber, L.A., Z.L. Bajdakova, A.N. Gardaš'jan, N.V. Konovalov, T.L. Bunina, and

E.M. Barabadze, "Study of the etiology of amyotrophic lateral sclerosis," *Bull WHO*, 29:449-456 (1961).

Zschoch, H., "Beitrag zur Todesursachenstatistik," *Deutsche Gesundh*, 19:311-314 (1964).

Zu Rhein, G.M., and S.-M. Chou, "Papova virus in progressive multifocal leukoencephalopathy," *Proc Assn Res Nerv Ment Dis*, 44:307-359 (1968).

INDEX

Afebrile seizures, 40, 308
Age
  blindness and
    in foreign countries, 268-269
    in U.S., 256, 257, 262
  convulsive disorder incidence rates by, 34, 35
  hearing impairment in U.S. and, 291, 292
  herpes zoster incidence rates by, 220
  Huntington's chorea and, 224, 225
  maternal, and Down's syndrome, 162, 163, 164
  mortality rates in U.S. by
    cerebral palsy, infantile, 235, 236
    Down's syndrome, 155-156
    epilepsy, 18-20
    malformations, congenital, of nervous system, 179-180
    muscular dystrophy, 131-133, 135-138
    myasthenia gravis, 146-147
    parkinsonism, 43-44, 50
    sclerosis, amyotrophic lateral, 112, 113, 117
    sclerosis, multiple, 69-71
  parkinsonism and, 59
Amyotrophic lateral sclerosis (ALS), see Sclerosis, amyotrophic lateral
Anencephaly
  incidence rates, 204, 205
    among births, 199-200
  secular trends in, 203-207
  summation, 313-315
Anomalies, see Malformations
Ataxias, hereditary, 228-229, 317
Atrophy, muscular, 215
  Charcot-Marie-Tooth peroneal, 317
  progressive, 108
    mortality rates in U.S., 112
    myelopathic, 108
Atrophy, optic, 247
Audiometric school surveys, 287-288

Bell's palsy, see Palsy, Bell's
Birth rates
  hydrocephalus and, congenital, 177
  monstrosity and, 177
  spina bifida and, 177
Blindness, 246-275
  definition, 246-247
  in foreign countries, 264-273
    by age and sex, 268-269
    causes, 269-273
    incidence rates, 264-265

  prevalence rates, 265-268
  MRA statistics, 251-264
    limitations, 263-264
    standards, 253-254
    value, 263-264
  schools for, 250-251
  summation, 318
  survival and, 247-248
  in U.S.
    by age, 256, 257, 262
    by color, 256, 262, 263
    incidence rates, 248-251, 254-260
    prevalence rates, 248-251, 255, 260-263
    by sex, 256, 262

Case series, 7-8
Cataract, definition, 247
Cerebral palsy, see Palsy, cerebral
Cerebral spastic infantile paralysis, see Palsy, cerebral, infantile
Charcot-Marie-Tooth peroneal muscular atrophy, 317
Children, school-age
  blindness among, 252
  hearing impairments in, 285-288
Chorea, see Huntington's chorea
Color
  blindness in U.S. by, 256, 262, 263
  Down's syndrome and, 164-166
  hearing impairments in U.S. by, 293-295
  mortality rates in U.S. by
    cerebral palsy, infantile, 236, 237, 238
    cerebral palsy, neonatal, 239-241
    Down's syndrome, 155, 156, 157
    epilepsy, 18-20, 21
    hydrocephalus, congenital, 186
    meningocele, 185
    monstrosity, 183
    muscular dystrophy, 132, 134-136
    myasthenia gravis, 146-147, 148, 149
    nervous system malformations, congenital, 179, 180-181, 188
    parkinsonism, 44, 45, 48, 49
    sclerosis, amyotrophic lateral, 112-114, 115, 116, 117
    sclerosis, multiple, 69-71
    spina bifida, 185
  neurologic disorders and, 326, 328, 329-330
Convulsive disorders, 15-40. See also Epilepsy; Seizures
  incidence, 31-36

431

prevalence rates, 28-31
summation, 307-308
Cord, spinal, affections, 210-215

Deafness, 276. *See also* Hearing impairments
etiology, 284, 296, 299-300
prelingual, prevalence, 280-285, 302
schools for, enrollment in U.S., 303
Death, *see* Mortality
Degeneration
hepatolenticular, 227-228
retinal, 247
Disease, diagnosis, 6-7
Down's syndrome, 153-168
cases, 162
color and, 164-166
familial frequency, 166-167
features, 163-167
incidence, 159-163
in Australia, 160
in Denmark, 161
in England, 160, 161
in Rochester, Minnesota, 160
maternal age and, 162, 163, 164
morbidity data, 159-167
mortality rates in U.S., 154-159
by age, 155-156
by color, 155, 156, 157
geographic distribution, 156-158
by sex, 155, 156, 157
trend, 154-155
by type of county, 157, 158-159
sex and, 163-164
summation, 312-313
twins with, 166
Duchenne muscular dystrophy, 129
Dystonia musculorum deformans, 230-231
summation, 317
Dystrophy, muscular, 128-140
cases and prevalence rates, 139
Duchenne type, 129
facioscapulohumeral type, 129
limb-girdle type, 129-130
morbidity data, 137, 139-140
mortality rates, international, 130, 131
mortality rates, in U.S., 131-137, 138
by age, 131-133, 135-138
by color, 132, 134-136
geographic distribution, 134-135
by marital status, 135, 137, 138
nativity and, 137, 138
by sex, 132-134, 136-138
trend, 131
by type of county, 135, 136
summation, 310-311
Dystrophy, myotonic, 140-141
cases, 140

prevalence rates, 140
summation, 311

Encephalitis and parkinsonism, 58-61
Epidemiology, 306-307
analytic aspect, 2
data
case series, 7-8
population-based rates, 9-13
population-oriented studies, 8-9
relative frequency, 8
types, 7-13
definition, 2-3
descriptive aspect, 2
experimental aspect, 2
genetics and, 5
historical note, 3-4
scope, 2-3
Epilepsy
incidence rates, 32, 35
mortality rates, international, 24, 25
mortality rates, population surveys, 24-28
mortality rates, in U.S., 17-24
by age, 18-20
by color, 18-20, 21
geographic distribution, 20-22
by marital status, 22-24
nativity and, 24
by sex, 18-20, 21
trend, 17-18
by type of county, 22
prevalence rates, 31
seizures, types, 15-16

Facioscapulohumeral muscular dystrophy, 129
Febrile seizures, 34, 36
Fibroplasia, retrolental, definition, 247

Genetic drift, 5-6
Genetics and epidemiology, 5
Geographic distribution, mortality rates in U.S.
cerebral palsy, infantile, 236-238
cerebral palsy, neonatal, 241
Down's syndrome, 156-158
epilepsy, 20-22
hydrocephalus, congenital, 186
monstrosity, 182-183
muscular dystrophy, 134-135
myasthenia gravis, 147-148
nervous system malformations, congenital, 182-191
parkinsonism, 44-47
sclerosis, amyotrophic lateral, 114-116
sclerosis, multiple, 69, 71-78
spina bifida, 184, 185
Geographic isolates, 5-6

Glaucoma, definition, 246-247
Goiter and deafness, 284, 299
Grand mal, 15-16
  primary, incidence rates, 33
Guam form of ALS, 123-125
Guillain-Barré syndrome, 221-223, 316

Hearing impairments, 276-304. *See also* Deafness
  audiometric school surveys, 287-288
  etiology, 284, 296, 298-300
  incidence, 278-280
  population estimates, 278-296
  prevalence in U.S., 289-296
    age and, 291, 292
    in school-age children, 285-288
    color and, 293-295
    economic conditions and, 295-296, 297
    geographic distribution and, 295
    sex and, 290, 291-293
  summation, 318-319
  treatment, 300-301
  trend, 301-304
Hepatolenticular degeneration, 227-228
Hereditary ataxias, 228-229, 317
Hereditary disorders, 223-231
Heredity and seizures, 36-38
Herpes zoster, 218-221
  incidence rates, 219-221
    by age, 220
    by sex, 219, 220
  summation, 316
Huntington's chorea, 223-227
  age at onset, 224, 225
  cases, 226
  duration, 224
  frequency, 225
  prevalence rates, 226
  summation, 316
Hydrocephalus, congenital
  birth rates, 177
  incidence rates among births, 198-199
  mortality rates in U.S., 177
    by color, 186
    geographic distribution, 186
    by sex, 186
    by type of county, 192-194
  summation, 313-315

Incidence rates, 9-10, 307. *See also* Morbidity rates; individual disorders
Infants
  cerebral palsy. *See* Palsy, cerebral, infantile
  neurologic disorders, incidence rates, 324
International mortality rates
  cerebral palsy, 233-234
  epilepsy, 24, 25
  malformations, congenital, of nervous system, 173-176
    by sex, 175
  motor neuron disease, 110, 111
  muscular dystrophy, 130, 131
  myasthenia gravis, 145-146
  parkinsonism, 50-52
  sclerosis
    amyotrophic lateral, 110
    multiple, 65-68

Jamaican neuropathy, 212-213
Japanese myeloneuropathy, 213-215

Keratitis, definition, 247

"Latency," in multiple sclerosis, 96-99

Malformations
  congenital, 169-170
  of muscle, inborn. *See* Dystrophy, muscular
  of nervous system. *See* Nervous system, congenital malformations
  of neural tube. *See* Neural tube defects
Marianas form of amyotrophic lateral sclerosis, 123-125
Marital status, mortality rates in U.S. by
  epilepsy, 22-24
  muscular dystrophy, 135, 137, 138
  parkinsonism, 49, 50
  sclerosis
    amyotrophic lateral, 116-117
    multiple, 78-80
Maternal age, and Down's syndrome, 162, 163, 164
Meningocele mortality rates in U.S.
  by color, 185
  by sex, 185
  by type of county, 193
Migration and multiple sclerosis, 96-99
MND, *see* Motor neuron disease
Model reporting area for blindness statistics, *see* Blindness, MRA statistics
Mongolism, *see* Down's syndrome
Monstrosity
  birth rates, 177
  mortality rates in U.S., 177
    by color, 183
    geographic distribution, 182, 183
    by sex, 183
    by type of county, 191-192
  summation, 313-315
Morbidity rates
  cerebral palsy, 241-244
  Down's syndrome, 159-167
  muscular dystrophy, 137, 139-140
  myasthenia gravis, 149-152

nervous system malformations, congenital, 195-207
sclerosis
  amyotrophic lateral, 118-121
  multiple, 82-94
Mortality rates, 9, 10-11, 112, 307. *See also* individual disorders and variables
Motor neuron disease, 108-127
  incidence rates, 119
  mortality rates, 109-118
  summation, 310
MRA, *see* Blindness, MRA statistics
Multiple sclerosis (MS), *see* Sclerosis, multiple
Myasthenia gravis, 144-152
  familial features, 152
  incidence rates, 150, 151
  morbidity data, 149-152
  mortality rates, international, 145-146
  mortality rates, in U.S., 145-149
    by age, 146-147
    by color, 146-147, 148, 149
    comparison with international rates, 145-146
    geographic distribution, 147-148
    nativity and, 149
    by sex, 146-147, 148, 149
    trend, 146
    by type of county, 148
  prevalence rates, 150-151
  summation, 311-312
Myeloneuropathy, Japanese, 213-215
Myelo-optico-neuropathy, subacute, 213-215
Myopathies, 142-143

Nativity, mortality rates in U.S. and
  epilepsy, 24
  muscular dystrophy, 137, 138
  myasthenia gravis, 149
  parkinsonism, 49-50
  sclerosis, amyotrophic lateral, 117-118
  sclerosis, multiple, 80-81, 82
Neonatal cerebral palsy, *see* Palsy, cerebral, neonatal
Nerves, trigeminal, neuralgia, 218, 316
Nervous system, congenital malformations, 169-209
  classification, 170-172
  distribution, by type of malformation, 171
  incidence rates among births, 195-201
  morbidity data, 195-207
  mortality rates, international, 173-176
    by sex, 175
  mortality rates, in U.S., 176-195
    by age, 179-180
    by color, 179, 180-181, 188
    comparison with international rates, 173-176

    geographic distribution, 182-191
    by sex, 179, 180, 181, 188
    trend, 176-178
    by type of county, 191-195
  sex ratios in, 201-203
  summation, 313-315
Neural tube defects, 197
Neuralgia, trigeminal, 218, 316
Neuroepidemiology, 305-332
Neurologic disorders, 210-231
  distribution, 319-324
  geographic variations, 330-331
  incidence rates, 322, 323
    in infants, 324
  mortality rates, 320-321
  prevalence rates, 322, 324, 325
  rate variations by color, 326, 328, 329-330
  rate variations by sex, 324, 326-329
  summation, 315-317
Neuronitis, infectious, *see* Guillain-Barré syndrome
Neuropathy
  acute, 215-223
  hereditary, 229
  Jamaican, 212-213
  subacute myelo-optico-, 213-215

Optic atrophy, 247

Palsy, Bell's, 215-217
  cases, 216
  incidence rates, 216
  summation, 316
Palsy, cerebral, 232-245
  incidence rates, 242
  infantile; *see below*
  morbidity rates, 241-244
  mortality rates, 232-241
    international, 233-234
  neonatal; *see below*
  prevalence rates, 243
  summation, 317-318
Palsy, cerebral, infantile, mortality rates in U.S., 235-238
  by age, 235, 236
  by color, 236, 237, 238
  geographic distribution, 236-238
  by sex, 235-236, 237
  trend, 234-235
  by type of county, 238
Palsy, cerebral, neonatal, mortality rates in U.S., 239-241
  by color, 239-241
  geographic distribution, 241
  by sex, 239, 240
  trend, 234-235
  by type of county, 241
Palsy, progressive bulbar, 108

Paralysis, *see* Palsy, cerebral, infantile
Parkinsonism, 41–63
  age and, 59
  classification, 41–42
  encephalitis and, 58–61
  familial features, 61–62
  incidence rates, 52–57
    in Rochester, Minnesota, 53, 54
  mortality rates, in Canada, 43
  mortality rates, international, 50–52
  mortality rates, in U.S., 43–50
    by age, 43–44, 50
    by color, 44, 45, 48, 49
    early, 43
    geographic distribution, 44–47
    by marital status, 49, 50
    nativity and, 49–50
    by sex, 44, 45, 49, 50
    by type of county, 48–49
  prevalence rates, 52–57
  summation, 308
Peroneal muscular atrophy, Charcot-Marie-Tooth, 317
Polymyositis, 141–142, 311
Population, rates based on, 8–13
Prevalence rates, 9, 10, 307. *See also* Morbidity rates; individual disorders

Relative frequency, 8
Retinal degenerations, 247
Retrolental fibroplasia, definition, 247

Schools
  audiometric surveys, 287–288
  for the blind, 250–251
  for the deaf, 303
Sclerosis, amyotrophic lateral, 108–127
  classic form, 121, 122
  classification, 121–125
  clinical features, 122
  familial form, 121–123
  Guam form, 123–125
  Marianas form, 123–125
  morbidity data, 118–121
  mortality rates, international, 109–110
  mortality rates, in U.S., 111–118
    by age, 112, 113, 117
    by color, 112–114, 115, 116, 117
    geographic distribution, 114–116
    by marital status, 116–117
    nativity and, 117–118
    by sex, 112–114, 116–117
    trend, 111
    by type of county, 116
  pathologic features, 122
  sporadic form, 121, 122
Sclerosis, dorsolateral, 212
  incidence rates, 213
  prevalence rates, 213
  summation, 315
Sclerosis, multiple, 64–107
  characteristics, 94–99
  differential features, 99–102
  duration, 94–95
  familial features, 95–96
  foci, 91
  incidence rates, 91–94
    by sex, 93
  infectious origin, 102–106
  "latency," 96–99
  migration and, 96–99
  morbidity data, 82–94
  mortality rates, international, 65–68
  mortality rates, in U.S., 68–82
    by age, 69–71
    by color, 69–71
    geographic distribution, 69, 71–78
    by marital status, 78–80
    nativity and, 80–81, 82
    by sex, 69–71
    trend, 68–69
    by type of county, 78
  prevalence rates, 83–91
    geographic distribution, 83–91
  summation, 309
  survival by years after onset, 95
Sclerosis, primary lateral, 109
Seizures. *See also* Convulsive disorders; Epilepsy
  afebrile, 40, 308
  febrile, 34, 36
  heredity and, 36–38
  types, 33–34
Sex
  blindness and
    in foreign countries, 268–269
    in U.S., 256, 262
  deafness and, prelingual, 281, 284
  Down's syndrome and, 163–164
  hearing impairments in U.S. and, 290, 291–293
  herpes zoster and, 219, 220
  mortality rates by, international, for congenital malformations of nervous system, 175
  mortality rates by, in U.S.
    cerebral palsy, infantile, 235–236, 237
    cerebral palsy, neonatal, 239, 240
    Down's syndrome, 155, 156, 157
    epilepsy, 18–20, 21
    hydrocephalus, congenital, 186
    meningocele, 185
    monstrosity, 183
    muscular dystrophy, 132–134, 136–138
    myasthenia gravis, 146–147, 148, 149
    nervous system malformations, congenital, 179, 180, 181, 188

parkinsonism, 44, 45, 49, 50
sclerosis, amyotrophic lateral, 112-114, 116-117
sclerosis, multiple, 69-71
spina bifida, 185
multiple sclerosis, incidence rates by, 93
neurologic disorders, rate variations by, 324, 326-329
ratios in neural malformations, 201-203
Shingles, *see* Herpes zoster
Source materials, 13-14
Spina bifida
  birth rates, 177
  incidence rates among births, 199
  mortality rates in U.S.
    by color, 185
    geographic distribution, 184, 185
    by sex, 185
    by type of county, 192, 193
  summation, 313-315
Spinal cord affections, 210-215
Syringomyelia, 210-211, 315

Thyroid dysfunction and deafness, 284, 299
Trigeminal neuralgia, 218, 316
Twins with Down's syndrome, 166
Type of county, mortality rates in U.S. by
  cerebral palsy, infantile, 239
  cerebral palsy, neonatal, 241
  Down's syndrome, 157, 158-159
  epilepsy, 22
  hydrocephalus, congenital, 192-194
  meningocele, 193
  monstrosity, 191-192
  muscular dystrophy, 135, 136
  myasthenia gravis, 148
  nervous system malformations, congenital, 191-195
  parkinsonism, 48-49
  sclerosis, amyotrophic lateral, 116
  sclerosis, multiple, 78
  spina bifida, 192, 193

Wilson's disease, 227-228, 316-317

NO LONGER THE PROPERTY
OF THE
UNIVERSITY OF R. I. LIBRARY